Lower Extremity Wounds

Lower Extremity Wounds

A Problem-Based Learning Approach

Edited by

Karen Ousey
University of Huddersfield

and

Caroline McIntosh
University of Huddersfield

John Wiley & Sons, Ltd

Other Wiley Editorial Offices

John Wiley & Sons Inc., 111 River Street, Hoboken, NJ 07030, USA

Jossey-Bass, 989 Market Street, San Francisco, CA 94103-1741, USA

Wiley-VCH Verlag GmbH, Boschstr. 12, D-69469 Weinheim, Germany

John Wiley & Sons Australia Ltd, 42 McDougall Street, Milton, Queensland 4064, Australia

John Wiley & Sons (Asia) Pte Ltd, 2 Clementi Loop #02-01, Jin Xing Distripark, Singapore 129809

John Wiley & Sons Canada Ltd, 6045 Freemont Blvd, Mississauga, ONT, L5R 4J3

Wiley also publishes its books in a variety of electronic formats. Some content that appears in print may not be available in electronic books.

Library of Congress Cataloging-in-Publication Data

Lower extremity wounds : a problem-based learning approach / edited by Karen Ousey and Caroline McIntosh.
        p. ; cm.
    Includes bibliographical references and index.
     ISBN 978-0-470-51266-1 (cloth) – ISBN 978-0-470-05908-1 (pbk.)
   1. Leg–Wounds and injuries–Treatment.   2. Leg–Ulcers–Treatment.   3. Wound healing.   I. Ousey, Karen.   II. McIntosh, Caroline.
     [DNLM: 1. Lower Extremity–injuries.   2. Problem-Based Learning.   3. Skin Diseases– therapy.   4. Wound Healing–physiology.   5. Wounds and Injuries–therapy.   WE 850 L9179 2007]
     RD560.L72 2007
     617.5'8044–dc22   2007022434

British Library Cataloguing in Publication Data

A catalogue record for this book is available from the British Library

ISBN 978-0470-51266-1 (HB) 978-470-05908-1 (PB)

Typeset in 10/14 pt Myriad by Thomson Digital, India
Printed and bound by Graphos SA, Barcelona, Spain
This book is printed on acid-free paper responsibly manufactured from sustainable forestry in which at least two trees are planted for each one used for paper production.

Contents

Foreword

Karen Ousey and Caroline McIntosh along with their fellow authors have sought in this book to bring to the attention of the reader the reality of lower limb wounds today. That reality is that these wounds are invariably complex in nature with multiple causes and that their effective management requires the input of a variety of healthcare professionals whose roles may overlap. Traditionally, textbooks have sought to present the facts in clear and concise bite size sections. Such presentation is appealing to both reader and publisher but can at times lead to a false representation of reality by oversimplifying the topics presented. However, in the real world a patient rarely presents with a single cause of their wound. Wounds of the lower limb often develop as a result of a number of combined pathologies many of which are likely to be chronic diseases which can only be managed, not cured. Thus, an understanding of the various disease processes and their effective management needs to be related to the overall plan of care. When the patient is considered in terms of their psycho-social lives another set of challenges or potential impediments to healing can be found. Once again, there are professionals who can assist the patient and thus improve the likelihood of a successful outcome. Traditionally the term non-compliant has been used to describe patients who fail in the eyes of the professional to comply with the treatment plans provided. Consideration of the psycho-social aspects of the patient's life outside the clinic or between visits from the healthcare professional could identify reasons why the treatment prescribed is inappropriate for or unacceptable to the patient.

Within plans of care or management there is ample room for the use of specialist input. This is an issue which is explored in this text, and the issue of communication between members of the multidisciplinary team is also raised. These are questions that lie at the heart of effective management, because communication breakdowns between professionals can often occur and the patient is oblivious to the missed opportunity. Missed opportunities for professionals to combine their talents and knowledge for the benefit of the patient can have a catastrophic effect on the patient with a lower limb wound. In this text the reader is challenged to recognize the limits of their knowledge, thus identifying when another opinion may be required or when the skills of another specialty may complement those practitioners already involved in the patient's care. The multidisciplinary team is an often misunderstood concept but within the UK we need to recognize it can take many forms. The use of the word 'team' can create the idea that everyone has to meet or work side by side regularly, which is not always the case. In many instances what it means is a group of professionals whose focus is patient-centric and who recognize and respect the abilities of their colleagues, colleagues who seek advice and opinions as dictated by the patient's condition and their own knowledge.

To be able to function effectively in such a team requires the practitioner to critically assess their own knowledge and within this book the authors encourage the reader to reflect upon their own practice and knowledge. This helps to enhance the reader's experience and ultimately will lead to improved practice and perhaps the identification of areas for further study. Patients have a right to expect that every practitioner they place their trust in is constantly striving to improve their practice and thus the outcome for the patient. I, like the vast majority of practitioners in the UK, believe that every day and every new patient represent the opportunity to improve in practice and to advance knowledge. Books such as this one support that process by bringing the challenge faced by patients with lower limb wounds into sharp focus. The key message for me is that every practitioner is part of the process and potentially has something to offer, and that each practitioner is required to strive constantly to improve so that the patient can be assured of the very best of service.

David Gray
Clinical Nurse Specialist
Department of Tissue Viability
Grampian Health Services
Aberdeen

Karen Ousey and Caroline McIntosh

Introduction

This purpose of this book is to consider best practice, based on current evidence, in the assessment and management of wounds commonly encountered on the lower limb. Lower extremity wound care requires a multiprofessional approach involving a number of different health care professionals in order to achieve optimum patient care. Nurses and podiatrists, in particular, are frequently involved in the assessment and management of lower extremity wounds, often working in partnership. This book is written by experienced nurses and podiatrists with expert knowledge in wound care, to highlight the importance of a multiprofessional collaboration, to encourage the crossing and dismantling of professional boundaries, increase understanding of each other's roles and ultimately ensure that the patient receives the best available evidence-based interventions during their health care journey.

The book is primarily aimed at undergraduate/pre-registration nurses and podiatrists and non-specialist registered nurses and podiatrists; however, any professional with an interest in lower extremity wounds may find the book of interest.

The book is divided into 10 discrete chapters. Chapter one, the need for a multiprofessional approach to wound care; chapter two, normal and altered wound healing; chapter three, skin changes in the at-risk limb; chapter four, infected wounds; chapter five, leg ulcers; chapter six, surgical wounds; chapter seven, pressure ulcers; chapter eight, diabetic foot ulcers; chapter nine, rheumatoid foot ulcers; and chapter ten examining and exploring toenail surgery wounds.

Each chapter follows a uniform theme; a problem-based learning approach to the care of a patient with a lower extremity wound. The problem-based learning format brings theory to life with the use of case scenarios allowing the reader to consider the information and images provided and make autonomous decisions to assist in bridging the theory to practice gap. Each chapter explores and discusses the case scenario presenting current evidence to support interventions. Throughout the chapters the reader is encouraged to consider clinical and theoretical areas relevant to the presented case.

At the end of each chapter the reader is encouraged to reflect upon knowledge learnt and how this will influence future practice. Integral to each chapter are references to current national guidelines and policies that the reader is encouraged to access.

Caroline McIntosh and Karen Ousey

Chapter 1

The Need for a Multiprofessional Approach in Wound Care

1.1 | Introduction

Many different terms are used to describe collaborative working between health care professionals such as "interprofessional collaboration", "multidisciplinary/interdisciplinary team working" and "multiprofessional collaboration" (Xyrichis and Lowton, 2007).

The optimum treatment of lower extremity wounds depends on a multiprofessional collaborative approach that allows the related or underlying aetiology of the wound to be addressed, thus promoting wound healing and a positive outcome (Zgonis and Roukis, 2005). Standardized care provided by a specialist team has many advantages: a higher degree of continuity in treatment, increased patient satisfaction, greater potential for education and training and improved possibilities for basic and clinical research in healing and care (Gottrup, 2004). The concept of a multiprofessional approach is not new; Edmonds et al. (1986) reported the benefits of establishing a specialized multiprofessional clinic for patients with diabetic foot ulcers. Over three years, detailed analysis revealed a high rate of ulcer healing and a reduction in the number of major amputations which were attributed to the team approach. The team included podiatrists, orthotists, nurses, physicians and surgeons. A large number of published studies that evaluate the effect of a multiprofessional approach focus on diabetic foot ulcers; Boulton et al. (2005) reviewed the economic burden of diabetic foot ulcers and found that one

Parisian clinic reported a 33 % reduction in hospital in-patient stay after the establishment of a multiprofessional approach.

Gottrup (2004) undertook an evaluation of clinical outcomes within a dedicated multidisciplinary wound care centre. Findings demonstrated improved rates of healing in patients with leg ulcers and a decreased necessity for major amputations. Similarly Meltzer *et al.* (2002) investigated clinical outcomes for diabetic foot ulcers managed by a specialist multiprofessional team and found the amputation rate was significantly decreased; furthermore, the amputations that were required were at a significantly more distal level.

Studies have also demonstrated the benefits of a multiprofessional approach in reducing surgical site infections. Webb *et al.* (2006) developed a multiprofessional approach, using a computerized process for pre-operative prophylactic antibiotic administration. Findings indicated that a team approach allowed timely administration of appropriate antibiotic therapy which resulted in a significant reduction in the incidence of surgical site infections.

Hensen *et al.* (2005) developed and implemented a clinical pathway for ambulatory treatment of chronic wounds utilized by a multiprofessional team, with a primary focus on quality and coordination of care. After one year an evaluation demonstrated the benefits of the implemented pathway in improving clinical care and outcomes. However, the multiprofessional team consisted of physicians and nurses with no involvement of other professional groups.

It is apparent that unified care is an effective approach for patients with complex wounds. However, within published literature and clinical guidelines there is often little information regarding which professions should be involved in the care of chronic lower extremity wounds. This chapter will discuss the need for multiprofessional learning, consider barriers to multiprofessional learning and working, and explore the contribution of a number of professions in the care of a patient with a lower extremity wound in order to promote a greater understanding of professional roles, highlight the benefits of a team approach to wound care and the need for a collaborative approach to optimize patient care.

1.2 | The Need for Multiprofessional Learning

Wound care is an area that is truly multiprofessional in nature and as such it is important that medics, nurses and allied health professionals have in-depth training and education into the subject area to allow a holistic approach to patient care, both during initial training and post-registration. Multiprofessional (interprofessional) education has long been advocated as a key method for tackling problems with collaboration (World Health Organization (WHO), 1988). It can provide both novice and expert practitioners with shared experiences and knowledge about the work of other health care professions and, according to Van der Horst *et al.* (1995), can enhance team working skills.

More recently, the National Institute for Clinical Excellence (NICE), in relation to wound care, stated that:

> An interdisciplinary approach to the training and education of health care professionals should be adopted (NICE, 2001, page 4).

The Department of Health (DH) (2000) presented their NHS workforce strategy calling for education and training to be "genuinely multiprofessional" promoting:

- Teamwork
- Partnership and collaboration between professions, between agencies and with patients
- Skill mix and flexible working between professions
- Opportunities to switch training pathways to expedite career progression
- New types of workers

1.3 | Multiprofessional Wound Care

Multiprofessional team working is essential to develop an integrated team approach to achieve optimum wound care. Xyrichis and Lowton (2007) explored factors that facilitate interprofessional team working in primary and community care settings. Findings suggest regular team meetings, shared team premises, greater occupational diversity and positive interprofessional relations, enhanced information transaction, facilitated communication and increased personal familiarity.

A number of professions play vital roles in the holistic care of a patient with a lower limb wound, some of which will be explored within this chapter. Figure 1.1 summarizes some of the key, generic, members of the multiprofessional team involved in lower extremity wound care.

1.4 | Barriers to Collaborative Working

The multidisciplinary team approach is the ideal in wound care. However, there are often barriers that prevent this ideal being met. Xyrichis and Lowton (2007) identified several barriers to multiprofessional working in primary and community care including:

- Separate bases or buildings. This can result in team members feeling less integrated within the team which can limit team function and effectiveness.
- Team size. Large teams may have lower levels of participation than smaller teams.
- Lack of understanding as to who leads the multiprofessional team can cause frustration to team members and poor decision making.
- Lack of organizational support has been attributed to feelings of concern and disappointment which can impact negatively on team working.

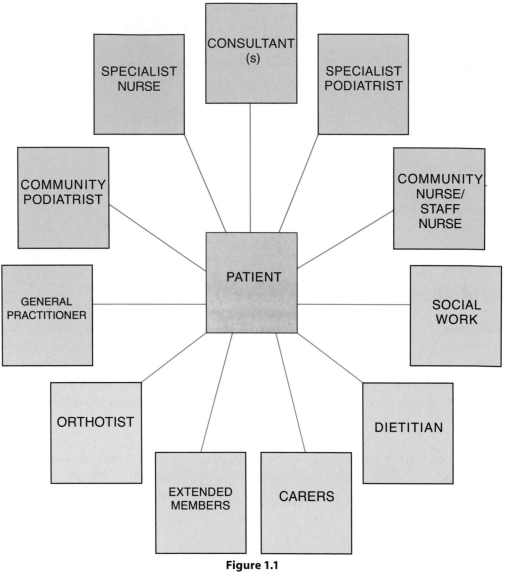

Figure 1.1
The lower extremity wound care multiprofessional team

- Lack of time. As a result, regular team meetings may not be feasible.
- Poor communication. A change to regimes without discussion could prove detrimental to patient care.
- Misunderstanding of each other's roles and professional stereotyping can promote professional conflict and personality differences among team members.
- Professional identity. Some professionals may be fearful that other professions are involved in their role and area of expertise.

Identification of potential barriers to effective team working can instigate change to overcome such barriers and enhance and maintain teamwork, which can improve quality of wound care provision.

1.5 | Case Scenario

The case details a multiprofessional team approach to the care of an amputee with chronic foot ulceration. It is recognized that this case can not address all professions involved in lower extremity wound care, so while the care of a person living with diabetic foot ulceration is exemplified, the multiprofessional team approach and individual professional roles for other lower extremity wounds will differ.

Case Scenario 1

Peter is a 58-year-old gentleman who has a history of chronic foot ulceration due to the chronic complications of diabetes mellitus. Peter was diagnosed with type 2 diabetes 12 years ago. He also has hypertension and dyslipidaemia and suffered a myocardial infarction three years ago. Peter underwent a below-knee amputation of the right limb two years ago and is fitted with a prosthetic limb. He has had a great toe amputation and a partial amputation of the fourth and fifth metatarsals in the last year. He currently has a large plantar ulcer on his left foot (see Figure 1.2). His remaining foot has significantly altered in shape, resulting in high pressure during gait; this corresponds with the site of ulceration. The wound has developed recurrent episodes of infection and Peter's blood glucose control is poor.

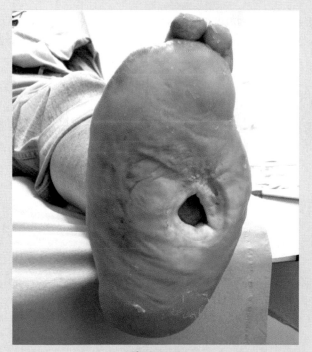

Figure 1.2
Planar ulceration on Peter's foot

Peter lives alone, having recently been moved to a warden-assisted bungalow in a small village. He feels isolated and has no family locally. Peter retired early on medical grounds. He previously enjoyed walking but he has lost confidence since his amputation and does not like going out alone.

Peter is at high risk of further amputation. It is therefore essential he receives integrated health and social care to prevent a further below-knee amputation.

Using the information provided within the chapter consider the following questions:

1. **Why is a multiprofessional approach needed?**

2. **Which members of the multiprofessional team need to be involved?**

3. **How can successful collaboration improve Peter's care?**

4. **Are there any potential barriers to collaborative care in Peter's case?**

The information provided within the chapter should enable you to answer the four questions posed above. The answers will be considered towards the end of the chapter.

1.6 | Multiprofessional Wound Care

In order to achieve optimum patient outcomes in wound care a multiprofessional approach is required with all team members working together in partnership. To improve working relations it is important that practitioners involved in wound care recognize that roles and responsibilities can overlap and cross professional boundaries. Many areas of wound care, such as patient-centred care, psychosocial support and structured education, require a shared responsibility from the team while other areas, such as wound debridement are only undertaken by a small number of professions in the wound care team.

To ensure referral to the most appropriate member of the multiprofessional team it is imperative to gain an appreciation of the role of each of the professions involved in lower extremity wound care, some of which are outlined in this chapter. It should be stressed that the roles outlined are specific to the case and may differ in individual clinical care settings. Local policy makers may develop their own protocols and with the advent of an extended scope of practice, professions such as nursing and podiatry are increasingly more autonomous.

1.6.1 | The Need for a Patient-Centred Approach

Previous studies have investigated patient perception to the care they receive (Callaghan and Williams, 1994; Ribu and Wahl, 2004). Findings suggest that patients prefer a person-centred approach with practitioners showing an interest in the patient, making them feel valued as an individual and keeping them well informed while ensuring consistency and continuity of care. The wound care multiprofessional team therefore has a shared responsibility to adopt a patient-centred approach to treatment ensuring continuity of care, regardless of the wound aetiology. It should be recognized that the patient plays a crucial role in the success of any management plan. The multi-professional team must therefore liaise with each other and with the patient when implementing care plans in order to ensure that they attempt to encompass best practice while also meeting the needs of the patient.

In Peter's case all members of the wound care multiprofessional team should appreciate that Peter must remain at the centre of the care plan designed to heal his complex wound.

> **It is important in Peter's case to establish his treatment goals. Peter was a keen walker prior to his amputation. He has since lost confidence and is reluctant to leave the house alone. All members of the team should ensure that any care plan addresses Peter's feelings and needs. Peter's primary goal, in terms of mobility, is to be able to walk to the local shop on his own.**

1.6.2 | Psychosocial Support

Psychosocial issues in wound care management are critical considerations when developing and implementing care plans, but they are frequently overlooked (Snyder, 2006). Increasingly, findings of qualitative studies that investigate health-related quality of life of those living with chronic wounds are being published in medical literature.

Published studies have investigated the impact of venous leg ulceration on health-related quality of life. Findings suggest that venous leg ulceration significantly reduces quality of life in the elderly, in patients who experience pain associated with venous leg ulceration, those who experience loss of sleep, itching, nonhealing and feelings of disappointment with treatment (Hareendran *et al.*, 2005; Snyder, 2006).

Similarly, the impact of pressure ulcers on heath-related quality of life has been explored. Hopkins *et al.* (2006) published patients' stories of living with a pressure ulcer in patients over the age of 65, with a grade 3 or 4 pressure ulcer with a minimum duration of one month. Common themes that emerged were feelings of a restricted life, restricted activities affecting themselves and their families, and endless pain which was exacerbated by pressure-relieving devices and dressing changes. These findings are supported by Spilsbury *et al.* (2007) who found pressure ulcers and their treatment affected peoples' lives emotionally, mentally, physically and socially. Specific aspects affecting quality of life were identified as pain, wound parameters such as appearance, smell and fluid leakage, and feelings of dependency on others for treatment. Yet it was perceived that the pain, discomfort and stress associated with living with a pressure ulcer was not acknowledged by nursing staff.

A large multicentre study compared health-related quality of life in patients with diabetic foot ulcers, with a nonulcerated diabetes group and the general population (Ribu *et al.*, 2007). Patients with diabetic foot ulcers reported significantly poorer health-related quality of life than those with diabetes without foot ulceration and the general population. Individuals living with diabetic foot ulceration reported role limitation, reduced physical functioning and emotional effects.

Although Peter lives in a warden-assisted bungalow he has stated that he feels isolated. When planning Peter's care the multiprofessional team has a responsibility to address not only his physical needs but also Peter's psychosocial issues. Members of the multiprofessional team should discuss with him these feelings of isolation and ascertain what measures may be implemented to overcome them. A package of care that includes integrated health and social care is important in achieving optimum outcomes in Peter's case; it is crucial that Peter is involved in the development of any care plan and agrees with the decisions made.

Peter can benefit from occupational therapy assessment. A key goal for the occupational therapist is to combat Peter's isolation. This could be achieved by exploring Peter's perceptions, his leisure interests and his psychological state. The establishment of leisure interests or goal/target setting could assist alongside access and referral to other agencies, e.g. day centres. Peter is keen to walk unassisted to the local shop. The occupational therapist, physiotherapist, podiatrist, orthotist and prosthetist must work collaboratively, with Peter, to make this goal a reality.

The social worker is an important member of the multiprofessional team. Social workers form relationships with people and assist them to live more successfully within their local communities by helping them find solutions to their problems. Social workers are knowledgeable about social, emotional and mental health needs of adults and can provide supportive counselling for Peter. Additionally social workers can discuss with Peter the availability of social care to assist him and coordinate community care. Social workers can also advise Peter on financial assistance that may be available to him.

Peter lives alone. He has no family members living locally but he is in a warden-assisted bungalow. It is therefore important that the warden is made aware of Peter's needs. For example, Peter may be referred to home care services by his social worker or general practitioner; the warden should be made aware so that they can ensure access to Peter's bungalow. The warden is also in a position to visit Peter throughout the day to attempt to overcome his feelings of isolation.

1.6.3 | The Delivery of Structured Education

All members of the multiprofessional team have a shared responsibility to offer structured education for individuals living with chronic wounds. National policy guidelines for differing wound types stress the importance of patient education to achieve concordance (agreement between the patient and practitioner) and patient empowerment (the process by which patients can take control of, and improve, their own health) (DH, 2001; NICE, 2005; Royal College of Nursing, 2006).

The Royal College of Nursing (2006) recommend patient education as a strategy to prevent recurrence of venous leg ulceration; specifically patients should be educated on concordance with compression hosiery, skin care, encouragement of mobility, exercise and elevation. Brooks *et al.* (2004) evaluated the effects of a structured nurse-led education programme that aimed to improve patient concordance and prevent venous leg ulcer recurrence. Findings suggest that those receiving structured education and usual care, versus usual care alone, experienced significantly less recurrence in one year.

The National Institute for Health and Clinical Excellence (NICE, 2005) published national policy guidance on pressure ulcer risk assessment and prevention. Recommendations include education and training for patients who are willing and able to be informed about risk assessment and prevention, including carers where appropriate. Specific recommendations include risk factors for pressure ulcer development, sites vulnerable to pressure damage, how to assess and recognize skin changes and when to refer to a health care professional.

The *National Service Framework* (*NSF*) *for Diabetes* (DH, 2001) has contributed to the focus on structured education in diabetes care. The *NSF for Diabetes* recommends structured education to improve patients' knowledge and understanding of their condition, thus encouraging empowerment (DH, 2001). The primary goal for all health care professionals and carers involved in Peter's care is therefore to enable him to manage his own diabetes and foot care as is reasonably practical.

1.6.4 | Effective Communication

One shared aspect of care that is critical to achieving optimum outcomes is effective communication between all members of the multiprofessional team. Members of the multiprofessional team must liaise with one another to achieve the implementation of agreed care plans, discuss any progress or deterioration in Peter's general and foot health and avoid offering conflicting advice to Peter.

A joint statement by the Department of Health, Universities UK, the Health Professions Council, the General Medical Council and the Nursing and Midwifery Council (DH, 2003) emphasize the importance of effective communication skills training in pre-registration and undergraduate education for health care professionals. At the point of registration and throughout professional careers health care students/professionals should:

- Be able to identify communication skills required in practice to improve patient care
- Have the ability to communicate effectively with fellow professionals and other health care staff
- Have the ability to recognize their communication skills limitations and be committed to personal development

While the Nursing and Midwifery Council (2004) stresses the importance of working as part of a team they maintain that all health care professions are personally accountable. Communication extends to the written form with onus on the individual health professional to document patient care accurately within their medical records. This is an essential component of patient care that forms a communication between professions that additionally addresses medicolegal issues. Barriers to effective communication between the multiprofessional team include poor written communication. Patient records may not be accessible to all members; some professions may not have access to the patient's medical records and as a result keep their own profession-specific patient records.

> **?** **What other barriers might exist that make communication between the multiprofessional team difficult?**

1.6.5 | Control Concomitant Medical Conditions

Many patients with chronic lower extremity ulceration will be living with concomitant medical pathologies that may be related or unrelated to the aetiology of the ulcer. Wound healing is likely to be impaired in the presence of a number of medical pathologies, e.g. peripheral arterial disease, diabetes mellitus and conditions leading to malnutrition (Morison, 2006). It is therefore important that concomitant disease processes are controlled to facilitate wound healing regardless of wound aetiology.

Other examples of concomitant diseases include rheumatologic and inflammatory diseases. Patients with these conditions are commonly prescribed drugs, such as nonsteroidal anti-inflammatory drugs and disease-modifying drugs that decrease inflammation and/or autoimmune response. These drugs can affect inflammation and local immune response required for wound healing and can ultimately delay healing. Busti *et al.* (2005) investigated the effects of periop-erative anti-inflammatory and immunomodulating therapy on surgical wound healing. Findings suggest that post-operative complications, such as wound dehiscence, infection and impaired collagen synthesis can occur as a consequence of these drugs and it may therefore be necessary to withdraw therapy prior to surgery. However, patients may experience exacerbation of symptoms. It is imperative that members of the multiprofessional team, in instances such as this, collaborate to establish risks and benefits, working with the patient to decide whether therapy should be discontinued. Medical practitioners, such as rheumatology consultants and general practitioners, play a key role in such decision making while other team members, such as nurses and therapists, can play a role in managing symptoms following withdrawal of therapy.

Achieving good metabolic control of blood glucose is essential to facilitate wound healing and prevent further complications of diabetes in individuals with diabetic foot ulceration. This can be achieved by reviewing current glycaemic control and initiating changes to therapy as required. Management of diabetes is further considered within Chapter 8. The diabetic specialist nurse can assess and closely monitor glycaemic levels and offer advice and support to Peter regarding maintenance of these levels. Diabetes specialist nurses work closely with the diabetologist to monitor and achieve tight control of blood glucose levels and arterial risk factors, such as hypertension and dyslipidaemia. In terms of local wound care the diabetes specialist nurse should liaise with podiatrists regarding dressing regimes, management of infection and wound bed preparation.

In Peter's case the diabetologist is involved in assessing and managing risk factors that could negatively impact on Peter's cardiovascular health. The United Kingdom Prospective Diabetes Study (UKPDS) (1998) demonstrated the benefits of tight control of dyslipidaemia (abnormal lipid levels in the blood) and meticulous management of blood pressure in reducing the risk of arterial pathology. This is particularly important to achieve in Peter's case as he has a history of coronary heart disease.

1.6.6 | Lower Limb Ischaemia

Ischaemia can contribute to wound chronicity and is commonly associated with diabetes, peripheral arterial disease and pressure ulcers among the elderly, and can contribute to the impaired healing of venous leg ulcers (Morison, 2006). Assessment of arterial perfusion is therefore imperative for all patients presenting with lower extremity wounds. This can be achieved by simple noninvasive tests by members of the multiprofessional team, e.g. nurses and podiatrists, but if significant ischaemia is identified a further, more detailed, vascular investigation is required and a referral must be made to the vascular team.

Within the vascular team the vascular specialist nurse takes a lead in the identification of arterial risk factors and liaises with the tissue viability nurse, ward nurses and podiatrists with clinical findings and subsequent care plans. Working closely with the vascular surgeon the vascular specialist nurse undertakes noninvasive vascular assessment identifying those who require additional investigation and intervention under the care of the consultant. The vascular surgeon can investigate arterial perfusion to the foot via more sophisticated methods such as angiography, to determine the need for revascularization surgery (Faries *et al.*, 2004). The vascular surgeon may be involved in revascularization of the lower limbs to facilitate healing of lower extremity wounds, including pressure ulcers, leg ulcers and diabetic foot ulcers.

Patients with diabetes mellitus present a unique challenge in lower extremity revascularization due to distal distribution of arterial occlusive disease and calcified vessel walls (Sumpio *et al.* 2003). Successful healing in Peter's case relies on an adequate arterial supply to the foot; he therefore requires assessments to determine his vascular status. This will inform a prognosis for wound healing and determine the need for a referral to the vascular surgeon for further assessment and revascularization.

What vascular tests might be appropriate in Peter's case?

1.7 | Nutritional Assessment and Management

Nutrition is a crucial aspect of a holistic approach to wound management, regardless of wound aetiology (Todorovic, 2002). Poor nutritional status can delay healing (Russell, 2001) and as such it is important that patients with wounds undergo nutritional assessment. All members of the multiprofessional team, but perhaps particularly nurses based in hospital and the community, play an important part in identifying patients who are nutritionally compromised. Nurses and dietitians may be involved in undertaking nutritional assessment. Dietitians are able to offer further in-depth advice on nutritional requirements. The dietitian can educate Peter regarding his nutritional requirements. Peter is able to maintain a balanced diet but in patients where this is not feasible nutritional requirements may need to be met through the use of nutritionally complete supplements (Todorovic, 2002).

1.8 | Rehabilitation Following Amputation

Members of the multiprofessional team involved in rehabilitation include physiotherapists, prosthetists, podiatrists and occupational therapists, all of whom need to be involved in Peter's rehabilitation. In Peter's case rehabilitation includes (1) assessing activities of daily living, (2) assessing mobility, (3) maintaining cardiovascular health, (4) assessing foot function and (5) maintaining foot health.

1.8.1 | Assessment of Activities of Daily Living

The occupational therapist can aim to establish how Peter is coping with activities of daily living and offer strategies and interventions to maximize Peter's quality of life. This might include assessment of personal activities: toileting, washing/bathing, dressing and stump care. The latter overlaps with nursing, podiatry and physiotherapy highlighting the need for liaison and notifying other professionals involved in Peter's care if problems arise. In terms of domestic activities Peter feels alone and isolated. The occupational therapist can assess how Peter is coping with basic tasks: home care, laundry, shopping, cooking, etc. Where possible equipment to assist Peter can be provided, energy management techniques taught and access to other services such as dietitians or social services could be established.

1.8.2 | Mobility

The overall aim of the physiotherapist is to maximize independence to minimize carer input. This can be achieved by liaison with the prosthetist to ensure the best fit of Peter's prosthesis to maximize weight-bearing capacity on his right limb. A prosthetist can assess and provide Peter with the most appropriate artificial limb, ensuring that the limb fits correctly and does not compromise his skin integrity. A prosthetist considers prosthetic function, usefulness, residual limb health and prosthetic appearance at fitting and review appointments.

It is essential that members of the team liaise with one another regarding Peter's care. The physiotherapist needs to be aware of Peter's weight-bearing status on his ulcerated foot. On occasion nonweight bearing may be advised to completely offload the wound and promote healing, but the risk of a decrease in cardiovascular fitness and respiratory reserve should be considered when rendering the patient immobile. It is important that the physiotherapist and podiatrist work together, with Peter, to determine the most appropriate offloading strategy for Peter's foot ulcer.

The occupational therapist can assess Peter's mobility both indoors and outdoors. This role overlaps with that of the physiotherapist involved in Peter's care, highlighting the need for effective communication. The assessment involves Peter's ability to transfer in the house, his ability to use his prosthesis and his access to transportation outdoors. Dependent on the findings, the occupational therapist can provide Peter with adaptive equipment to assist his mobility, provide pressure relief in consultation with the podiatrist and physiotherapist, and investigate and establish access to services to assist Peter's transportation. An assessment of seating can also be undertaken with provision of pressure-relieving devices to prevent pressure damage on the sacrum or on the contralateral limb.

1.8.3 | Risk of Deterioration of Cardiorespiratory Fitness

The physiotherapist plays a key role in maintaining and improving Peter's cardiorespiratory function so that he can maintain present mobility and cope with extra demands should a second amputation take place. Transfers for a bilateral amputee are more demanding in terms of cardiovascular fitness. This is achieved by teaching wheelchair manoeuvres to increase cardiorespiratory fitness and prophylactic respiratory exercises to maintain respiratory reserve.

1.8.4 | Assessment of Foot Function

The presence of foot deformity is a known risk factor for foot ulcers, particularly rheumatoid foot ulcers and diabetic foot ulcers. The International Diabetes Federation Clinical Guidelines Task Force (2005) recommends that the foot should be inspected for hammer or clawed toes and bony prominences that could be subject to high pressure and trauma. In Peter's case he has established Charcot's neuroarthropathy which has caused significant foot deformity (please refer to Chapter 8 for further details). Peter has also undergone amputation of the great toe and partial amputations of the forefoot. As a result foot function is significantly impaired. The podiatrist can assess foot function and undertake gait analysis, including measurement of foot pressures. Measurement of foot pressure allows the podiatrist to identify sites of high pressure on the foot, so appropriate management strategies that offer pressure relief can then be implemented.

In the case of established foot deformities, e.g. secondary to rheumatoid arthritis, orthopaedic surgeons may undertake corrective surgery to prevent primary episodes of ulceration or prevent recurrence of foot ulceration.

Therapeutic footwear and total contact insoles can reduce plantar pressure in Peter's case. The podiatrist must work with the orthotist to achieve the best outcomes for Peter. This can be achieved by assessing the mechanics of the foot, identifying problems with foot function and producing insoles to correct foot function and relieve pressure. Additionally the orthotist can assess and measure Peter's foot for therapeutic footwear that can provide extra depth and width to accommodate insoles, while minimizing the risk of pressure, shear and friction on his already compromised foot.

1.8.5 | Maintenance of Foot Health

Podiatrists play a key role in maintaining foot health. Podiatric care, including nail care and management of skin pathologies such as callosities, has been shown to reduce the risk of foot ulceration and therefore reduce the prevalence of lower extremity amputation (Ronnemaa *et al.*, 1997; Plank *et al.*, 2003).

Peter requires regular foot care to prevent new episodes of ulceration. Community or hospital-based podiatrists can provide regular skin and nail care.

1.9 | Wound Care

A number of members of the multiprofessional team are involved in lower extremity wound care and are involved in assessing wound characteristics and striving to achieve microbiological control.

The main treatment objectives in Peter's case are to promote wound healing and prevent adverse outcomes, such as infection and tissue necrosis, that could precede further amputation.

1.9.1 | Microbiological Control

All members of the multiprofessional team should assess wounds for signs of infection. However, the podiatrist or nurse are often the professionals involved in local wound care and therefore the first to observe clinical signs of infection. Shank and Feibel (2006) suggest that broad-spectrum antibiotics and meticulous local wound care may achieve remission of mild-to-moderately severe infections and should be included in all treatment regimens complicated by mild-to-moderately severe infections. It is imperative that communication is maintained between members of the multiprofessional team, particularly with the evolution of extended-scope practice for nurses and professions allied to medicine. Traditionally doctors have prescribed antibiotic therapy for wound infections; however, dependent on demonstrable training and qualification, nurses and podiatrists have access to medication, including broad-spectrum antibiotics.

Infection can spread rapidly in the diabetic foot with devastating consequences; if infection is not recognized or treatment is delayed diabetic foot ulcers can become limb and life threatening (Sheppard, 2005). It is important that all members of the multiprofessional team involved in local wound care monitor Peter's wound for further episodes of infection. Prompt management of infection in the diabetic foot is imperative. In the case of severe infection the diabetologist must admit the patient to the ward for intravenous antibiotics and urgent assessment of the need for surgical drainage and debridement (Edmonds, 2006). In the case of severe infection, particularly when complicated by the presence of ischaemia, an aggressive surgical approach may be required (Shank and Feibel, 2006). In this case the orthopaedic surgeon may be involved in bone resection, correction of deformity or amputation.

1.9.2 | Wound Debridement

Wound debridement is an essential aspect of wound care that is required to remove dead and devitalized tissue from the wound bed to facilitate wound healing. There are many methods of debridement available to the practitioner; therefore it is important to discuss these options with the patient so they are involved in decision making and can give their informed consent (Anderson, 2006). Anderson (2006) states that nurses should be aware of professional requirements for competence and refers to the Tissue Viability Association's guideline (2005) for conservative sharp debridement.

Podiatrists are ideally placed to offer skilled debridement of foot ulcers having undergone extensive training in sharp debridement. Additionally, scalpel work forms a major part of a podiatrist's daily workload and so scalpel techniques are developed to a high level of skill with experience (Baker, 2002).

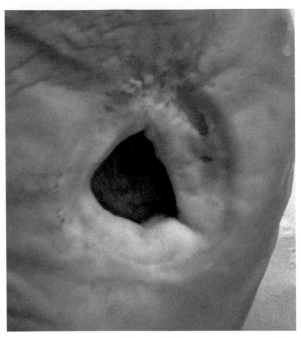

Figure 1.3
Macerated callus surrounds the wound

Peter's wound has macerated callused margins requiring regular sharp debridement (Figure 1.3).

1.9.3 | Instigate Dressing Regimens

Different professionals in the multiprofessional team may be involved in the instigation of dressing regimens; typically nurses and podiatrists are involved in dressing selection. At present there is no one ideal wound dressing for all stages of healing. With a plethora of wound dressings available to the practitioner this task can prove challenging and, not surprisingly, can lead to disagreement within the team. However, it is important to ensure continuity of care and avoid conflict within the team. Dressing choice should not be altered without prior discussion with other members of the multiprofessional team.

1.9.4 | Implement Offloading Strategies

Achieving effective pressure relief (offloading) is considered key to promoting healing of foot ulcers. Many methods have been suggested, including bed rest, wheelchair, crutches, total contact casting, felted foam and therapeutic shoes (Boulton *et al.*, 2004) with much research focusing on offloading diabetic foot wounds (Chapter 8). Effective pressure relief is equally as important for all foot ulcers, e.g. rheumatoid foot ulcers (Chapter 9).

Achieving effective offloading is challenging in Peter's case. Peter has already undergone a below-knee amputation. He is ambulant with his prosthetic limb and crutches but offloading his residual limb via crutches is not feasible. It is essential that the podiatrist liaises with other members of the multiprofessional team, including physiotherapy and occupational therapy, when selecting offloading strategies. It is important that Peter remains mobile to encourage his rehabilitation and preserve cardiovascular health, so in this case a wheelchair is not an option.

1.10   Case Study Revisited

1. **Why is a multidisciplinary approach needed?**
   A multiprofessional approach is needed to ensure that all of Peter's physical and psychosocial needs are addressed. No one member of the wound care team can address all elements. Therefore a team approach is warranted to ensure that Peter receives a holistic care plan tailored to meet his needs while optimizing outcomes and preventing further amputation.

2. **Which members of the multidisciplinary team need to be involved?**
   Ward nurses, community nurses, specialist nurses, podiatrists, specialist podiatrists, occupational therapists, physiotherapists, general practitioners, dietitians, consultants, prosthetists, orthotists, social workers and Peter are all required to work in partnership.

3. **How can successful collaboration improve Peter's care?**
   Successful collaboration can optimize Peter's care as a team approach improves planning, assessment, implementation and evaluation of Peter's care, and addresses his physical and psychosocial needs. The team can discuss his care and ensure that the best available evidence-based care is delivered. As the team are collaborating together this can reduce the risk of aspects of his care being missed and enhance effective care planning, ensuring that he has access to appropriate services to meet his needs.

4. **Are there any potential barriers to collaborative care in Peter's case?**
   Barriers to effective collaborative care include professionals having a lack of knowledge and understanding of the role of other professions, a lack of communication within the team, inadequate referral to the correct profession and each profession writing its notes in separate medical/nursing notes, leading to repetition and poor communication and conflicting opinions in terms of care strategies. In Peter's case, care was largely community based. Regular team meetings proved difficult as there were no single team premises and time was perceived as a barrier. Communication was largely via written notes and telephone calls rather than personal contact.

1.11 | Conclusion

This chapter has identified, discussed and explored the role of the wound care multiprofessional team and the importance of collaborative working. The role of each member of the wound care multiprofessional team has been explored and how they contribute to Peter's care has been highlighted. Peter's case has been used as a focus throughout the chapter and has exemplified how an effective multiprofessional approach to patient care can benefit the patient's health care and clinical outcomes.

Reflection

Take time to reflect upon your learning from this chapter. Ask yourself:

1. What knowledge did I possess prior to reading this chapter?

2. How has my knowledge developed?

3. How will I implement this into my future practice?

References

Anderson, I. (2006) Debridement methods in wound care. *Nursing Standard*, **20**(24), 65–6, 68, 70, *passim*.

Baker, N. (2002) Debridement of the diabetic foot: a podiatric perspective. *Lower Extremity Wounds*, **1**(2), 87–92.

Boulton, A.J.M., Connor, H. and Cavanagh, P.R. (2004) *The Foot in Diabetes* 3rd edn, John Wiley & Sons, Ltd, Chichester, p. 66.

Boulton, A.J.M., Vileikyte, L., Ragnarson-Tennvall, G. and Apelqvist, J. (2005) The global burden of diabetic foot disease. *The Lancet*, **366**, 1719–23.

Brooks, J., Ersser, S.J., Lloyd, A. *et al.* (2004) Nurse led education sets out to improve patient concordance and prevent recurrence of leg ulcers. *Journal of Wound Care* **13**(3), 111–6.

Busti, A.J., Hooper, J.S., Amaya, C.J. *et al.* (2005) Effects of perioperative antiinflammatory and immunomodulating therapy on surgical wound healing. *Pharmacotherapy*, **25**(11), 1566–91.

Callaghan, D. and Williams, A. (1994) Living with diabetes: issues for nursing practice. *Journal of Advanced Nursing*, **20**(1), 132–9.

Department of Health (2000) *A Health Service of All the Talents: Developing the NHS Workforce*, Department of Health, London.

Department of Health (2001) *National Service Framework for Diabetes: Standards*, Department of Health (online), Available at: http://www.dh.gov.uk/PublicationsAndSLatistics/Publications/PublicationsPolicyAndGuidance/PublicationsPolicyAndGuidanceArticle/fs/en?CONTENT_ID=4002951&chk=09Kkz1, Accessed 28 January 2007.

Department of Health (2003) Statement of Guiding Principles relating to the commissioning and provision of communication skills training in pre-registration and undergraduate education for healthcare professionals (online), Available at: http://www.dh.gov.uk/en/Publicationsandstatistics/Lettersandcirculars/Dearcolleagueletters/DH_4093504, Accessed 12 april 2007.

Edmonds, M. (2006) Diabetic foot ulcers: practical treatment recommendations. *Drugs*, **7**, 913–29.

Edmonds, M.E., Blundell, M.P. and Morris, M.E. (1986) Improved survival of the diabetic foot: the role of a specialised foot clinic, *Quarterly Journal of Medicine*, **60**(232), 763–71.

Faries, P.L., Teodoresau, V.J. Morrisey, N.J. *et al.* (2004) The role of surgical revascularisation in the management of diabetic foot wounds. *American Journal of Surgery*, **187**(5A), 34S–37S.

Gottrup, F. (2004) A specialized wound healing center concept: importance of a multidisciplinary department structure and surgical treatment facilities in the treatment of chronic wounds. *American Journal of Surgery*, **187**(5), Suppl. 1, 385–435.

Hareendran, A., Bradbury, A. and Budd, J. (2005) Measuring the impact of venous leg ulcers on quality of life. *Journal of Wound Care*, **14**(2), 53057.

Hensen, P., Ma, H.L., Luger, T.A. *et al.* (2005) Pathway management in ambulatory wound care: defining local standards for quality improvement and interprofessional care. *International Wound Journal*, **22**, 104–11.

Hopkins, A., Dealey, C., Bale, S. *et al.* (2006) Patients stories of living with a pressure ulcer. *Journal of Advanced Nursing*, **56**(4), 345–53.

International Diabetes Federation (IDF) Clinical Guidelines Task Force (2005) *Global Guidance for Type 2 Diabetes*, International Diabetes Federation, Brussels.

Meltzer, D.D., Pels, S., Payne, W.G. *et al.* (2002) Decreasing amputation rates in patients with diabetes mellitus: an outcome study. *Journal of the American Podiatric Medical Association*, **92**(8), 425–8.

Morison, M. (2006) *Chronic Wounds*, An educational booklet (sponsored by Smith & Nephew), Wounds UK Publishing, Aberdeen.

National Institute for Clinical Excellence (2001) *Pressure Ulcer Risk and Assessment Recommendations 2001*, Royal College of Nursing, London.

National Institute for Health and Clinical Excellence (2005) *Pressure Ulcers: The Management of Pressure Ulcers in Primary and Secondary Care: A Clinical Guideline*, CG029, NICE, London.

Nursing and Midwifery Council (2004) *Code of Professional Conduct*, NMC, London.

Plank, J., Haas, W., Rakovac, I. *et al.* (2003) Evaluation of the impact of chiropodist care in the second-ary prevention of foot ulcerations in diabetic subjects. *Diabetes Care*, **26**(6), 1691–5.

Ribu, L. and Wahl, A. (2004) How patients with diabetes who have foot and leg ulcers perceive the nursing care they receive. *Journal of Wound Care*, **13**(2), 65–8.

Ribu, L., Hanestad, B.R., Moum, T. *et al.* (2007) A comparison of the health related quality of life in pa-tients with diabetic foot ulcers, with a diabetes group and a non-diabetes group from the general population, *Quality of Life Research*, **16**(2), 179–89.

Ronnemaa, T., Hamalainen, H., Toikka, T. *et al.* (1997) Evaluation of the impact of podiatrist care in the primary prevention of foot problems in diabetic subjects. *Diabetes Care*, **20**, 1833–7.

Royal College of Nursing (2006) Clinical Practice Guidelines: the nursing management of patients with venous leg ulcers (online), Available at: `http://www.rcn.org.uk/publications/pdf/ guidelines/venous_leg_ulcers.pdf`, Last accessed 11 april 2007.

Russell, L. (2001) The importance of patients' nutritional status in wound healing. *British Journal of Nursing*, **10**(6), Suppl., S42, S44–9.

Shank, C.F. and Feibel, J.B. (2006) Osteomyelitis in the diabetic foot: diagnosis and management. *Foot and Ankle Clinics*, **11**(4), 775–89.

Sheppard, S.J. (2005) Antibiotic treatment of infected diabetic foot ulcers. *Journal of Wound Care*, **14**(6), 260–3.

Snyder, R.J. (2006) Venous leg ulcers in the elderly patient: associated stress, social support, and coping. *Osteomyelitis and Wound Management*, **52**(9), 58–66.

Spilsbury, K., Nelson, A., Cullum, N. *et al.* (2007) Pressure ulcers and their treatment and effects on quality of life: hospital in-patient perspectives. *Journal of Advanced Nursing*, **57**(5), 494–504.

Sumpio, B.E., Lee, T. and Blume, P.A. (2003) Vascular evaluation and arterial reconstruction of the diabetic foot. *Clinical Podiatric Medical Surgery*, **20**(4), 689–708.

Tissue Viability Nurses Association (2005) Conservative Sharp Debridement Procedure, Competencies and Training. http://www.tvna.org/generic_forms/sharp_debridement_revise.pdf (12 September 2007).

Todorovic, V. (2002) Foods and wounds: nutritional factors in wound formation and healing. *British Journal of Community Nursing*, **9**, Wound Suppl., 43–54.

United Kingdom Prospective Diabetes Study (UKPDS) (1998) Intensive blood-glucose control with sulphonylureas or insulin compared with conventional treatment and risk of complications in patients with type 2 diabetes (UKPDS 33). *The Lancet*, **352**(9131), 837–53.

Van der Horst, M., Turpie, I. and Nelson, W. (1995) St Joseph's Community Centre model of community based inter-disciplinary health care team education. *Health Society Care Community*, **3**, 33–42.

Webb, A.L.B., Flagg, R.L. and Fink, A.S. (2006) Reducing surgical site infection through a multidisciplinary computerised process for pre-operative prophylactic antibiotic administration *American Journal of Surgery*, **192**(5), Special Issue, 663–8.

World Health Organization (1988) *Learning Together to Work Together for Health*, WHO, Geneva.

Xyrichis, A. and Lowton, K. (2007) What fosters or prevents interprofessional team-working in primary and community care? A literature review. *International Journal of Nursing Studies* (online), Available at: `http://www.sciencedirect.com/science?_ob=ArticleURL&_udi=B6T7T-4NBRFWN1&_user=495973&_coverDate=03%2F26%2F2007&_rdoc=1&_fmt=&_orig=search&_sort=d&view=c&_acct=C000024198&_version=1&_urlVersion=0&_userid=495973&md5=487544a44c1ac6446684e189cbd9e8eb`, Last accessed 12 april 2007.

Zgonis, T. and Roukis, T.S. (2005) A systematic approach to diabetic foot infections. *Advances in Therapy*, **22**(3), 244–62.

Karen Ousey and Caroline McIntosh

Chapter 2

Physiology of Wound Healing

2.1 | Introduction

The skin is the largest organ in the human body, accounting for approximately 15 % of body weight and receiving a third of the circulating blood volume. Protection is one of the major homeostatic functions of the skin as it is constantly exposed to the trauma of its external environment (Flanagan and Fletcher, 2003). The skin plays a crucial role in the sustenance of life through the regulation of water and electrolyte balance, thermoregulation, and by acting as a barrier to external noxious agents including micro-organisms. When this barrier is disrupted due to any cause, e.g. pressure damage, burns or trauma, these functions are no longer adequately performed. It is therefore vital to restore its integrity as soon as possible.

A wound can be defined as a break in the epithelial integrity of the skin. The disruption to skin integrity could, however, extend deeper to the dermis, subcutaneous fat, fascia, muscle or bone. The development of a wound may be described as an assault on the body's environment from external sources. This can be due to a number of extrinsic factors:

- Surgical incision
- Accidental damage/ trauma
- Pressure damage
- Heat, e.g. thermal burn
- Excessive cold, e.g. frostbite
- Chemical damage

Additionally, the risk of damage to the skin from external sources, such as those listed above, is elevated in the presence of certain intrinsic factors, such as vascular disease, neuropathy and some medication.

When considering causation and aetiology of wounds on the lower extremities, an essential pre-requisite for accurate assessment and optimum wound management is a sound understanding of the natural structure of the skin and an appreciation of the stages of wound healing.

Wound healing involves a complex and dynamic, but superbly orchestrated, series of events leading to the repair of injured tissues. A completely healed wound, usually seen after simple injury, is defined as one that has returned to its normal anatomical structure, function and appearance within a reasonable period of time. It is also defined as one that has attained complete skin closure without drainage or dressing requirements. In contrast, some wounds fail to heal in a timely and orderly manner, resulting in chronic, nonhealing wounds (Enoch and Price, 2004).

This chapter has two main objectives:

1. To discuss the natural structure and function of the skin
2. To consider the normal stages of wound healing

2.2 | Case Scenario

Case Scenario 2

Julie is a 35-year-old lady who has a history of painful hallux abductovalgus (bunion deformity) on her left foot. She is generally fit and healthy with no relevant medical history but Julie smokes 20 cigarettes per day. Julie is under the care of a consultant podiatric surgeon and has undergone corrective surgery.

The wound is due to a surgical incision (Figure 2.1). The wound has been sutured (Figure 2.2) and as such will heal by primary intention (a form of healing whereby the skin edges are held together to facilitate the healing process).

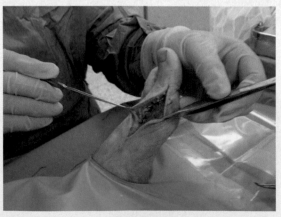

Figure 2.1
Surgical incision on the dorsum aspect of the left foot

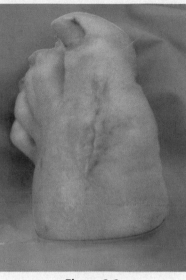

Figure 2.2
Sutured wound

? Consider the following questions prior to reading this chapter:

1. **What is the normal function of the skin?**

2. **What is the natural structure of the skin?**

3. **How do wounds heal?**

4. **How long should wound healing take in this case?**

5. **Which members of the multiprofessional team need to be involved?**

The information provided within the chapter should enable you to answer the five questions posed above. The answers will be considered towards the end of the chapter.

2.3 | Skin Physiology

In order to gain an appreciation of the physiology of wound healing it is important to first gain an appreciation of the skin's normal physiology and the natural structure of the skin. The skin has several important functions, which are listed below (adapted from Graham-Brown and Burns, 2004; Tortora et al., 2004; Butcher and White, 2005):

1. Regulation of body temperature. In response to a high environmental temperature the evaporation of sweat from the skin surface helps to lower an elevated body temperature to normal. Alternatively, in response to a low body temperature the production of sweat is decreased to aid in the conservation of heat.
2. Protection. The skin covers the body, providing a protective barrier that protects the underlying tissues from abrasions, bacterial invasion, dehydration and ultraviolet radiation.
3. Sensation. The skin contains many nerve endings and receptors that detect stimuli related to touch, pressure, pain and temperature.
4. Excretion. In addition to removing heat and some water from the body sweat also acts as the vehicle for excretion of a small amount of salts and several organic compounds.
5. Immunity. Certain cells of the epidermis are important components of the immune system.
6. Blood reservoir. The dermis of the skin houses extensive networks of blood vessels that carry 8–10% of the total blood flow in a resting adult. In moderate exercise skin blood flow may increase, which helps dispel heat from the body. During hard exercise the skin blood vessels constrict and more blood is able to flow to the contracting muscles.
7. Synthesis of vitamin D. Vitamin D synthesis begins with activation of a precursor molecule in the skin by ultraviolet rays in the sunlight. Enzymes in the liver and kidneys then modify the molecule, finally producing calcitriol, which is the most active form of vitamin D. Calcitriol contributes to the homeostasis of body fluids by aiding absorption of calcium in foods.

2.4 | Structure of the Skin

The skin acts as a barrier to entry for the body. It is the largest organ of the body and in its normal state is home to a variety of bacteria. These bacteria, known as skin commensals, are classed as normal flora which live in warm, moist sites and generally cause no problems on intact skin. When the skin is broken the resultant wound may become inhabited with the skin's own bacteria or bacteria from the environment without host reaction; this is known as colonization (Kingsley, 2001). If the bacterial burden in the wound increases a host reaction ensues; this is known as infection. Infection may be characterized by the classic signs of redness, pain, swelling, raised temperature and fever (Calvin, 1998).

The skin is composed of two types of tissue:

1. Surface epidermis
2. Underlying dermis

2.4.1 | Epidermis

The cells of the basal cell layer act as stem cells from which the rest of the epidermis is formed (Figure 2.3). From this layer, cells are pushed towards the surface by the formation of new cells by the stem cells. It takes approximately two weeks for the cells to reach the surface. As the cells

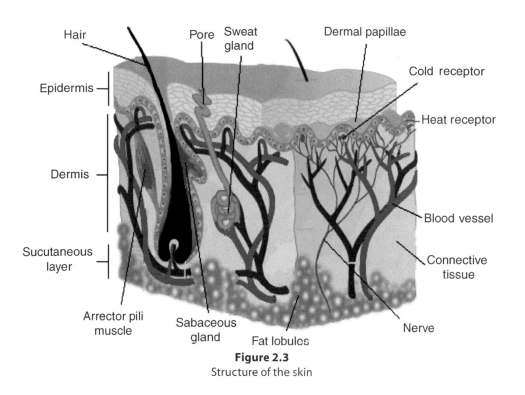

Figure 2.3
Structure of the skin

migrate they change structure and activity so that they eventually form the keratin layer of the stratum corneum (Kindlen, 2003).

The epidermis is the uppermost layer of skin and consists of layered (stratified) epithelium (surface tissue). It is only 0.1–1.5 millimetres thick and is made up of five layers:

1. Basal cell layer (stratum germinativum). This is the innermost layer of the epidermis and houses the basal cells. These cells constantly divide, with the new cells pushing the older ones upwards towards the surface of the skin. The basal cell layer also contains melanocytes that produce melanin.
2. Squamous cell layer (stratum spinosum). This is the thickest layer of the epidermis. These cells are held together with spiny projections. Here the basal cells have been pushed upwards, with the mature cells now being called squamous cells or keratinocytes. They produce keratin, a protective protein that makes up the structure of the skin, hair and nails. Also contained in this layer are the Langerhan cells, these cells alert the immune system to invading antigens.
3. Stratum granulosum. Cells become flattened, filled with granules of keratohyalin and die.
4. Stratum lucidum. In this layer the keratohyalin in the dead cells become translucent eleidin.
5. Stratum corneum. These layers work together to rebuild the surface of the skin. This is the outermost, most visible part of the epidermis. In this layer, under the influence of secretion from lysosomes, the eleidin becomes keratin, a horny material that is continually rubbed off (Rowett, 1996).

2.4.2 | Dermis

The dermis is the inner and thicker layer of the skin (Figure 2.3), which lies beneath the epidermis. The dermis consists mainly of a fibrous network of two kinds of protein: collagen and elastin. These proteins are formed and secreted by cells including fibroblasts. Collagen fibres give strength to the skin while elastin provides flexibility. Secretory glands, sensory receptors and defence cells are situated in the dermis. Collier (2002) states that the dermis consists of fibrous and elastic connective tissue containing blood and lymphatic vessels, nerves and their end organs, sebaceous and sweat glands, ducts and hair follicles, as seen in Figure 2.3. Furthermore, the dermis is highly vascular and well supplied with sensory receptors to pain, temperature and touch. It contains blood capillaries, sebaceous glands, hair follicles and lymphatic capillaries.

Sweat glands

Sweat glands are located within the dermis and are present over the majority of the body. There are estimated to be 2.5 million sweat glands on the skin surface. The glands are composed of coiled tubes which secrete a watery substance and are classified into two different types: eccrine and apocrine (Gawkrodger, 1997).

Eccrine glands

These sweat glands are found all over the skin, especially in the palms, soles, axillae and forehead, but are not present in mucous membranes. Eccrine glands are under psychological and thermal control and are innervated by sympathetic (cholinergic) nerve fibres. The watery fluid that the glands secrete contains chloride, lactic acid, fatty acids, urea, glycoproteins and mucopolysaccharides (Gawkrodger, 1997).

Apocrine glands

These are large sweat glands, the ducts of which empty out into the hair follicles. They are present in the axillae, anogenital region and areolae. They become active at puberty and produce an odourless, protein-rich secretion that gives out a characteristic odour when acted upon by skin bacteria. The apocrine glands are a phylogenetic remnant of the mammalian sexual scent gland. Wax in the ears is produced by a modified version of the same gland. Apocrine glands are also present on the eyelids. These glands are under the control of the sympathetic (adrenergic) nerve fibres (Gawkrodger, 1997).

Hair follicles are embedded in the dermis and occur all over the body, except on the soles, palms and lips. Each hair follicle has a layer of cells at its base that continually divides, pushing overlying cells upwards inside the follicle. These cells become keratinized and die, like the cells in the epidermis, but here form the hair shaft which is visible above the skin. A sebaceous gland opens into each hair follicle and produces sebum, helping to repel water, damaging chemicals and microorganisms. Attached to each hair follicle are small erector pili muscle fibres. These muscle fibres contract in cold weather and sometimes in fright (Kindlen, 2003).

The dermis connects the epidermis to the underlying structures. It consists of a dense, tough, but elastic connective tissue with nerves and blood vessels. The boundary between the epidermis and the dermis contains protruding dermal papillae, which help to hold the layers together (Rowett, 1996).

2.4.3 | Subcutaneous Layer

The subcutaneous layer separates the dermis from the deeper structures of the deep fascia, muscle and bone. It varies in thickness and is dependent upon body type, gender and the location of the skin on the body. This is due to the deposition of fat cells in various parts of the body. Fat cells are arranged in lobules that are separated by bands of connective tissue known as the interlobular space (Woolf, 1998). It has looser connective tissue with fat deposits in adipose cells. This allows insulation against heat loss and acts as storage and padding.

2.4.4 | Deep Fascia

The deep fascia lies beneath the subcutaneous layer and is an avascular, inelastic membrane that covers muscle and muscle groups. It is resistant to pressure and is the last line of protection for vulnerable muscle tissue (Morison, 2001).

2.4.5 | Blood Vessels

There are three interconnected networks of blood vessels associated with the skin:

- Capillary network beneath the epidermis
- Arterioles and venules in the dermis
- Larger arteries and veins in the subcutaneous tissue

The regulation of blood flow and capillary permeability play a central role in the inflammatory process. Arterioles are highly muscular, which enables changes to their diameters. They branch into a network of metarterioles, which have a structure midway between arterioles and capillaries, consisting of smooth muscle fibres that encircle the blood vessel at intermediate points rather than a continuous muscle coat (Guyton, 1997).

The metarterioles further subdivide into capillaries. The large ones are called preferential channels and the small ones are known as true capillaries. The capillaries are composed of a single layer of highly permeable endothelial cells surrounded by a basement membrane. Between each endothelial cell is a small channel known as an intercellular cleft. Within the endothelial cells are plasmalemmal vesicles. These structures are important in the exchange of nutrients and other substances between the blood and interstitial fluid (Guyton, 1997). Blood enters the venules after passing through the capillaries returning to general circulation.

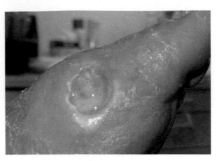

Figure 2.4
Wound requiring healing by secondary intention

2.5 | Process of Wound Healing

Wound healing is a complex physiological process that occurs in response to trauma. All tissues in the body are capable of healing by one of two mechanisms: regeneration and repair. Regeneration is the replacement of cells with identical cells; this only occurs in a limited number of cells such as liver cells, nerves cells and epidermal cells. The main mechanism for the healing of wounds is repair where damaged tissue is replaced by connective tissue, which then forms a scar (Flanagan, 2000).

The healing process of wounds is generally categorized into three sections:

1. Healing by primary intention. This is a wound that normally heals with no problems. The edges are held together by sutures, staples or glue, as in Julie's case. There is little blood loss and epithelization is rapid.
2. Healing by secondary intention. A wound healing by secondary intention involves repair of tissue loss (Figure 2.4). Wounds healing in this manner will take a longer period of time to heal and have an elevated risk of infection. As seen in Figure 2.4, a wound healing by secondary intention requires a large amount of tissue repair. Epithelialization occurs once granulation tissue fills the wound bed. New epithelial cells, which have a translucent appearance and are usually whitish-pink in colour, originate from either the wound margin or from the remnants of hair follicles, sebaceous glands or sweat glands. They divide and migrate along the surface of the granulation tissue until they form a continuous layer (Garrett, 1998).
3. Healing by tertiary intention. Healing by tertiary intention, also known as delayed primary intention, involves leaving a wound open for an extended period of time, usually because of complications such as infection. Once the problem has been resolved the wound edges are brought together to achieve closure.

?   **By which process is Julie's wound healing?**

2.5.1 | Four Stages of Wound Healing

It is important to remember that the stages of wound healing to be discussed are for descriptive purposes only and are essentially more relevant to the acute wound healing process. Winter's seminal work (1962) on partial thickness wounds identified that a moist wound healing environment was the most effective process to heal a wound. A moist environment enables epithelial cells to migrate easily, thus accelerating the wound healing process. Myers (1982) states that the progress of epithelial migration is significantly reduced in the presence of either necrotic tissue or a scab, as epithelial cells are forced to burrow underneath the eschar, which forms a mechanical obstruction in the wound bed. The mitotic activity of cells within a wound is sensitive to local fluctuations in temperature and is slowed down at temperature extremes.

Wound healing is typically described as having four stages (Flanagan, 2000):

1. Haemostasis
2. Inflammation
3. Proliferation
4. Maturation

It should be remembered that these stages do not operate in isolation; rather there is often considerable overlap between them. Careful assessment should help to identify each stage and treatment objectives should reflect the stage of wound healing (Flanagan, 2000). A summary of the stages of wound healing is provided in Figure 2.5.

Stage 1: Haemostasis
If damage to the skin affects more than the epidermis, bleeding will occur. Tissue injury is characterized by microvascular injury and therefore extravasation of blood into the wound. Injured vessels constrict rapidly and the coagulation cascade is activated to limit blood loss, leading to clot formation and platelet aggregation (Enoch and Price, 2004). The blood clot consisting of a fibrin mesh will eventually become a scab that closes the wound and vasodilatation of the vessels begins (Figure 2.6).

Platelets
Platelets have several functions in the healing process, including the cessation of bleeding. The platelets join together to form a plug to stop the blood loss. The damaged smooth muscle of the blood vessels constricts in response to the autonomic nervous system and constrictors, such as serotonin, are released by the platelets. The narrowing of the blood vessels temporarily reduces blood loss and increases the stability of the platelet plug. Further platelet aggregation is stimulated by the release of platelet factors, causing local vasoconstriction and the formation of a clot.

Platelets control the bleeding and assist the wound to enter the inflammatory stage, stage 2 of the wound healing process. When the clot is no longer useful it is removed by the enzyme plasmin, which breaks down the fibrin matrix (Monaco and Lawrence, 2003).

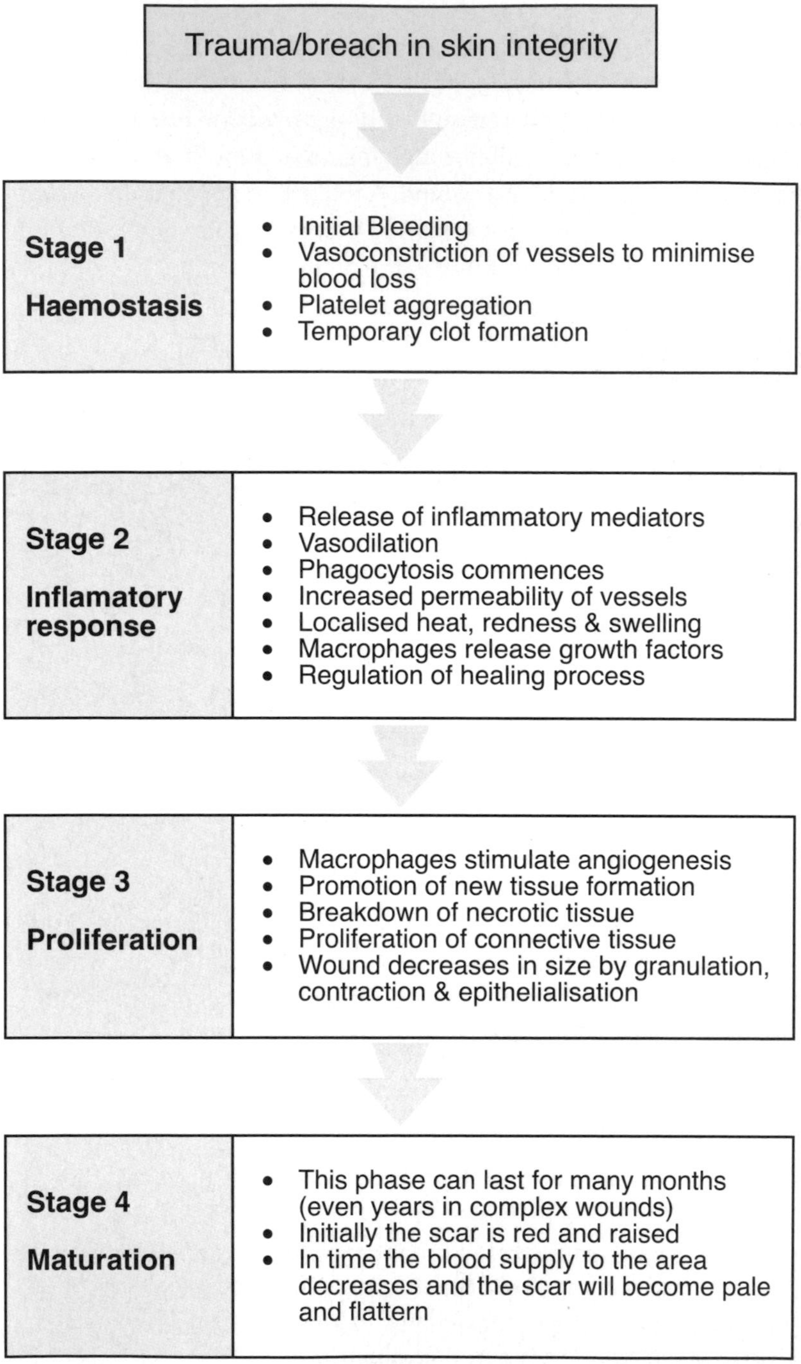

Trauma/breach in skin integrity

Stage 1

Haemostasis

- Initial Bleeding
- Vasoconstriction of vessels to minimise blood loss
- Platelet aggregation
- Temporary clot formation

Stage 2

Inflamatory response

- Release of inflammatory mediators
- Vasodilation
- Phagocytosis commences
- Increased permeability of vessels
- Localised heat, redness & swelling
- Macrophages release growth factors
- Regulation of healing process

Stage 3

Proliferation

- Macrophages stimulate angiogenesis
- Promotion of new tissue formation
- Breakdown of necrotic tissue
- Proliferation of connective tissue
- Wound decreases in size by granulation, contraction & epithelialisation

Stage 4

Maturation

- This phase can last for many months (even years in complex wounds)
- Initially the scar is red and raised
- In time the blood supply to the area decreases and the scar will become pale and flattern

Figure 2.5
Four stages of wound healing

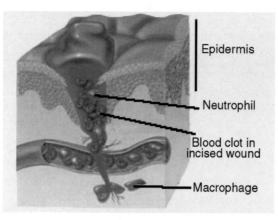

Figure 2.6
Haemostasis (adapted from Marieb, 2004, p. 143)

Stage 2: Inflammation

This stage protects the body from further damage dealing with toxins and killing bacteria. Phago-cytosis commences, which is the ingestion of foreign material by the neutrophils and monocytes. In acute wounds the inflammatory stage will last approximately 3–5 days, but in chronic wounds the process is prolonged. Injury to the dermis causes bleeding, with the damaged blood vessels constricting to minimize the blood flow and to commence the clotting process. This is accelerated due to platelet aggregation and the release of growth factors required for tissue repair. The activa-tion of clotting factors stimulates the release of inflammatory mediators such as histamine, which cause local blood vessels to become more permeable and dilated (Flanagan and Fletcher, 2003).

This inflammatory response is normal and required to initiate the rest of the healing process. The clinical signs are similar to those of infection but care should be taken not to confuse them. Flana-gan and Fletcher (2003) state that the inflammatory response can be observed around an injured area by the presence locally of:

- Oedema
- Erythema
- Heat
- Discomfort
- Loss of movement

Neutrophils

Neutrophils will migrate to the wound site in large numbers and are regarded as the first line of defence against infection. They release cytokine factors that attract other leucocytes and proteo-lytic enzymes that assist in cleaning the damaged tissue. Monocytes are stimulated by a number of platelet and leucocyte factors to release mediators and stimulate the macrophages. The monocytes will increase in number as the neutrophils decrease, taking over the sequence of healing events.

Monocytes

Some of the monocytes will mature into macrophages that continue to clean the wound bed during the inflammatory stage. It is during this stage that erythema, heat, oedema, discomfort and functional disturbance around the wound area may be observed. These are due to an increase in blood flow and an accumulation of fluid in the soft tissues. They are a normal part of the inflammatory process and should not be confused with infection.

Macrophages

The macrophages are not only able to destroy bacteria and remove tissue debris but they can also produce growth factors that stimulate the formation of fibroblasts, the synthesis of structural protein collagen and the process of angiogenesis (Kindlen, 2003).

This stage may last for up to four days, during which time the wound lacks tensile strength. If the wound is infected this stage may be prolonged. This phase is critical to the wound healing process, but some patients may be unable to produce this stage due to drug therapies, cancer or advanced age and the wound will therefore not heal.

Stage 3: Proliferation

During this stage the wound begins to replace lost tissue and form collagen fibres that will give the wound its strength. Key to this stage are fibroblasts that form the extracellular matrix by producing fibronectin and proteoglycans. The fibres support the capillary loops and new capillary buds that form the base for the new granulation tissue across the wound, promoting an increased supply of oxygen to the wound (Figure 2.7).

Angiogenesis

Angiogenesis is stimulated by several factors including PDGF (PDGF is produced from cells other than platelets) and new blood vessels start to infiltrate the wound. New capillary loops are rapidly

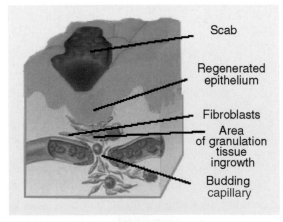

Figure 2.7
Proliferation (adapted from Marieb, 2004, p. 143)

growing structures but are fragile and easily destroyed; at this stage great care must be taken during dressing change to prevent damage (Frubeck and Salvador, 2000).

The hormone leptin acts as a growth factor and promotes the vascular response. Epithelization will now commence and takes place from the wound margins towards the centre of the wound. Epithelial cells will then begin to migrate across the wound surface providing they have a moist environment and viable granulation tissue.

Epithelialization

Restoration of injured epithelium is crucial to re-establish the barrier functions of the skin. Incisional injuries with a minimal epithelial gap, such as Julie's wound (Figure 2.1), typically re-epithelialize within 24–48 hours after initial injury (Monaco and Lawrence, 2003). In epithelialization, basal cells situated at the wound margins migrate across the wound bed. Epithelial appendages, such as hair follicles and sweat glands, also contribute migratory epithelial cells to assist the healing process (Monaco and Lawrence, 2003). When advancing epithelial cells from opposing wound borders meet, cellular movement begins to cease (Garrett, 1998). In contraction, the wound is made smaller by the action of myofibroblasts. A myofibroblast is a form of fibroblast cell that has differentiated partially towards a smooth muscle phenotype. It can contract by using some of the cytoskeletal proteins that are normally found in smooth muscle cells, in particular a form of actin called alpha-smooth muscle actin. These cells are then capable of speeding wound repair by contracting the edges of the wound. The myofibroblasts establish a grip on the wound edges and contract themselves using a mechanism similar to that in smooth muscle cells (Garg, 2000).

Wounds that are granulating will appear bright red and moist. As epithelialization occurs, the wound becomes a paler pink and less moist in appearance.

Stage 4: Maturation

This is the final stage of the wound healing process and may continue for over 12 months from the initial injury. In healthy individuals this stage generally commences 20 days following injury. The wound regains its strength and function, but the wound never fully regains its pre-injury strength. During this stage scarring occurs. Mature scar tissue is avascular and contains no hairs, sebaceous glands or sweat glands, as seen in Figures 2.8 and 2.9. Remodelling of scar tissue is stimulated by macrophages and results in the reorganization of collagen fibres to maximize tensile strength (Flanagan, 2000). The tensile strength of scar tissue is approximately 80 % compared to normal skin (Brown, 1988).

2.6 | The Physiology of Chronic Wounds

Unfortunately, wounds do not always follow an orderly pattern of healing, as outlined in Section 2.5.1, and can become chronic in nature. A chronic wound is defined as one in which the normal process of healing is disrupted at one or more points in the phases of haemostasis, inflammation,

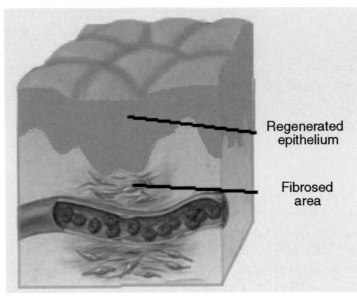

Figure 2.8
Maturation (adapted from Marieb, 2004, p. 143)

proliferation and remodelling (Lazarus *et al.*, 1994). In most chronic wounds, however, the healing process is thought to be "stuck" in the inflammatory or proliferative phase. As growth factors, cytokines, proteases, and cellular and extracellular elements all play important roles in different stages of the healing process, alterations in one or more of these components could account for the impaired healing observed in chronic wounds (Lazarus *et al.*, 1994).

Morison (2006) discusses the significant differences in the cellular and molecular environments of healing and nonhealing wounds, as highlighted in Table 2.1.

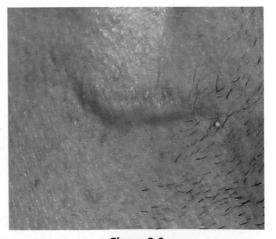

Figure 2.9
Scar tissue 10 months following acute trauma

	Healing wounds	Nonhealing wounds
Level of cell mitosis	High	Low
Macrophage activity	Occurs normally	Suppressed
Fibroblast proliferation	Increased	Decreased
Migration of keratinocytes over the wound bed	Occurs normally	Impaired
Presence of inflammatory cytokines in wound exudate	Low	High
Protease production and activity	Low	High

Table 2.1
Physiological differences between healing and nonhealing wounds (adapted from Morison, 2006)

2.6.1 | Factors that Impair Wound Healing

There are a number of local and systemic factors that can disrupt the delicate balance of wound healing, as highlighted in Table 2.2. If wound healing does not proceed as expected it is important that practitioners explore all aspects of the patient's medical and social history to identify factors that may contribute to delayed healing. Many of the factors listed in Table 2.2 are further considered throughout the chapters contained in this book.

Systemic factors	Local factors
Ageing	Infection
Poor nutritional status	Necrotic tissue
Chronic disease (e.g. diabetes mellitus (Chapter 8) and rheumatoid arthritis (Chapter 9))	Foreign bodies
Medication	Mechanical injury
Compromised perfusion	Local pressure/shear and friction
Smoking	

Table 2.2
Factors that impair wound healing (adapted from Krasner, 1995, and Morison, 2006)

Ageing

Desai (1997) argues that ageing results in changes to the skin structure and its ability to maintain its normal function. There is a reduction in the barrier function of the stratum corneum that results in an increased susceptibility to infection and increased risk of skin irritation. A reduction in the numbers of sensory receptors, thinning of the epidermis and changes in the basement membrane make the skin more susceptible to trauma. Within the basement membrane there is a flattening of the structure and consequent reduction in the surface area in contact with the dermis. This leads to an increased risk of the epidermis being sheared off the dermis by either trauma or friction. The reduction in contact between the two layers can lead to a slowdown in the rate of cell division and replacement, thus increasing the healing time of wounds in the older person.

Nutritional status

Adequate nutrition is essential for health. During wound healing it is important that essential nutrients are available as they form the building blocks for repair. Poor nutritional status can compromise wound healing due to an overall deficiency of intake, due to nonavailability or due to the inability of the patient to adequately absorb nutrients (Reynolds, 2001). Gray and Cooper (2001) stress the benefits of nutritional screening and assessment in wound care. This identifies patients who are malnourished or at risk of becoming malnourished, so dietary needs should be considered and addressed.

Chronic disease

Wound healing is likely to be impaired by a number of medical pathologies. This can include endocrine disorders such as diabetes mellitus (Chapter 8), inflammatory disorders such as rheumatoid arthritis (Chapter 9) and impaired circulation (Chapter 5) (Morison, 2006). As people live longer the number of individuals presenting with multiple concurrent health problems is likely to increase. This problem can be further confounded by unhealthy lifestyle factors, such as poor diet and smoking (Morison, 2006).

Julie smokes approximately 20 cigarettes per day. What impact might this have on wound healing?

Three days post-operatively Julie complains of a "sharp burning pain" around her wound site. On examination the wound is oozing green exudate and the surrounding skin is red and inflamed. Julie has a fever (pyrexia) with a raised body temperature of 38° Celsius.
What additional signs and symptoms would lead you to assume Julie had developed a wound infection?

Wound infection

A wound infection is a problem as it will delay the normal wound healing process by:

1. Prolonging the inflammatory stage by delaying collagen synthesis and causing granulation tissue to become more fragile and prone to bleeding (Flanagan, 1998).
2. Depleting the components of the complement cascade.
3. Disrupting the normal clotting mechanism, promoting disordered leukocyte function and ultimately preventing the development of new blood vessels and the formation of granulation tissue (Robson *et al.*, 1990).

Invasion of bacteria

When bacteria attack the tissue an inflammatory response is initiated and neutrophils are mobilized. If the body's immune system is compromised the micro-organisms will multiply and an infection will develop.

Signs of infection

There may be inflammation, increased amounts of exudate, pain and a malodorous discharge. There may also be the systemic response of fever, increased production of immature white blood cells and neutrophils, as well as a positive wound culture. An increased amount of exudate is due to underlying capillaries dilating as a part of the inflammatory response to allow white cells to migrate to the source of the infection. The capillaries become permeable and allow greater quantities of plasma to leak out. Cutting *et al.* (2005) produced consensus criteria for recognizing signs of infection, which are further explored within Chapter 4.

Body's response

When an infection occurs in a wound the body responds by releasing a variety of chemicals to cause vasodilation and to increase capillary permeability. This improves access to the site of injury for the defending cells and increases the delivery of soluble factors and vital nutrients. The increased blood supply raises the temperature of the tissue, so that the site feels warm and appears red in colour. The increased capillary permeability allows for the influx of cells, fluids and chemical mediators to the site of injury. The accumulation of fluid causes tissue swelling and, combined with the action of mediators on nerve endings, pain is often felt (Kindlen, 2003).

2.7 | The Future of Wound Healing

As understanding of the wound healing physiology improves and the science of wound healing continues to advance, the future of wound healing is promising. One exciting area focuses on the role of growth factors in healing.

2.7.1 | Growth Factors

Growth factors, or cytokines, are polypeptide proteins that occur naturally in the body. Growth factors are, in simple terms, chemical messengers that enable a wound to progress through the stages of wound healing (Edwards, 2001). Following injury, growth factors are thought to be centrally involved in stimulating and controlling all aspects of the wound healing process, including inflammatory cell recruitment, re-epithelialization, fibroplasia, angiogenesis and the maturation of new dermal tissue to form a scar (Hart, 1999).

Garrett and Garrett (1997) state that wound healing growth factors are produced by many cells including platelets and macrophages, and act as chemical messengers throughout the healing process. Hart (1999) described a variety of growth factors that had been subjected to clinical evaluation. These include basic fibroblast growth factor (bFGF), transforming growth factor-ß2 (TGF-ß2), platelet-derived growth factor-BB (PDGF-BB), epidermal growth factor (EGF) and interleukin-1ß.

Xiaobing et al. (2004) argue that several growth factors have been identified as regulatory polypeptides that coordinate wound healing as a dynamic biological process consisting of a complex interaction of cellular and biochemical events. The average wound healing time in acute skin wounds can be shortened when locally treated with growth factors.

Indeed, Folkman et al. (2001) state that platelets carry over 20 growth factors, including platelet-derived growth factor-BB (PDGF-BB), epidermal growth factor (EGF), transforming growth factor-b (TGF-b), and vascular endothelial growth factor (VEGF), with Kirchner et al. (2003) maintaining that they have all been shown to improve wound healing in healing-impaired animal models and in human chronic wounds.

In relation to the wound healing process, as discussed earlier in this chapter, platelets accumulate in the wound. The platelets release PDGF, transforming growth factor-ß1 (TGF-ß1), and other peptides (Falanga, 1992). These growth factors can stimulate the synthetic activity of fibroblasts and provide the wound with a provisional matrix essential to the migration of other cells. The clinical application of growth factors is based on an assumption that chronic wounds need a trigger to stimulate the healing process (Edwards, 2001). As such, various products containing growth factors have been produced to provide this trigger for chronic wounds.

Slavin et al. (1994) maintain that a growth factor cannot compensate for poor basic wound care, inadequate blood supply or sensory loss, but if a defined aspect of wound repair is missing the pharmacological manipulation may enhance the outcome. However, Kingsley (2002) suggests by using knowledge of the wound healing process and appropriately preparing the wound bed, nurses and other clinicians should be able to focus their choice of dressing product and wound care interventions on unblocking barriers to the wound healing cascade.

While the development of products containing growth factors is an exciting development for the future of wound healing, further research is required into this particular aspect of wound care.

2.8 | Case Scenario Revisited

You should now be able to answer the initial questions posed by reviewing the content of this chapter.

1. **What is the normal function of the skin?**
    The skin has a number of important functions: regulation of body temperature, protection, sensation, excretion, immunity, blood reservoir and synthesis of vitamin D.
2. **What is the natural structure of the skin?**
    The skin is composed of two types of tissue: the surface epidermis and underlying dermis. A subcutaneous layer lies beneath the dermis which separates the dermis from the deeper structures such as deep fascia, muscle and bone.
3. **How do wounds heal?**
    Wound healing physiology involves four stages: haemostasis, inflammation, proliferation and maturation. Julie's wound is a surgical wound healing by secondary intention. It would be expected that her wound would follow the four stages of wound healing and heal uneventfully.
4. **How long should wound healing take in this case?**
    Wounds healing by primary intention would normally be expected to follow the orderly pattern of wound healing as outlined. Julie's wound will now take longer to heal due to the presence of infection. If the infection does not improve then it may be necessary for the wound closure to be reopened and to allow the wound to heal by secondary intention.
5. **Which members of the multiprofessional team need to be involved?**
    As the consultant podiatric surgeon undertook the procedure it is important that the overall responsibility for Julie's post-operative care be resumed. The need for effective communication between other members of the multiprofessional team is essential in order to ensure optimum patient care. Nurses and podiatrists might be involved in regular redressings; Julie's GP might be involved in prescribing antibiotics for the infection. It may also be necessary to refer Julie to the dietician to offer advice on a healthy eating plan. All health care professionals will be involved in the promotion of smoking cessation. Dependent on how well she mobilizes post-operatively, it may be necessary to involve the physiotherapist in Julie's care.

2.9 | Conclusion

This chapter has identified the many functions of the skin and its natural structure. In addition, normal wound healing physiology has been discussed. Julie was admitted for a surgical procedure and the wound would have normally healed by primary intention. However, due to her developing a wound infection the wound will take substantially longer to heal and it may be necessary for it to heal by secondary intention. Now take time to reflect upon the knowledge you have gained and how this will affect your future practice.

> **? Reflection**
>
> **Take time to reflect upon your learning from this chapter. Ask yourself:**
>
> 1. **What knowledge did I possess prior to reading this chapter?**
> 2. **How has my knowledge developed?**
> 3. **How will I implement this into my future practice?**

References

Brown, G.L. (1988) Acceleration of tensile strength with EGF and TGF. *Annals of Surgery*, **208**, 788–94.

Butcher, M. and White, R. (2005) The structure and functions of the skin, in *Skin Care in Wound Management* (ed. R. White), Cromwell Press, Trowbridge, Wiltshire, pp. 13–14.

Calvin, M. (1998) Cutaneous wound repair. *Wounds*, **10**(1), 12–32.

Collier, M. (2002) Caring for the patient with a skin or wound care need, in *Watson's Clinical Nursing and Related Sciences* (ed. M. Walsh), Baillière Tindall, Edinburgh, pp. 925–59.

Cutting, K.F., White, R.J., Mahoney, P. and Harding, K.G. (2005) Understanding wound infection, in Identifying Criteria for Wound Infection, European Wound Management Association (EWMA) Position Document, MEP Ltd, London, pp. 2–5.

Desai, H. (1997) Ageing and wounds: Part 2: healing in old age. *Journal of Wound Care,* **6**(5), 237–9.

Edwards, J. (2001) Growth factors: the healing messengers. *Journal of Community Nursing*, **15**(7), 14–21.

Enoch, S. and Price, P. (2004) Cellular, molecular and biochemical differences in the pathophysiology of healing between acute wounds, chronic wounds and wounds in the aged, http://www.world-widewounds.com/2004/august/Enoch/Pathophysiology-Of-Healing.html, Last accessed 30 September 2006.

Falanga, V. (1992) Growth factors and wound repair. *Journal of Tissue Viability*, **2**(3), 100–4.

Flanagan, M. (1998) The characteristics and formation of granulation tissue. *Journal of Wound Care*, **7**(10), 508–10.

Flanagan, M. (2000) The physiology of wound healing. *Journal of Wound Care*, **9**(6), 299–300.

Flanagan, M. and Fletcher, J. (2003) Tissue viability: managing chronic wounds, in *Nursing Adults: The Practice of Caring* (eds C. Brooker and M. Nicol), Mosby, London.

Folkman, J., Browder, T. and Palmblad, J. (2001) Angiogenesis research: guidelines for translation to clinical application. *Thrombosis and Haemostasis*, 2001, **86**, 23–33.

Frubeck, G. and Salvador, J. (2000) Is leptin involved in the signalling cascade after myocardial infarction and reperfusion? *Circulation*, **101**, 194.

Garg, H.G. (2000). *Scarless Wound Healing*, Marcel Dekker, Inc., New York, Electronic book.

Garrett, B. (1998) Re-epithelisation. *Journal of Wound Care*, **7**(7), 358–9.

Garrett, B. and Garrett, S. (1997) Healing messengers. *Nursing Times*, **93**(46), 79–82.

Gawkrodger, D.J. (1997) *Dermatology: An Illustrated Colour Text*, 2nd edn, Churchill Livingstone, London.

Graham-Brown, R. and Burns, T. (2004) *Lecture Notes on Dermatology,* 8th edn, Blackwell Publishing, Oxford, pp. 1–8.

Gray, D. and Cooper, P. (2001) Nutrition and wound healing: what is the link? *Journal of Wound Care*, **10**(3), 86–9.

Guyton, A.C. (1997) *Human Physiology and Mechanisms of Disease*, 6th edn, W.B. Saunders, London.

Hart, J. (1999) Growth factors, in *Wound Management Theory and Practice* (eds M. Miller and D. Glover), NT Books, London.

Kindlen, S. (2003) *Physiology for Health Care and Nursing*, Churchill Livingstone, London.

Kingsley, A. (2001) A proactive approach to wound infection. *Nursing Standard*, **15**(30), 50–8.

Kingsley, A. (2002) Wound healing and potential therapeutic options. *Professional Nurse*, **17**(9), 539–44.

Kirchner, L.M., Meerbaum, S.O. and Gruber, B.S. (2003) Effects of vascular endothelial growth factor on wound closure rates in the genetically diabetic mouse model. *Wound Repair and Regeneration*, **11**(2), 127–31.

Krasner, D. (1995) Minimising factors that impair wound healing *Osteomyelitis and Wound Management*, **41**(1), 22–30.

Lazarus, G.S., Cooper, D.M., Knighton, D.R. *et al.* (1994) Definitions and guidelines for assessment of wounds and evaluation of healing. *Archives of Dermatology*, **130**(4), 489–93.

Marieb, E. (2004) *Human Anatomy and Physiology*, 6th edn, Benjamin Cummings, San Francisco, California, p. 143.

Monaco, J.L. and Lawrence, W.T. (2003) Acute wound healing: an overview. *Clinics in Plastic Surgery* **30**, 1–12.

Morison, M. (2001) *The Prevention and Treatment of Pressure Ulcers*, Mosby, London, pp. 19–21.

Morison, M. (2006) *Chronic Wounds,* An educational booklet (sponsored by Smith & Nephew), Wounds UK, Aberdeen, Publishing pp. 4–9.

Myers, J.A. (1982) Wound healing and the use of a modern surgical dressing. *Journal of Clinical Investigation,* **2**, 103–4.

Reynolds, T.M. (2001) The future of nutrition and wound healing. *Journal of Tissue Viability,* **11**(1), 5–11.

Robson, M.C., Stenberg, B.D. and Heggers, J.P. (1990) Wound healing alterations caused by infection. Clinics in Plastic Surgery, 1990 (July), **17**(3), 485–92.

Rowett, H.G.O. (1996) *Basic Anatomy and Physiology,* 3rd edn, John Murray Publishers, London, pp. 80–1.

Slavin, J., Unemori, E., Hunt, T.K. *et al.* (1994) Transforming growth factor beta (TGF-beta) and dexomethasone have direct opposing effects on collagen metabolism in low passage human dermal fibroblasts *in vitro. growth Factors,* **11**(3), 205–13.

Tortora, G.J., Grabowski, S.R. and Reynolds, S. (2004) *Introduction to the Human Body: The Essentials of Anatomy and Physiology,* 6th edn, Wiley Publications, London.

Winter, G. (1962) Formulation of the scab and the rate of epithelisation in the skin of the domestic pig. *Nature,* **193**, 293–4.

Woolf, N. (1998) *Pathology Basic and Systemic,* W.B. Saunders, London.

Xiaobing Fu, Xiaokun Li, Biao Cheng *et al.* (2004) Engineered growth factors and cutaneous wound healing: success and possible questions in the past 10 years. *Wound Repair and Regeneration,* **13**(2), 122–30, (doi: 10.1111/j.1067-1927.2005.130202).

Caroline McIntosh and Kimberley Martin

Chapter 3

Skin Changes in the At-Risk Limb

3.1 | Introduction

The skin is the largest organ in the human body, providing approximately 10% of body mass (Butcher and White, 2005) which, as discussed in Chapter 2, has a number of important functions to sustain well-being. Intact skin is the body's first line of defence against the invasion of micro-organisms and harmful chemicals and trauma (Bryant and Rolstad, 2001; Bale, 2005). An essential, yet basic, aspect of patient care is therefore the maintenance of healthy intact skin (Bryant, 2002).

Various medical conditions increase the risk of skin changes that can place the lower limb "at risk". An at-risk limb can be defined as a limb with reduced tissue viability, an increased risk of infection, ulceration, necrosis and amputation (Dawber *et al.*, 2001). This is usually due to a number of intrinsic factors such as:

- Systemic disease
- Peripheral neuropathy
- Peripheral vascular disease
- Inflammatory arthropathy
- Immunosuppression

As a result a small breach in skin integrity can have devastating consequences; e.g. a simple abrasion from poorly fitting footwear could result in ulceration in the at-risk limb.

This chapter aims to explore intrinsic factors that result in skin changes in the lower extremities, consider a systematic approach to skin assessment and discuss management strategies for both the prevention and management of skin changes.

3.2 | Case Scenario

Case Scenario 3

Consider the following case scenario. Brenda, a 67-year-old lady, presents with a lesion on the dorsum aspect of the right foot (Figure 3.1). The patient reports that the lesion developed a week ago and has increased in size. She has observed increased swelling on the top of the foot and reports mild pain.

This patient has a history of hypertension, coronary heart disease and varicose veins. There is no previous history of lower extremity ulceration. Figures 3.1(a) and (b) illustrate the presenting lesion.

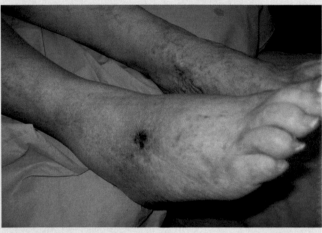

(a)

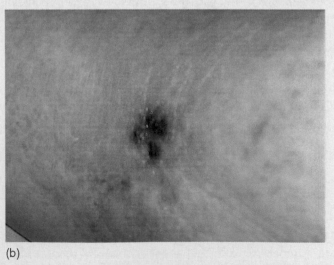

(b)

Figure 3.1
The presenting lesion

?   **Consider the following questions in relation to this case:**

1. **What is the possible cause of the skin lesion?**

2. **Identify which factors in the patient's history increase the risk of foot ulceration.**

3. **What assessments should be undertaken before implementing a management plan?**

4. **Outline management strategies appropriate for this case.**

5. **Who should be involved in this patient's care?**

The information provided within the following sections should enable you to answer the five questions posed above. The answers to the case will be further considered towards the end of the chapter.

3.3 | Skin Assessment

A systematic skin assessment can provide baseline information, an indication of ulceration risk in the at-risk limb and can allow measurement of the effectiveness of preventative care plans (Clark and Stephen-Haynes, 2005). When undertaking skin assessment Dawber *et al.* (2001) recommend staging the process:

1. History taking. A detailed history is essential to allow an accurate diagnosis. The patient's age, gender, past and present medical history, current or previous medication, family history and social history should be explored and accurately documented.
2. Physical examination. A thorough examination is essential to allow an accurate diagnosis and inform management planning. Assessment of the lower limb and feet is best performed with the leg exposed to the knee, and both limbs should be assessed simultaneously so that subtle changes become apparent.
3. Accurate documentation and monitoring outcomes. Accurate documentation in the patient's medical records is an essential aspect of the primary assessment. This provides a foundation for future care planning, a form of communication between health care professionals and meets minimum standards of care in terms of professional accountability. Accurate documentation should therefore include:

- Exact anatomical location
- Duration and cause of the lesion, if known
- Size (height, width, surface area and depth) of the lesion
- A description of the appearance, including colour, borders, inflammation, whether the lesion is dry or moist, and the state of the surrounding skin

- Description of any discharge: colour, consistency and volume
- Symptoms, e.g. itching, burning, pain
- Any notable changes such as increasing size or bleeding
- Any previous management of the lesion

At each patient consultation it is imperative to reassess any skin changes, using the above format, and monitor and document outcomes. Appropriate health outcome measures include: simple measurement of the lesion, lesion charts that allow tracing of the lesion dimensions, photography and visual analogue scales for pain assessment.

3.4 | The Ageing Skin

As the most visible organ of the human body, signs of ageing are often apparent. Optically the skin becomes more transparent with age, allowing veins, tendons and muscles to be easily seen, as illustrated in Figure 3.2 (Marks, 1999).

The incidence of chronic wounds, as highlighted in Chapter 2, has been partially attributed to an ageing population. Older patients are at greater risk of ulceration due to structural changes of the skin secondary to the ageing process. Ageing is reported as the most common cause of an overall thinning of the epidermis (skin atrophy), especially after the age of 70 years (Desai, 1997; Savin *et al.*, 1997). Normal total skin thickness in adults is 1.0–1.2 mm and 0.8–1.0 mm in men and women respectively; however, at the age of 70 there is a decreased thickness, with measurements becoming similar for both genders, 0.7–0.9 mm (Marks, 1999). Structural changes, secondary to the ageing process, result in fragile tissue that has increased susceptibility to disease and damage (Copson, 2006). Specifically, changes at the dermoepidermal junction mean that tissue is less resistant to shearing forces, a significant risk factor for the development of pressure ulcers and diabetic foot ulcers.

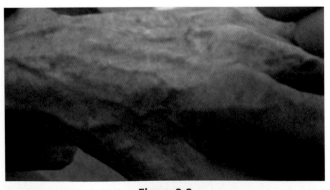

Figure 3.2
Translucency of ageing skin

Some of the effects of ageing on the skin and wound healing are outlined below (Burr and Penzer, 2005; Copson, 2006; Morison, 2006):

- The dermis becomes thinner and skin is more susceptible to trauma.
- Collagen loses elasticity so the skin does not return to its usual state, seen visually as wrinkles and skin folds.
- There is a reduced turnover of keratinocytes in the epidermis.
- The rate of epithelialization declines.
- There is an impaired ability to form granulation tissue.
- Dehydration occurs due to loss of water content.
- Decreased sensation is common.
- Reduced sebum production results in anhydrotic skin more prone to skin fissuring.

All of the structural and functional changes outlined have the capacity to impede the skin's primary function of protection, rendering the individual more susceptible to tissue damage and infection. Additionally, the likelihood of comorbidities is high in the older population. Optimizing skin health in the elderly will therefore help maintain skin integrity, and as such should be a fundamental aspect of wound prevention (Fore, 2006).

3.5 | Diabetes Mellitus

Effects of prolonged hyperglycaemia (high blood glucose levels) due to diabetes mellitus are associated with arterial disease and nerve dysfunction, as discussed in Chapter 8.

It has been suggested that as many as 30% of patients with diabetes will develop skin changes during the course of their disease (Ahmed and Goldstein, 2006). Skin manifestations of diabetes often occur following a diagnosis of diabetes but it may be that skin changes are the first signs of the disease prior to a diagnosis being made. McIntosh and Newton (2005) list several skin conditions specific to diabetes mellitus that practitioners working in the field of diabetes should be aware of:

- Necrobiosis lipoidica diabeticorum. Barnes and Davies (2005) define necrobiosis lipoidica diabeticorum as a disorder of collagen degeneration with a granulomatous response. Typically there is thickening of blood vessel walls and fat deposition. The exact cause of necrobiosis lipoidica diabeticorum is unknown, but it is thought that it is due to diabetic microangiopathy. Other theories suggest trauma, inflammatory changes or metabolic changes.
- Granuloma annulare. Granuloma annulare is a benign, asymptomatic self-limited eruption that classically presents as groups of round firm, skin-coloured papules frequently occurring on the lateral or dorsal surfaces of the hands and feet (Cyr, 2006).
- Acanthosis nigricans. Acanthosis nigricans is a skin condition characterized by a dark, warty, hyperpigmentated thickening of the skin. Multiple warty papillomata may be profuse and may affect the palms of the hands and plantar aspects of the feet. Acanthosis nigricans is reportedly

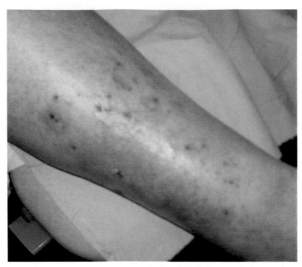

Figure 3.3
Diabetic dermopathy

a reliable predictor of hyperinsulinaemia, a known precursor for type 2 diabetes. Early screening for the signs of acanthosis nigricans has been advocated to identify individuals at risk of type 2 diabetes so that preventative strategies can be implemented (Stoddart *et al.*, 2002).

- Diabetic dermopathy (spotted leg syndrome). This skin condition is characterized by small brown lesions on the shins of some patients with diabetes (illustrated in Figure 3.3), thought to be a consequence of diabetic microangiopathy (Graham-Brown and Burns, 2004). Differential diagnoses for this condition include age spots and trauma. If a patient presents with spotted shins, without a history of diabetes, testing for diabetes is advisable.

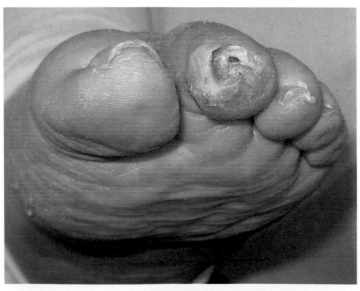

Figure 3.4
Lipoatrophy of the fibrofatty padding

- Diabetic bullae. This rare blistering condition results in subepidermal bullae occurring on the hands and feet of individuals with diabetes (Graham-Brown and Burns, 2004).
- Waxy skin syndrome.
- Lipoatrophy. Lipoatrophy is associated with partial or generalized thinning of the fatty cutaneous layer of the skin. Figure 3.4 illustrates lipoatrophy of the plantar fibrofatty padding. In patients with diabetes it is thought that lipoatrophy occurs due to insulin resistance (Graham-Brown and Burns, 2004).

3.6 | Peripheral Neuropathy

Peripheral neuropathy, or nerve dysfunction, is commonly observed in patients with diabetes mellitus but can also arise due to other systemic conditions, such as human immunodeficiency virus (HIV) and acquired immunodeficiency syndrome (AIDS), chronic alcoholism, vitamin deficiency, stroke, spinal trauma and other neurological conditions such as multiple sclerosis and spina bifida.

Sensory loss is a major risk factor for ulceration. Neuropathic ulcers typically occur on weight-bearing areas of the foot. The characteristic features of neuropathic ulceration include deep ulceration with hyperkeratosed edges, usually painless, highly exudative and sloughy, irregular borders, and the surrounding skin may be macerated as seen in Figure 3.5 (Dawber *et al.*, 2001).

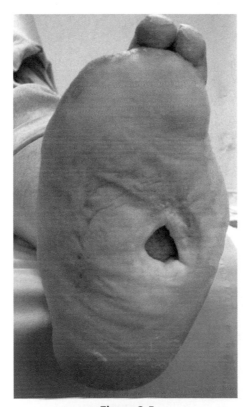

Figure 3.5
Neuropathic foot ulceration

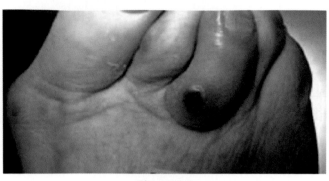

Figure 3.6
Extravasated callus (capillary bleeding into callus)

In the presence of sensory loss, inadvertent trauma and skin lesions such as callosities can occur unbeknown to the patient. Callus and corn are identified as independent risk factors for ulceration. In the neuropathic foot callus occurs at sites of high shear and pressure. Extravasated/ haemorrhagic callus (capillary bleeding into callus) forewarns of high pressure and vulnerability for ulceration (McIntosh and Newton, 2005). Figure 3.6 illustrates extravasated callus on the dorsal aspect of the toe. Evidence suggests that sharp debridement of such lesions decreases localized pressure (Young *et al.*, 1992; Murray *et al.*, 1996). Callus should therefore be debrided, by an appropriately trained and skilled practitioner, to minimize the risk of tissue breakdown. Additionally debridement allows practitioners to reveal the true extent of the lesion, often revealing ulceration as seen in Figures 3.7(a) and (b).

Skin changes associated with autonomic neuropathy include anhidrosis (dry skin) and decreased sweating, the combination of which can exacerbate callus formation and leave skin prone to fissuring (McIntosh and Newton, 2005).

Patients presenting with peripheral neuropathy are at increased risk of foot ulceration. Management strategies should therefore focus on prevention, including structured education to empower patients to manage their own foot health, regular assessment by a trained health care professional and podiatric management of foot pathologies.

3.7 | Peripheral Vascular Disease

The term peripheral vascular disease is an umbrella term that encompasses pathology of the arterial, venous or lymphatic systems.

3.7.1 | Peripheral Arterial Disease

Lower limb arterial perfusion has a direct correlation with lower limb tissue viability. In the presence of a diminished arterial supply the skin on the lower limbs and feet may show classic changes associated with arterial deficit, as illustrated in Figure 3.8:

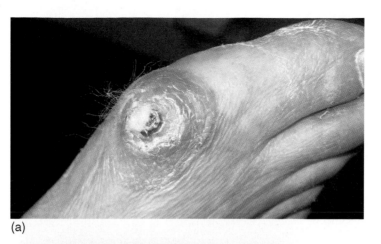

(a)

(b)

Figure 3.7
(a) Extravasated callus pre-debridement. (b) Ulceration is revealed post-debridement

- Atrophic (thin) skin
- Anhydrotic (dry) skin
- Pale skin
- Hair loss
- Thickened toenails (onychauxis) or fungal toenails (onychomycosis)
- Loss of fibrofatty padding on the plantar aspect (sole) of the foot

Peripheral ischaemia is a risk factor for lower limb ulceration. Ischaemic ulcers typically occur on the anterior shin of the leg, the heel, the lateral border of the foot and on the toes, as seen in Figure 3.8.

The characteristic features of ischaemic ulcers include either necrotic eschar, as seen in Figure 3.8, or a punched-out appearance, as seen in Figure 3.9. Dull granulation tissue, dry base of wound,

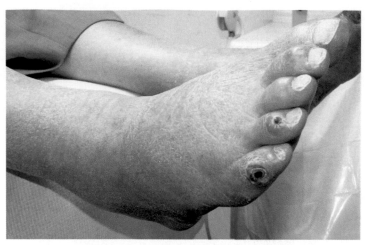

Figure 3.8
Lower limb ischaemia and necrosis of the fourth and fifth digits

minimal hyperkeratosis to the wound edges, little exudate or slough and ischaemic ulcers are generally painful for the patient (Dawber *et al.*, 2001).

3.7.2 | Venous Disease

Classic skin changes associated with venous dysfunction in the lower limb include:

- Haemosiderosis. Haemosiderosis occurs due to leakage of red blood cells from capillaries, causing a characteristic brown/orange discoloration, as seen in Figure 3.10, (Graham-Brown and Burns, 2004).

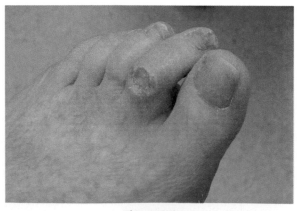

Figure 3.9
Ischaemic ulceration

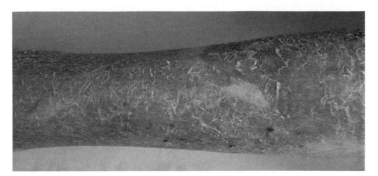

Figure 3.10
Haemosiderosis

- Telangiectasia. Characterized by permanent dilation of superficial vessels that are usually blue/mauve in appearance, telangiectasia can be an indication of venous hypertension (Savin *et al.*, 1997; Marks, 1999). Telangiectasia is usually asymptomatic but it can be a cause of concern for patients due to the aesthetic appearance.
- Varicose veins. Varicose veins are a common manifestation of venous dysfunction in the lower extremities. They appear as dilated, elongated or tortuous superficial veins. Incompetence of veins can cause venous hypertension which leads to hyperpigmentation and increased risk of ulceration (Evans *et al.*, 1999).

Review Brenda's case. Brenda has a history of varicose veins as seen in Figure 3.11 below. What impact might this have in Brenda's case?

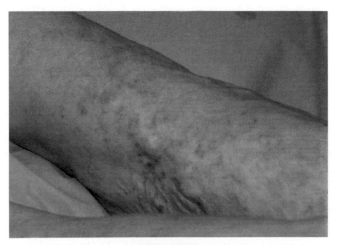

Figure 3.11
Varicose veins

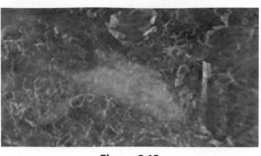

Figure 3.12
Atrophie blanche

- Atrophie blanche. These are porcelain white depressed macules thought to be due to skin infarcts (Marks, 1999), as seen in Figure 3.12.
- Cyanosis. Cyanosis is the term used to describe a bluish discoloration to the skin due to tissue hypoxia.
- Varicose eczema. Although the exact aetiology of varicose eczema remains unknown, the disorder is related to varicose veins. Typically varicose eczema occurs on the lower legs and is seen clinically as atopic, discoid, seborrhoeic eczema (Quartey-Papafio, 1999). Quartey-Papafio (1999) stresses the importance to differentiate between varicose eczema and cellulitis, an acute bacterial infection affecting the subcutaneous layers of the skin. Both are characterized by erythematous inflammation but the management of these conditions differs significantly and hence accurate diagnosis is imperative. Varicose eczema typically causes small vesicles that may leak serous fluid.
- Oedema. Oedema can be defined as an accumulation of fluid in interstitial tissues of the body. In the lower limbs oedema typically occurs at the ankle or on the dorsum of the foot, and can arise as a direct consequence of venous or lymphatic insufficiencies.

> **?** **Brenda has oedema on the dorsum of the foot, as seen in Figure 3.1. What factors might cause oedema in Brenda's case?**

Venous dysfunction is a significant risk factor for leg ulceration and delayed wound healing. Tissue viability is adversely affected due to venous incompetence, skin atrophy is common and ulceration of the skin can arise secondary to minor trauma. Typically venous ulceration occurs around the gaiter region of the leg. Venous ulcers are classically large shallow lesions, highly sloughy and exudative with irregular borders (Dawber *et al.*, 2001). Chapter 5 provides a comprehensive guide to venous leg ulceration.

Rarely in long-standing venous ulceration malignant changes known as Marjolin's ulceration can occur (Graham-Brown and Burns, 2004).

3.7.3 | Lymphatic Disease

Lymphoedema is a chronic medical condition in which the most prominent feature is swelling of an extremity due to insufficiency of the lymphatic system. Poor skin condition is common in people with lymphoedema and frequent recurrent episodes of infection, such as cellulitis, are common, resulting in further damage to the skin and exacerbation of existing swelling (Bogan *et al.*, 2007).

Classic skin changes, termed elephantiasis, are associated with lymphoedema. These include:

- Lipodermatosclerosis, thickening of the skin, is a regular occurrence in chronic venous disease and lymphoedema due to tissue damage, deposition of fibrin and hypoxia (Marks, 1999).
- Excessive swelling of the tissues can lead to deep skin folds, particularly around the ankles and toes, which can predispose to infection.
- Anhydrotic skin.
- Papillomatosis is characterized by wart-like growths.
- Stemmer's sign, an inability to pick up a fold of skin, on the dorsal aspect, at the base of the second toe, is a diagnostic sign of lymphoedema (Williams, 2003).

As the lymphatic system plays an important role in immunity individuals with lymphatic dysfunction are susceptible to infection. Meticulous skin care is essential to minimize infection risk and maintain tissue viability.

3.8 | Rheumatic Diseases

Dermatological manifestations are common in rheumatoid arthritis (RA). This has been attributed to the side effects of drug therapy used to treat the disease and direct effects from the disease (Douglas *et al.*, 2006). Chapter 9 explores the manifestation of lower limb pathology, specifically rheumatoid-related ulceration, in greater depth. However, cutaneous involvement in RA is summarized below:

- Rheumatoid nodules. The most widely recognized skin lesion in RA is the rheumatoid nodule (Magro and Crowson, 2003). Rheumatoid nodules are subcutaneous nodules of connective tissue occurring in approximately 20–30 % of cases, typically arising over bony prominences, often on the hands, but they can occur on the feet (Burton and Lloyd, 2006).
- Vasculitic lesions. Vasculitis is inflammation of blood vessel walls. The clinical features of vasculitis are variable, depending on the site and type of blood vessel affected (Savage *et al.*, 2000). However as the layers of the skin are highly vascular, manifestations of vasculitis often first appear on the skin (Savin *et al.*, 1997). Skin changes associated with vasculitis include hypoxia (diminished oxygen levels), hypercapnia (elevated carbon dioxide levels), ischaemia, necrosis and ulceration (Dawber *et al.*, 2001). Digital vasculitis may produce small infarcts around the nail folds (Bywater's lesions) or in some cases more severe ulceration (Graham-Brown and Burns, 2004).

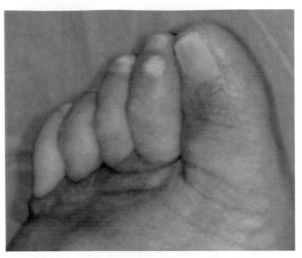

Figure 3.13
Gouty tophi on the second digit

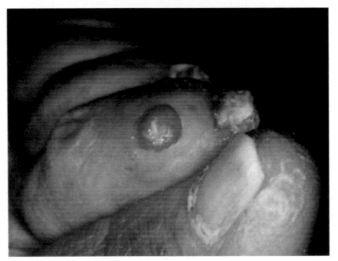

Figure 3.14
Ulcerated gouty tophi

Other noninflammatory rheumatologic conditions can also result in prototypic cutaneous lesions. For example gout, a crystal arthropathy, can give rise to tophaceous deposits around affected joints. In the lower limbs gouty tophi can occur on the toes and act as a precursor for ulceration. Figure 3.13 shows gouty tophi on the left second digit that subsequently ulcerated (see Figure 3.14).

3.9 | Immunosuppression

In order to gain an appreciation of the effects of immunosuppression on the skin and the resultant impact on wound healing it is important to review facets of the immune system. Bennett and

Baker (2001) discuss two branches of the immune system, the nonspecific (innate) and the specific (adaptive or acquired):

- Nonspecific immunity. Nonspecific immunity includes physical barriers such as microbial flora on the skin and destructive mechanisms such as the complement system and certain white blood cells, specifically neutrophils and macrophages, which do not change with repeated exposure to an antigen.
- Specific immunity. Specific immunity consists of humoral and adaptive specific immunity, and is required when antigens bypass nonspecific immune mechanisms. In humoral immunity antibodies bind to antigens activating the complement system. In adaptive specific immunity, large numbers of activated T-lymphocytes form to destroy the foreign agent.

In recent years significant advances have been made in understanding the immunological function of the skin. When a breach in skin integrity occurs, an immunological response involving Langerhans cells is mounted; this is key to preventing infection. However, it is increasingly recognized that certain conditions either result in unnecessary immunological responses so that, in effect, the body mounts an immunological response against itself (e.g. psoriasis and eczema) or the immune response is diminished due to immunosuppression (Burr and Penzer, 2005) and the body is therefore unable to prevent infection.

The hallmark of the immunosuppressed patient is an increased susceptibility to infection. The infections are often persistent and refractory to treatment, with an increased likelihood of reoccurrence. As the immune system has been impaired the patient is at risk of opportunistic infections, which are caused by organisms that are usually not pathogenic but are able to multiply and cause disease (Petrov, 1998). The clinically significant pathogens encountered when treating the lower limb are traditional tissue-borne or air-borne pathogens such as bacteria or fungi (Cope, 1995).

3.9.1 | Bacterial Infections of the Lower Limb

Traditionally, bacterial infections are responsible for substantial ill health, a decline in the quality of life and are a leading cause of mortality (Gould, 2004). In the health care setting the bacteria commonly found are:

- *Staphylococcus aureus* is normally present on the skin and mucous membrane and is the most common cause of boils and abscesses.
- *Pseudomonas* is found in decomposing organic matter and is able to cause wound infections.
- *Streptococcus* usually colonizes in the nose but can be readily spread via the hands of health care professionals. *Streptococcus* can cause infections of the urinary tract, infections of the respiratory tract and infections of the skin (Daly and Dickson, 1998).

Bacterial skin infections are virtually always curable but if left untreated or misdiagnosed can lead to severe problems such as carditis, arthritis, sepsis or bacteraemia, and in some cases be fatal (Scanlon, 2005; Mohammedamin *et al.*, 2006).

A bacterial infection commonly seen in the lower limb is cellulitis; this occurs when bacteria (usually *Staphylococcus* and/ or *Streptococcus*) invade the soft tissues through a break in the skin. Cellulitis can present as a localized infection from a wound or a more diffuse infection involving the whole leg. Involvement of the whole leg is a common medical emergency which could lead to septicaemia. Anybody with a break in the skin is liable to be at risk of soft tissue infection but some people are more prone to infection than others; people with a prior history of cellulitis, ulceration, oedema, peripheral vascular disease and/or tinea pedis are some of those considered to be at greater risk (Baxter and McGregor, 2001).

The type and number of bacteria (bacterial bioburden) may influence wound healing. Many wounds are colonized with bacteria such as *Staphylococcus aureus*, including methycillin-resistant *Staphylococcus aureus* (MRSA), but these bacteria do not always have an adverse affect on wound healing. Colonization is a normal state where bacteria in the wound multiply without reaction or clinical symptom. Infection occurs where the bacteria have multiplied to such vast numbers that they engulf the wound's defences and cellulitis occurs. The transformation from colonization to infection is specific to each person and dependent on the bacteria found in the wound at the time (Scanlon, 2005).

3.9.2 | Fungal Infection of the Lower Limb

The immunosuppressed patient is more susceptible to fungal infection. The skin normally has fungi present and an infection will manifest when the fungus overgrows to a critical level (Blenkinsopp *et al.*, 2003). The most common cause of fungal infections are dermatophytes, which are confined to the stratum corneum. The fungi are drawn to keratin and colonize keratinocytes, hair and nails, digesting keratin (Smoker, 1999). The most common fungal infections associated with the feet are onychomycosis (fungal nail infection) and tinea pedis (athlete's foot) caused most frequently by the dermatophyte *Trichophytan rubrum*. Some nail infections may be caused by the yeast *Candida albicans*. Candidiasis initially invades the nail bed in the area of the hyponychium (see Chapter 10, Figure 10.3) (Loveland, 1998; Smoker, 1999; Woodfolk, 2005). Generally onychomycotic nails tend to be thickened, dystrophic with subungual hyperkeratosis, onycholysis (loosening of the nail plate) and yellow brown discoloration (see Figure 3.15). Onychomycosis is classified according to the nail's clinical appearance, i.e. distal subungual, white superficial, proximal white subungual and *Candida* (Loveland, 1998; Smoker, 1999).

The treatment of onychomycosis has improved in recent years and many patients can now expect a complete and lasting cure. However, for up to 25 % of patients, persistent disease remains a problem, thus presenting a particular challenge to the clinician. For these patients, it is important to ensure that a correct diagnosis of onychomycosis has been made, as misdiagnosis will inevitably jeopardize the perception of therapeutic effectiveness (Scher and Baran, 2003).

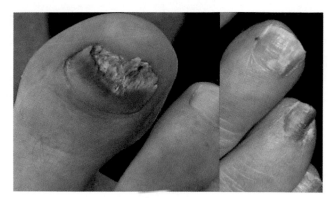

Figure 3.15
Examples of onychomycosis of the toenails

Tinea pedis often starts as in itchy, dry scaly rash between the fourth and fifth digits before extending to the plantar aspect of the foot, presenting in a moccasin distribution usually due to *Trichophytan rubrum* (Savin *et al.*, 1997; Smoker, 1999). In severe cases the risk of contracting a secondary bacterial infection is increased as the skin can peel and start to bleed (Smoker, 1999). Figure 3.16 shows a neuropathic ulcer on the plantar aspect of the heel, where examination of the surrounding skin shows a widespread fungal infection.

3.9.3 | Viral Infection of the Lower Limb

The main variety of viral infection on the foot is due to the wart virus, human papilloma virus (HPV). HPV manifests on the skin as verrucae and is limited to the epithelial layer of the skin (see Figure 3.17). The differentiated epithelial cells replicate in the upper epidermal levels while viral particles can occasionally be found in the basal layer (Watkins, 2006). Any immunocompromised person is at a greater susceptibility to HPV infection. In older patients, particularly those who are immunocompromised, HPV infection can lead to squamous cell carcinoma (Dawber *et al.*, 2001).

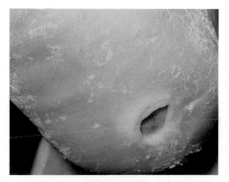

Figure 3.16
A diabetic foot ulcer with notable fungal skin infection present

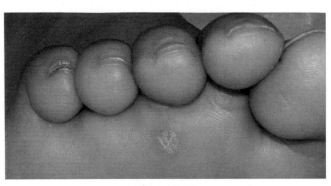

Figure 3.17
Plantar verrucae

3.10 | Human Immunodeficiency Virus/AIDS

Human immunodeficiency virus (HIV) is an immunodepressive disease that progresses to severe depletion of CD4 T-lymphocytes with a resultant deficiency in cell mediated immunity, thus leading to an increased susceptibility to opportunistic infections (Petrov, 1998; Zipfel and Badenhorst, 2002). The CD4 cell count estimates the number of CD4 T-lymphocytes per cubic millimetre (cells/mm^3) found in the peripheral blood; this important laboratory test monitors the tendency of the CD4 T-lymphocytes over time to increase and decrease, therefore calculating disease progression and response to treatment. Healthy individuals who are not immunosuppressed will, on average, have a CD4 cell count in the region of 600–1200 cells/mm^3 (Pratt, 2003). There is no documented average CD4 count expected in patients with HIV/AIDS but there is a decline of approximately 60–80 cells/mm^3 over the year if an average person with HIV was left untreated; when the CD4 count falls to 200 or below there is an increased risk of opportunistic infections.

Dermatological problems may have unusual or severe presentations in patients with HIV (Kouba and Martins, 2003). Patients with HIV portray an increased number of fungal, bacterial and viral infections that present in the skin (Petrov, 1998). With the widespread introduction of highly active antiretroviral therapies (HAART) in the mid 1990s, the cutaneous manifestations associated with HIV and acquired immunodeficiency syndrome (AIDS) have altered. With the continual advances in the treatment for HIV/AIDS the cutaneous manifestations associated with the disease will continue to evolve. Cutaneous manifestations that were commonly associated with the onset of HIV infection dramatically improved following the commencement of HAART (Mirken, 2000; Zancanaro *et al.*, 2006). HAART is a combination of three or more antiviral medications to help slow progression of the disease and each HAART regimen is tailored to suit each individual need (Tinkle, 1995; Petrov, 1998). Prior to HAART the majority of dermatological problems were due to *Staphylococcal* infections, which were more common in patients with HIV and more severe and resistant to treatment (Mirken, 2000).

3.10.1 | Fungal Infections and HIV

Fungal infections are no more common in patients with HIV but the character of the infection changes.

- The most common fungus is *Tinea*, especially *Tinea pedis*, caused by dermatophyte fungi.
- The next most common fungus is *Candida albicans*, which causes a yeast infection (Loveland, 1998)

Lesions associated with fungal infection may be more widespread and resemble psoriasis or eczema; the resultant breakdown in the skin predisposes to bacterial infection. Fungal infections generally respond poorly to treatment and the recurrence rate is high (Kouba and Martins, 2003).

Onychomycosis is not the most severe infection to affect patients with HIV but again is more extensive and refractory to treatment. Onychomycosis usually spreads rapidly but stays localized at the nails and evolves into a systemic infection (Loveland, 1998; Petrov, 1998). *Trychophytum rubrum* and *Candida albicans* are the causative organisms of onychomycosis. It is also important to consider the possibility that onychomycosis may mask or be the causative factor of a secondary infection or pathological process. The most common type of onychomycosis associated with HIV is proximal white subungual, while distal subungual and white superficial onychomycosis are more commonly associated with AIDS (Tinkle, 1995; Loveland, 1998; Petrov, 1998). There is an increased prevalence of ingrowing toenails with associated paronychia (soft tissue infection of the nail fold) in patients with HIV. This is thought to be either due to immunodeficiency or as a direct result of the HAART regime. Other skin conditions often related to antiretroviral therapy are anhydrosis and itching (Mirken, 2000).

3.10.2 | Psoriasis

Psoriasis associated with HIV/AIDS reduced in frequency by the mid 1990s even before the onset of HAART. It is more treatment resistant in patients with HIV. Abrupt development without a history of disease could be the first manifestation of HIV infection. There may be localized or generalized lesions characterized by erythematous plaques with thick silvery scales which detach easily, revealing a pink area. The most common areas for these psoriatic plaques are found on the hands, feet and scalp (Kouba and Martins, 2003).

3.10.3 | Kaposi's Sarcoma

Kaposi's sarcoma is a neoplasm and is the most common form of tumour associated with HIV/AIDS (Tinkle, 1995; Galantino *et al.*, 1998; Petrov, 1998). Kaposi's sarcoma is mainly reported in patients who have contracted HIV via sexual transmission and is more common in homosexual men (Tinkle, 1995; Mirken, 2000; Princeton, 2003). Clinical manifestations present as brown/red or red/purple indurated papules, macules and plaques following skin tension lines. They can range in size from a couple of millimetres to about 10 cm (Mirken, 2000; Princeton, 2003; Sanders *et al.*, 2004), sometimes rapidly progressing to form subcutaneous nodules and tumours. The clinical course is unpredictable, ranging from localized and indolent to widespread and aggressive with a fatal outcome. Kaposi's sarcoma can be found anywhere on the body but with a predilection to the leg and foot (Mirken, 2000; Sanders *et al.*, 2004). Differential diagnoses include verrucae, melanoma, granuloma or purpura (Tinkle, 1995; Galantino *et al.*, 1998; Petrov, 1998).

3.10.4 | Molluscum Contagiosum and Eosinophilic Folliculitis

Molluscum contagiosum and eosinophilic folliculitis were originally thought of as the markers for HIV disease. Molluscum contagiosum present as smooth waxy bumps with navel-like indentations, not usually painful or itchy. The CD4 count is usually less than 100 cells/mm^3. Eosinophilic foliculitis is a foliculitis specific to HIV that presents as a red, itchy acne-like skin eruption. The CD4 count is usually less than 200 cells/mm^3 (Parker *et al.*, 2006). The human papilloma virus (HPV), seen as warts and verrucae, are a common problem associated with HIV and are usually increased in number and size, with the mosaic type being the most common (Petrov, 1998). These are usually difficult to eradicate but flourish in patients with HIV not affected by the HAART regime (Mirken, 2000).

3.11 | Skin Allergies

When undertaking a patient history it is important to enquire regarding skin allergies. Allergic contact dermatitis is an eczematous reaction that can occur at the site of contact with an agent to which the individual has hypersensitivity (Marks, 1999). In the at-risk limb, allergic contact dermatitis can lead to severe anhydrosis, skin fissuring and secondary bacterial infection due to breached skin integrity.

3.12 | State of Continence

Older patients, as discussed in Section 3.5, are more vulnerable to skin damage. As the proportion of the older population increases protection of skin is a critical component in preventing tissue damage. Incontinence is an area of particular concern when caring for older individuals. Incontinence dermatitis in old age heightens the risk of damage when the skin is in prolonged contact with urine and faecal matter and is frequently washed (Bale *et al.*, 2004). The normal pH of the skin is 4.0–5.5; this slightly acidic environment is known to play a role in the body's natural defence mechanisms by inhibiting the growth of bacteria on the skin (Copson, 2006). A mixture of urine and faeces on the skin alters the normal pH, making the skin surface more alkaline and an ideal environment for bacterial proliferation. Prolonged exposure to urinary and faecal incontinence can cause significant problems: tissue excoriation, contact dermatitis, irritation, increased risk of pressure ulceration and episodes of infection (Copson, 2006). While incontinence is often a major issue in the management of sacral pressure ulcers, urinary incontinence can also complicate lower extremity wounds and should be considered and addressed, where required, in a comprehensive management plan.

3.13 | Skin Management Strategies

Promotion and maintenance of skin integrity is a common challenge for nurses and podiatrists involved in tissue viability. Morris (2005) suggests that maintenance of healthy skin depends on a number of factors: moisture, nutritional status and mechanical stress.

Skin care protocols are essential to maintain skin integrity. Bale (2005) advises that skin assessment should incorporate:

- Regular inspection for signs of tissue damage or skin conditions, such as dermatitis, that could predispose the individual to tissue breakdown and/ or infection
- Assessment of the state of continence including appropriate management strategies to prevent tissue damage
- Optimum skin care strategies including skin cleansing, drying, moisturising and the use of skin barrier products

Bale *et al.* (2004) explored the benefits of implementing skin assessment care protocols in nursing homes. The skin care protocol comprised the use of skin cleansers, barrier cream and barrier film in conjunction with structured education. Findings suggest that staff adherence to the protocol was good, skin condition was maintained or improved and the prevalence of grade 1 pressure ulcers and incontinence dermatitis was found to significantly reduce. These findings are supported by Thompson *et al.* (2005) who evaluated a skin care protocol for pressure ulcers and incontinent patients. Findings suggest that the implementation of skin care protocols that included body wash and a skin protectant reduced the incidence of grade 1 and grade 2 pressure ulcers and accelerated healing times in established wounds.

While these studies addressed skin care in relation to sacral pressure ulcers it is apparent that basic care, cleansing, drying and emollient use can contribute significantly to the prevention of ulceration in the at-risk limb. Management plans for individuals identified at risk of lower limb complications should address strategies to promote tissue viability and maintain skin integrity. People considered to be at risk of lower limb ulceration should be advised on the need for meticulous daily skin care to minimize risk status and ultimately maintain skin integrity.

3.14 | Case Study Revisited

1. **What is the possible cause of the skin lesion?**

    There are potentially a number of factors that could have caused the lesion in this case. It is important that practitioners consider possible differential diagnoses in order to arrive at a preferred diagnosis. In this case it is important to consider the potential for malignant changes. If in doubt it is imperative that dermatological opinion is sought. Brenda reported increased oedema in her right foot. This swelling consequently increased the size of her foot, which resulted in difficulties with footwear. Increased pressure on the dorsum aspect of the foot from tight footwear has led to a breach in skin integrity in this case.

2. **Identify which factors in the patient's history increase the risk of foot ulceration.**

    Brenda has a number of factors in her history that increase ulceration risk. Primarily this is due to venous insufficiency: varicose veins, telangiectasia and oedema (visible in Figure 3.1). Venous incompetence has a direct impact on tissue viability, increasing the risk of venous ulceration and chronicity of the wound.

3. **What assessments should be undertaken before implementing a management plan?**

    It is important to assess arterial blood supply to the feet to inform a prognosis for wound healing. Additionally, testing neurological status and venous function can inform management planning.

4. **Outline management strategies appropriate for this case.**

    It is important to remove the cause of the lesion. In this case ill-fitting footwear was causing pressure. A referral was made to the orthotist for therapeutic footwear and temporary soft boots were issued for the interim period. The patient's GP was consulted to review current medication and diuretic therapy was initiated to reduce lower limb oedema. Findings from vascular investigations revealed no significant arterial problems so compression therapy was deemed appropriate in this case to improve venous function. Local wound care was initiated and the patient was reviewed regularly until healing had occurred.

5. **Who should be involved in this patient's care?**

    It is imperative that a team approach is adopted. The podiatrist was involved in the assessment of footwear and liaised directly with the orthotist. Additionally, the podiatrist undertook vascular assessments and worked with the nurse to provide optimum wound care. The nurse was involved in compression bandaging to facilitate wound healing and the GP prescribed medication to reduce oedema.

3.15 | Conclusion

Butcher and White (2005) describe the skin as the "window to the soul". Many systemic pathologies have cutaneous manifestations; thus practitioners can readily assess general health and disease state by regularly undertaking dermatological assessment. Early recognition of skin changes that increase the risk of lower limb ulceration can contribute to timely prevention of lower extremity ulceration. All practitioners involved in the assessment of the lower limb should therefore have sufficient knowledge to recognize dermatological manifestations on the at-risk limb and recognize when referral for specialist assessment and management is warranted.

Reflection

Take time to reflect upon your learning from this chapter. Ask yourself:

1. **What knowledge did I possess prior to reading this chapter?**

2. **How has my knowledge developed?**

3. **How will I implement this into my future practice?**

References

Ahmed, I. and Goldstein, B. (2006) Diabetes mellitus. *Clinics in Dermatology*, **24**(4), 237–46.

Bale, S. (2005) Incontinence care, in *Skin Care in Wound Management* (ed. R. White), Wounds UK Publishing, Wiltshire, pp. 107–21.

Bale, S., Tebble, N., Jones, V. *et al.* (2004) The benefits of implementing a new skin care protocol in nursing homes. *Journal of Tissue Viability*, **14**(2), 44–50.

Barnes, C.J. and Davies, L. (2005) Necrobiosis Lipoidica *eMedicine* (online), Available at: http://www.emedicine.com/derm/topic283.htm, Last accessed 31 October 2006.

Baxter, H. and McGregor, F. (2001) Understanding and managing cellulitis. *Nursing Standard*, **15**(44), 50–6.

Bennett, C. and Baker, K. (2001) HIV and AIDS: an overview. *Nursing Standard*, **15**(24), 45–52.

Blenkinsopp, A., Paxton, P. and Blenkinsopp, J. (2003) Fungal Infections 1- Athletes Foot *Primary Health Care*, **13**(1), 31–2.

Bogan, L.K., Powell, J.M. and Dudgeon, B.J. (2007) Experiences of living with non-cancer related lymphoedema: implications for clinical practice *Qualitative Health Research*, **17**(2), 213–24.

Bryant, R. (2002) Maintaining skin integrity *Caring*, **21**(6), 34–6.

Bryant, R.A. and Rolstad, B.S. (2001) Examining threats to skin integrity. *Ostomy Wound Manage*, **47**(6), 18–27.

Burton, S. and Lloyd, M. (2006) An overview of rheumatoid arthritis *Nursing Standard*, **20**(24), 46–9.

Butcher, M. and White, R. (2005) The structure and functions of the skin in *Skin Care in Wound Management* (ed. R. White), Wounds UK Publishing, Wiltshire, pp. 1–16.

Burr, S. and Penzer, R. (2005) Promoting skin health *Nurs Stand*, **19**(36), 57–65; quiz 66.

Clark, M. and Stephen-Haynes, J. (2005) Superficial pressure ulcers, in *Skin Care in Wound Management* (ed. R. White), Wounds UK Publishing, Wiltshire, pp. 17–46.

Cope, R.K. (1995) Guidelines for the prevention of HIV transmission in the podiatric medical practice. *Journal of the American Podiatric Medical Association*, **85**(8), 428–33.

Copson, D. (2006) Management of tissue excoriation in older patients with faecal incontinence. *Nursing Standard*, **21**(7), 57–8, 60, 62.

Cyr, P.R. (2006) Diagnosis and management of granuloma annulare *American Family Physician*, **74**(10), 1729–34.

Daly, T. and Dickson, K. (1998) Biological hazards *Nursing Standard*, **13**(3), 43–9.

Dawber, R., Bristow, I. and Turner, W. (2001) *Text Atlas of Podiatric Dermatology*, Martin Dunitz Ltd, London.

Desai, H. (1997) Ageing and wounds. Part 2: healing in old age. *Journal of Wound Care*, **6**(5), 237–9.

Douglas, K.M., Ladoyanni, E., Treharne, G.J. *et al.* (2006) Cutaneous abnormalities in rheumatoid arthritis compared with non-inflammatory rheumatic conditions. *Annals of Rheumatic Disease*, **65**(10), 1341–5.

Evans, C.J., Fowkes, F.G.R. and Ruckley, C.V. *et al.* (1999) Prevalence of varicose veins and chronic venous insufficiency in men and women in the general population: Edinburgh Vein Study. *Journal of Epidemiology Community Health*, **53**, 149–53.

Fore, J. (2006) A review of skin and the effects of aging on skin structure and function. *Osteomyelitis and Wound Management*, **52**(9), 24–35.

Galantino, M.L., Jermyn, R.T., Tursi, F.J. and Eke-Okoro, S. (1998) Physical therapy management for the patient with HIV/lower extremity challenges. *Clinics in Podiatric Medicine and Surgery*, **15**(2), 329–43.

Gould, D. (2004) Bacterial infections: antibiotics and decontamination, *Nursing Standard*, **18**(40), 38–42.

Graham-Brown, R. and Burns, T. (2004) *Lecture Notes on Dermatology*, 8th edn, Blackwell Publishing, Oxford.

Kouba, D.J. and Martins, C.R. (2003) *A Clinical Guide to Supportive and Palliative Care for HIV/AIDS*, pp. 177–206.

Loveland, L.J. (1998) Onychomycosis in HIV-positive patients. *Clinics in Podiatric Medicine and Surgery*, **15**(2), 305–15.

McIntosh, C. and Newton, V. (2005) Superficial diabetic foot ulcers, in *Skin Care in Wound Management: Assessment, Prevention and Treatment* (ed. R. white), Wounds UK Publishing, Aberdeen, pp. 47–73.

Magro, C.M. and Crowson, A.N. (2003) The spectrum of cutaneous lesions in rheumatoid arthritis: a clinical and pathological study of 43 patients. *Journal of Cutaneous Pathology*, **30**, 1–10.

Marks, R. (1999) *Skin Disease in Old Age*, 2nd edn, Martin Dunitz Ltd, London, pp. 245–50.

Mirken, B. (2000) HIV skin complications in the age of HAART. An interview with Toby Maurer MD, AIDS Foundation, San Francisco, California (online), Available from `http//www.thebodypro.com`, Last accessed 27 March 2007.

Mohammedamin, R.S.A., Van der Wouden, J.C., Koning, S. *et al.* (2006) Association between skin diseases and severe bacterial infections in children: case control study, BMC Family Practice (online), Available from `http://www.biomedcentral.com/1471-2296/7/52`, Last accessed 19 January 2007.

Morison, M. (2006) *Chronic Wounds*, An educational booklet (sponsored by Smith & Nephew), Wounds UK Publishing, Aberdeen, pp. 6–7.

Morris, C. (2005) Skin trauma, in *Skin Care in Wound Management*: *Assessment, Prevention and Treatment* (ed. R. White) Wounds UK Publishing, Aberdeen, pp. 74–06.

Murray, H.J., Young, M.J., Hollis, S. *et al.* (1996) The association between callus formation, high pressures and neuropathy in diabetic foot ulceration. *Diabetes Medicine*, **13**, 979–82.

Parker, S.R., Parker, D.C. and McCallco, S. (2006) eosinophilic foliculitis in HIV infected women: case series and review. *American Journal of Clinical Dermatology*, **7**(3), 193–200.

Petrov, O. (1998) The podiatric examination. *Clinics in Podiatric Medicine and Surgery*, **15**(2), 249–80.

Pratt, R.J. (2003) *HIV and AIDS: A Foundation for Nursing and Healthcare Practice*, 5th edn, BookPower, London, pp. 366–73 and 432.

Princeton, D.C. (2003) *Manual of HIV AIDS Therapy*, 2003 edn, Current Clinical Strategies Publishing, California, pp. 36, 53, 82–5.

Quartey-Papafio, C.M. (1999) Lesson of the week: importance of distinguishing between cellulitis and varicose eczema of the leg. *British Medical Journal*, **318**(7199), 1672–3.

Sanders, C.J.G., Canninga-van Dijk, M.R. and Borleffs, J.C. (2004) Kaposi's sarcoma. *The Lancet*, **364**(9444), 1549–52.

Savage, C.O.S., Harper, L., Cockwell, P. *et al.* (2000) Vasculitis, in *ABC of Arterial and Venous Disease* (eds R. Donnelly and N.J.M. London), BMJ Publishing Group, London, pp. 38–41.

Savin, J.A., Hunter, J.A.A. and Hepburn, N.C. (1997) *Skin Signs in Clinical Medicine*, Mosby Wolfe, London, pp. 13–8.

Scanlon, E. (2005) Wound infection and colonisation. *Nursing Standard*, **19**(24), 57–67.

Scher, R.K. and Baran, R. (2003) Onychomycosis in clinical practice: factors contributing to recurrence. *British Journal of Dermatology*, **149** (Suppl. 65), 5–9.

Smoker, A. (1999) Fungal infections. *Nursing Standard*, **13**(17), 48–56.

Stoddart, M.L., Blevins, K.S., Lee, E.T., *et. al.* (2002) Association of acanthosis nigricans with hyper-insulinaemia compared with other selected risk factors for type 2 diabetes in Cherokee Indians. *Diabetes Care*, **25**(6),1009–14.

Thompson, P., Langemo, D. and Anderson, J. (2005) Skin care protocols for pressure ulcers and incontinence in long term care: a quasi-experimental study. *Advances in Skin Wound Care*, **18**(8), 422–9.

Tinkle, J.T. (1995) AIDS and the podiatric medical practice. *Journal of the American Podiatric Medical Practice*, **85**(8), 420–7.

Watkins, P. (2006) Identifying and treating plantar warts. *Nursing Standard*, **20**(42), 50–54.

Williams, A. (2003) An overview of non-cancer related chronic oedema – a UK perspective. *World Wide Wounds* (online), Available at: `http://www.worldwidewounds.com/2003/april/Williams/Chronic-Oedema.html`, Last accessed 19 January 2007.

Woodfolk, J.A. (2005) Allergy and dermatophytes. *Clinical Microbiology Reviews*, **18**(1), 30–43.

Young, M. Cavanagh, P.R., Thomas, G. *et al.* (1992) The effect of callus removal on dynamic foot pressures in diabetic patients. *Diabetes Medicine*, **9,** 55–7.

Zancanaro, P.C.Q., McGirt, L.Y., Mamelak, A.J., Nguyen, R.H.N. and Martins, C.R. (2006) Cutaneous manifestations of HIV in the era of highly active antiretroviral therapy: an institutional urban clinic experience. *Journal of the American Academy of Dermatology*, **54**(4), 581–8.

Zipfel, B. and Badenhorst, G. (2002) Attitudes and knowledge about AIDS among podiatry students in South Africa. *Australasian Journal of Podiatric Medicine*, **36**(2), 39–44.

Nicoletta Frescos and Tabatha Rando

Chapter 4

Infected Wounds

4.1 | Introduction

Wound infection is diagnosed clinically and can compound illness, increase patient discomfort and anxiety, and can lead to death. Second only to urinary tract infection, wound infection in hospitals is the most common form of health care-related infections, accounting for 10–16 % of all nosocomial infections (Emmerson *et al.*, 1996; Crow, 1998; Kingsley, 2001; Dumpis *et al.*, 2003; Morris *et al.*, 2003; Davies, 2004). The cost to the National Health Service for surgical site infections alone has been noted at almost one billion pounds per annum (Nosocomial Infections National Surveillance Service (NINSS), 2002).

In the United Kingdom, wound infection accounts for up to 10 % of admissions to infection units and can increase a patient's length of hospital stay by 6.5 days (Plowman, 2000; Fron *et al.*, 2003). In particular, the infected diabetic foot wound is the most common reason for hospitalization among patients with diabetes and accounts for approximately one-quarter of all diabetes-related admissions in the US and UK (Wu and Armstrong, 2005).

The identification, management and prevention of wound infection are essential components of wound care. The consequence of a wound infection is reliant upon a complex interplay between the host, the potential pathogen(s) and the environment (Cooper, 2005).

The ability to prevent wound infection, implement risk-minimizing strategies and support the host is crucial. The wound practitioner must know of the wound infection continuum, including the early identification of signs of a pending or actual wound infection. The management of wound infection with antibiotics and the judicial use of topical antimicrobial therapies are also vital. This chapter will discuss the clinical identification, management and prevention of wound infection with particular emphasis on the lower limb.

4.2 | Case Scenario

Case Scenario 4

Consider the image and information provided for the following case scenario. All information provided is based on a case seen in a primary care setting.

Mary is a 65-year-old lady who has been discharged from a medical ward post-inpatient treatment for pneumonia one week ago. She has a past history of a cerebral vascular accident (with minimal reduction in sensory and motor function of her left side), type 2 diabetes mellitus and chronic right medial malleolus leg ulcer that has been present for six months and was initially caused by trauma (see Figure 4.1). Prior to Mary's hospitalization her carer had been changing her wound dressings twice weekly. Mary has recently lost weight, usually mobilizes with a four-pronged stick and is on the following medications:

- Oral hypoglycaemic agent – Metformin 500 mg BD
- Antithrombotic agent – Aspirin 100 mg daily
- Antihypertensive agent – Captopril 12.5 mg BD
- Analgesia – Paracetamol 1 g QID

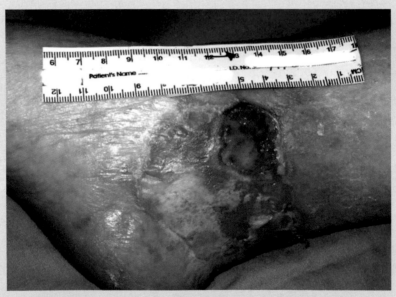

Figure 4.1
Mary's wound

On examination she appears anxious, short of breath and is complaining about pain in her leg ulcer (6/10 visual analogue scale). She has had several wound infections in this leg ulcer during the past six months and is concerned she is developing another.

Local wound assessment conducted by the district nurse during the past week notes:

- Malodour
- An increase in purulent exudate
- Some friable granulation tissue present
- No change in wound dimensions
- An increase in slough (was 30% and is now 70%) and a minimal increase in peri-wound erythema noted during the past week
- No compression currently being worn
- Leg ulcer pain has increased since compression therapy was ceased one week ago by her carer, believing it would be more comfortable without bandages

? What do I need to know?

To determine why the wound is not healing and why there is an increase in pain there is a need to reassess Mary's wound holistically and review her wound management regimen. Make a list of the concerns and factors that you need to think about which may be causing the delay in healing.

- Is Mary feeling unwell?
- Is the wound pain today different from her usual wound pain?
- What usually resolves the wound pain?
- What factors may be causing an increase in wound pain?
- What have Mary's blood glucose levels been during the past week?
- What is Mary's ankle brachial pressure index and has she been treated with judicious compression for her leg ulcer? If so, where is the compression and why is it not being used?
- Is Mary taking paracetamol regularly, which may be masking a temperature?
- What is Mary's haemoglobin and serum albumin?
- What type of wound dressing regimen has been used?
- What antibiotics was Mary prescribed for her pneumonia and when were they ceased?
- Is Mary's wound infected?
- What diagnostics should be considered, if any?

4.3 | Prevalence and Cost of Wound Infection

Wound infections are costly, are associated with increased mortality and reduced quality of life, and may lead to morbidity. The incidence of wound infection has been estimated to be 5–10% in the UK (Kingsley, 2001). A true prevalence of infected wounds is difficult to obtain as most studies are based on hospital admissions, thus omitting episodes of wound infection treated in the community or outpatient setting, and the criteria for infection varies between studies. Of those hospital-based studies, surgical wounds and skin infections were found to be two of the largest categories of infection (Kingsley, 2001).

As a wound moves through the various stages of wound infection it becomes more complicated and the costs of treatment increase substantially due to the higher daily costs of treatment and the longer episode of care. Costs associated with the complications of infected wounds include dressings, antibiotics, diagnostics tests and extended inpatient length of stay. However, the indirect costs to the patient, such as the lost days from work, travel costs, carer costs and treatment of complications such as scarring, are often forgotten (International Committee on Wound Management (ICWM), 1995). Infected wounds are also associated with variable intensities of pain, which adversely affects the quality of life (QoL) in patients, by disturbing sleep, impairing mobility and having a negative psychological effect (Heinen *et al.*, 2004; Persoon *et al.*, 2004). Suffering and emotional pain cannot be financially identified but come at a personal cost to the patient and their carers.

A study by Bennett *et al.* (2004) on the cost of pressure ulcers found that the additional cost of a single episode of cellulitis in a grade 3 or 4 pressure ulcer compared to normal healing costs was £1920 and £16 500 for osteomyelitis. The total cost to treat infected pressure ulcers ranges from £8270 to £24 214 per episode. Furthermore, a systematic review by Nelson *et al.* (2006) on infected diabetic foot ulcers identified a study from 1994 that calculated the cost of treatment per hospital admission as £1451 and an extrapolated annual cost of £17 million. Today this figure will be much higher as the costs of health services have substantially increased over the past decade due to advances in biotechnology, which are expanding the range of diagnostic tools and interventions, and the growth in pharmaceutical expenditure.

4.4 | What Is Wound Infection?

All wounds are contaminated by bacteria (Fleck, 2006a). Contamination of wounds occurs when bacteria enter the wound through external sources, such as:

1. Direct contact, e.g. transfer from equipment, hands of the carer, poor hand washing techniques of health care practitioners during patient care
2. The environment, e.g. micro-organisms deposited from the surrounding air
3. Self-contamination, e.g. the patient's own skin, hands or body fluids (Sibbald and Orsted, 2004; Sibbald *et al.*, 2006)

It is important to understand that not all wounds containing bacteria are infected. Wound healing and infection are influenced by the relationship between the ability of the bacteria to create a flourishing and prosperous bacterial community within the wound and the ability of the host resistance to control the bacterial community. Host resistance is defined as the ability of the body's local and systemic defence mechanisms to resist bacterial invasion and damage (Sibbald *et al.*, 2006).

Bacterial infection of wounds depends on three factors: dose, virulence and host resistance (Dow *et al.*, 1999). This can be illustrated as an equation:

$$\text{Infection} = \frac{\text{dose} \times \text{virulence}}{\text{host resistance}}$$

The dose is the measurement of the bacterial bioburden present in the wound. This is measured by quantity and number of different species of micro-organisms present. Virulence is the power of micro-organisms to produce disease/tissue damage (Mosby, 1983). Host resistance is the most important determinant of whether a wound will become infected. Host resistance can be affected by local or systemic factors (Table 4.1).

A systemically adequate blood supply is required for wound healing. An inadequate blood supply increases the risk of infection as it favours bacterial proliferation, thus increasing the bacterial

Local	Systemic	Behavioural	Medication
Wound size	Vascular disease	Nonadherence to advice regimen	Immunosuppressive drugs
Depth	Oedema	Smoking	Cytotoxic drugs
Duration	Diabetes mellitus	Drug and alcohol abuse	
Anatomic location	Renal failure	Nutrition and diet	
Blood perfusion	Immunodeficiency	Depressive illness	
Mechanism of injury (contaminated penetrating objects)	Inherited neutrophil defects	Lack of sleep and exercise	
Presence of necrotic tissue	Rheumatoid arthritis diseases		
Presence of foreign bodies			

Table 4.1
Factors that increase the risk of infection (Schultz *et al.*, 2003)

bioburden, which delays wound healing. Arterial or venous insufficiency and uncontrolled diabetes mellitus all interfere with tissue perfusion. Local factors that increase the risk of infection include large wound size, anatomic location, such as distal extremities and perineal, and the presence of foreign bodies such as prostheses (Schultz *et al.*, 2003).

> **?** **Are there any other factors in the case provided that may increase the risk of infection in Mary's wound? Make a list of these.**

A clear understanding of terms related to the bacterial involvement in a wound is essential. These terms include:

- Wound contamination. The presence of bacteria within a wound without a host reaction (Collier, 2004).
- Wound colonization. The presence of bacteria within the wound which multiply or initiate a host reaction (Ayton, 1985) but do not cause any harm or injury to the host. This occurs in all chronic wounds and is a normal microbiological state of a healing wound where the growth and death of micro-organisms is at a healthy balanced level (Kingsley *et al.*, 2004; Fleck, 2006b).
- Critical colonization. Multiplication of bacteria causing a delay in wound healing, usually associated with an exacerbation of pain not previously reported but still with no overt host reaction (Kingsley, 2001). There is an inability to maintain a balance between the increasing numbers of bacteria and host resistance (Fleck, 2006b). This is a stage between colonization and infection, which if left unchecked may progress to invasive wound infection. It has been described as being on the "brink of infection" (Cutting and White, 2005). A critically colonized wound is commonly described as covert where the presence of signs and symptoms is subtle or silent.
- Wound infection. The deposition and multiplication of bacteria which invade the tissue and elicit an associated marked host reaction (Ayton, 1985), leading to nonhealing or a decline in the wound (Fleck, 2006b). The infected wound is commonly described as overt where the wound presents with classic signs and symptoms of infection.
- Bioburden. The quantity of the bacteria present (Fleck, 2006a).
- Biofilm. Communities of bacteria attached to unstable wound surfaces and encased in slime (Figure 4.2). This offers protection against phagocytes, antibiotics and antimicrobial agents (White, 2003). Biofilms can lead to local infection or weakening of the collagen matrix in a recently healed wound, causing breakdown and re-ulceration (Sibbald *et al.*, 2003).
- Bacterial synergy. The process in which agents work simultaneously to enhance the function and effect of one another (Mosby, 1983).

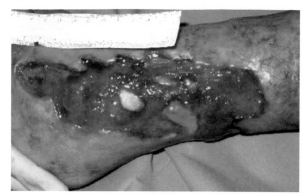

Figure 4.2
Biofilm on the wound surface. Note the shiny slimy surface and friable granulation tissue

- Quorum sensing. The process by which micro-organisms communicate within a mixed community of organisms to enable them to coordinate their activities and enhance their pathogenicity and ability to cause disease (Percival and Bowler, 2004).

4.5 | Wound Infection Continuum: Bacterial Balance

Over the past few years there has been an evolving consolidation between microbiological theory and clinical signs and symptoms. The wound infection continuum is an assessment tool that describes the clinical states and varying levels of microbial growth in the wound. It provides a framework to enable the clinician to recognize factors that lead to infection in order to aid clinical decision making (Kingsley *et al.*, 2004).

As the bacterial load increases, the wound shows increasing severity of clinical and microbiological states. The progression of these states is known as the wound infection continuum, of which there are four stages (see Figure 4.3) (Kingsley *et al.*, 2004):

- Contamination
- Colonization
- Critical colonization
- Infection

Each stage of the continuum involves an increase in the quantity of microbes, the arrival of new species of pathogens, an increase in the quantity of virulent organisms and an increase in the virulence of the collective organisms through microbial interactions known as bacterial synergy (Bowler *et al.*, 2001). Basically, the greater the bioburden, the greater the likelihood of wound deterioration or delayed wound healing.

<u>Contamination/colonization:</u> Bacteria are present in the wound surface Low level of bacterial load Bacterial balance	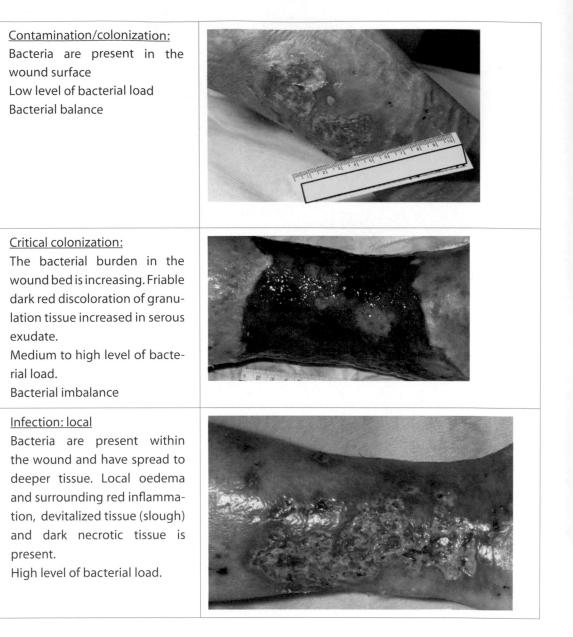
<u>Critical colonization:</u> The bacterial burden in the wound bed is increasing. Friable dark red discoloration of granulation tissue increased in serous exudate. Medium to high level of bacterial load. Bacterial imbalance	
<u>Infection: local</u> Bacteria are present within the wound and have spread to deeper tissue. Local oedema and surrounding red inflammation, devitalized tissue (slough) and dark necrotic tissue is present. High level of bacterial load.	

Figure 4.3
Wound infection continuum: progression of bacterial balance to bacterial damage

Figure 4.4 shows the importance of the host–bacterial balance, combining the different wound infection concepts: the wound infection continuum (White, 2003) and the bacterial bioburden balance and infection staging system (Vowden and Cooper, 2006).

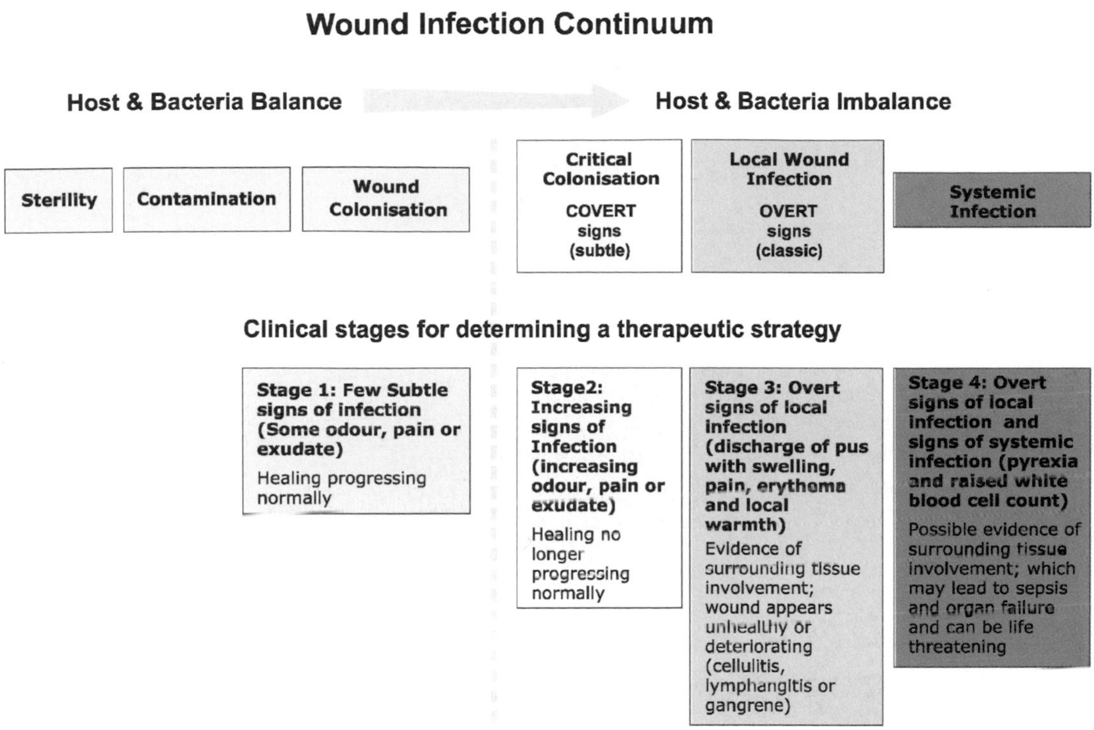

Wound Infection Continuum

Host & Bacteria Balance ⟹ **Host & Bacteria Imbalance**

Sterility	Contamination	Wound Colonisation	Critical Colonisation COVERT signs (subtle)	Local Wound Infection OVERT signs (classic)	Systemic Infection

Clinical stages for determining a therapeutic strategy

Stage 1: Few Subtle signs of infection (Some odour, pain or exudate) Healing progressing normally	Stage 2: Increasing signs of Infection (increasing odour, pain or exudate) Healing no longer progressing normally	Stage 3: Overt signs of local infection (discharge of pus with swelling, pain, erythema and local warmth) Evidence of surrounding tissue involvement; wound appears unhealthy or deteriorating (cellulitis, lymphangitis or gangrene)	Stage 4: Overt signs of local infection and signs of systemic infection (pyrexia and raised white blood cell count) Possible evidence of surrounding tissue involvement; which may lead to sepsis and organ failure and can be life threatening

Figure 4.4

An overview of the wound infection conceptual framework (adapted from Vowden and Cooper (2006) and White (2003)

4.6 | Common Wound Pathogens

All wounds contain micro-organisms, but the majority of these wounds are not infected. The wound care clinician should be aware of the types of common wound pathogens that can cause wound infections. These micro-organisms include bacteria, fungi, protozoa and viruses (see Table 4.2).

Other bacteria have been demonstrated to have a positive effect on wound healing, such as skin commensals *Staphylococcus epidermidis* and *Corynebacterium flora* which are often present in wounds (Schultz *et al.*, 2003).

Infected wounds of less than one month duration tend to have a high percentage of Gram positive (+ve) bacteria. Wounds of greater than one month have Gram negative (−ve) bacteria present followed by anaerobes (Sibbald *et al.*, 2003). Delayed wound healing is not dependent on the presence of one specific organism or a group of bacteria; evidence shows that it is caused by the effect of multiple species of four or more micro-organisms (Trengrove *et al.*, 1996).

Type of pathogen	Causative organism
Gram negative aerobic rods	• *Pseudomonas aeruginosa*
Gram negative facultative rods	• *Escherichia coli* • *Enterobacter* species • *Klebsiella* species • *Proteus* species
Gram positive cocci	• Beta haemolytic *Streptococci (Streptococcus pyogenes)* • *Enterococci* • *Staphylococci aureus*/MRSA
Anaerobes	• Bacteroides • *Clostridium*
Fungi	• Yeasts *(Candida)* • *Aspergillus*

Table 4.2
Most common causative organisms associated with wound infections (adapted from Collier, 2004)

Infected wounds have been considered as those with $>10^5$ colony-forming units (CFUs) per gram of viable tissue or wounds containing any amount of β-haemolytic *Streptococcus* (Gardner *et al.*, 2001; Fleck, 2006b). However, current evidence shows that chronic wounds can contain higher levels of bacteria or greater numbers of different species of bacteria before infection is clinically evident and healing is delayed (Carville, 2005).

Antibiotic-resistant bacteria

Bacteria are extremely diverse. Each strain within each pathogen can have quite different abilities to cause disease or variable sensitivity to antibiotics. Due to the overuse of antibiotics, new strains of antibiotic-resistant bacteria have emerged. A patient can develop a drug-resistant infection either by contracting resistant bacteria or by having a resistant microbe emerge in the body once antibiotic treatment begins. These antibiotic-resistant bacteria are predominately hospital-acquired infections that are commonly known as "superbugs" as they are difficult to treat, often associated with prolonged hospital stay, cause complications and can increase the risk of death.

Strains of *Staphylococcus aureus* have evolved to become resistant to certain drugs. Examples of these strains include methicillin-resistant *Staphylococcus aureus* (MRSA) (also known as golden *Staphylococci*) and methicillin-susceptible *Staphylococcus aureus* (MSSA). If an immunocompromised individual is exposed, an MRSA infection can result without an apparent open wound. The symptoms can range from skin boils to necrotizing fasciitis, popularly known as "flesh-eating disease".

New strains that are emerging are *Clostridium difficile* and vancomycin-resistant *Enterococcus* (VRE), which can be acquired while taking antibiotics while in hospital (Johnson *et al.*, 2005).

4.6.1 | Pathophysiology

The most common microbes that cause wound infection are bacteria. They produce endotoxins which cause an elevation of proinflammatory cytokines or chemical messengers, which in turn delays wound repair. Matrix metalloproteases are released in response to these cytokines and growth factor production subsequently decreases (Warriner and Burrell, 2005).

Good blood perfusion is required for wound healing; it allows oxygen, nutrients and cells to be delivered to the wound and limits the opportunity for microbes to colonize (Bowler *et al.*, 2001). The continuous presence of virulent pathogens and a high bioburden may lead to a prolonged inflammatory phase, which increases the risk of cellular dysfunction and biochemical imbalances. The prolonged inflammatory response destroys cells by localized thrombosis and releases vaso-constricting metabolites which leads to tissue hypoxia (Dow *et al.*, 1999). This condition creates ideal conditions for bacterial proliferation and synergy. Bacterial synergy increases the pathogenic effect through quorum sensing, thus increasing their power (virulence) to destroy cells by com-peting for available oxygen and releasing toxins and metabolic products that damage tissue (Kingsley, 2003). Not all wounds with an increased bacterial load will become critically colonized or infected.

The first sign of critical colonization or local infection may be delayed wound healing after pre-vious signs of healing progress (Dow, 2003). Exudate increases as a result of the inflammatory reaction to surface tissue damage. Atrophy of granulation tissue occurs often with discolora-tion to a pale grey or deep red hue and the tissue becomes more friable due to an increase of vascular endothelial growth (Sibbald *et al.*, 2003). There is an excessive increase in exudate. The exudate produced may be serous rather than purulent due to lysis of neutrophils by bacterial toxins (Dow, 2003).

A critically colonized wound can extend to an invasive infection, which can directly damage surrounding healthy tissue and further delay wound healing. The wound increases in size and satellite areas of breakdown may occur. More extensive bacterial damage results in deeper and surrounding skin infection. Surrounding tissue infection is referred to as cellulitis and is associated with increased pain on palpation, erythema and oedema (Sibbald *et al.*, 2006). Local infection presents with a surrounding red inflammatory ring and the spreading infection is greater than 2 cm with increased pain (Kingsley *et al.*, 2004). If a deep proportion of the wound probes to bone, osteomyelitis may be present. A probe to the bone is usually a reliable sign of osteomyelitis, especially in people with neuropathy and foot ulcers as they do not always present with the typical signs and symptoms of infection (Zgonis and Roukis, 2005) (Figure 4.5). Radiographic imaging should be conducted to confirm the diagnosis.

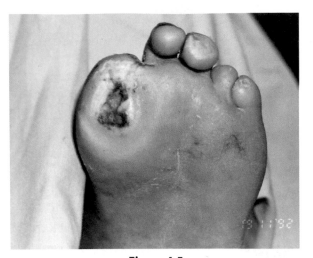

Figure 4.5
Deep tissue diabetic foot wound with associated undermining, probing to bone (courtesy of the
Department of Podiatry, Caulfield Medical Centre, Australia)

4.7 | Clinical Identification of Wound Infection

Wound infection and delayed healing present a challenge to the clinician in the diagnosis of
clinical infection and appropriate management. There is considerable debate within the literature
as to whether the diagnosis of infection should be based on clinical signs and symptoms, and/or
laboratory analysis of microbiological specimens.

4.7.1 | Signs and Symptoms

Clinical signs and symptoms are important indicators of infection for the timely identification
and management of chronic wound infection. The "classic" signs of increasing pain, erythema,
oedema, heat and purulent exudate have been traditionally used to identify wound infection.
However, it is important to recognize that chronic wounds do not necessarily present with
these signs and symptoms of infection (Gardner *et al.*, 2001). Infected chronic wounds tend to
display additional clinical signs and symptoms which are expressed more frequently than the
classic signs and symptoms. These additional signs reflect infection-induced alteration to
the proliferative phase of wound healing, such as serous exudate plus inflammation, delayed
healing, discoloration, friable granulation tissue, foul odour and wound breakdown (Cutting
and White, 2005).

A number of assessment tools exist to guide the clinical diagnosis of wound infection. The two
tools presented here are basic, effective and user friendly. One provides a description of the
established common signs and symptoms of wound infection and the other categorizes these into
the stages of infection. The "Clinical Signs and Symptoms Checklist" developed by Gardner *et al.*
(2001) contains descriptors of each clinical sign and symptom to identify localized chronic wound

infection (Table 4.3). The checklist incorporates the "classic" and secondary signs specific to wounds healing by secondary intention. This is a simple and descriptive tool for the novice practitioner to use for gaining experience in identifying signs of infection.

Classic signs of infection

Increasing pain in the ulcer area: subject's subjective report of perceived increase in level of peri-ulcer pain since the ulcer developed

Erythema: presence of bright or dark red skin or darkening of normal ethnic skin colour immediately adjacent to the ulcer

Oedema: presence of shiny, taut skin or pitting impression in the skin adjacent to the ulcer but within 4 cm from the ulcer margin. Assess pitting oedema by firmly pressing the skin within 4 cm of ulcer margin with a finger, release and waiting 5 seconds to observe indentation

Heat: detectable increase in skin temperature of the skin adjacent to the ulcer within 4 cm of the ulcer margin as compared to the skin 10 cm proximal to the wound, assess the difference in skin temperature using the back of the examiner's hand or wrist

Purulent exudate: presence of tan, creamy yellow or green thick fluid on a dry gauze dressing removed from the ulcer one hour after placement

Signs specific to wounds healing by secondary intention

Serous exudate and inflammation: presence of thin watery fluid on a dry gauze dressing removed from the ulcer one hour after placement

Delayed healing of the ulcer: subject or caregivers report no change or an increase in the volume or surface area of the ulcer over the past 4 weeks. Ask subject or caregiver if the ulcer has filled with tissue or is smaller than it was 4 weeks before today

Discoloration of granulation tissue: granulation tissue that is pale, dusky or dull in colour

Friable granulation tissue: bleeding of granulation tissue when gently manipulated with a sterile cotton-tipped applicator

Pocketing at base of wound: presence of smooth nongranulating pockets of ulcer tissue surrounded by beefy red granulation tissue

Foul odour: putrid or distinctively unpleasant smell as assessed by the examiner

Wound breakdown: small open area in newly formed epithelial tissue not caused by re-injury or trauma

Table 4.3
Clinical Signs and Symptoms Checklist (CSSC) (Adapted from Gardner *et al.*, 2001)

Bacterial bioburden (critical colonization)	Local wound infection	Systemic infection
Nonhealing	Pain	Fever
Bright red granulation tissue	Swelling induration	Rigors
Friable and exuberant granulation tissue	Erythema	Chills
New areas of breakdown or necrosis on the wound surface (slough)	Increased peri-wound temperature	Hypotension
Increased exudate that may be translucent or clear before becoming purulent	Wound breakdown	Multiple organ failure
Smell or unpleasant odour	Increased size or satellite areas	
	Undermining	
	Probing to bone	

Table 4.4
Clinical signs and symptoms of wound infection (Sibbald *et al.*, 2003)

A more applied assessment tool collated by Sibbald *et al.* (2003) provides differentiation of the levels of wound infection and the related clinical signs and symptoms (Table 4.4). Consideration of the "balance of bacteria" within the wound is important in early detection of infection and determining appropriate antimicrobial management of the wound. It is important to remember that the focus of assessment should include not only the bacteria but also the wound management regime.

? **Look at the photograph of Mary's leg wound again and review her presenting symptoms. Using the wound infection assessment tools, list the clinical signs and symptoms present in Mary's wound. What stage of the wound continuum do you think it is?**

4.7.2 | The Role of Microbiology Culture

General consensus is that only wounds that have been clinically diagnosed or suspected of infection or those that have no clinical signs of infection but are deteriorating (i.e. diabetic ulcers) should be sampled (Bowler *et al.*, 2001). Bacterial culture can help to determine antimicrobial sensitivities for the selection of oral or parenteral antibiotic treatment and to identify colonization with resistant organisms such as MRSA. If infection is present the clinician needs to determine whether quantitative tissue biopsy or qualitative swab techniques should be conducted (Dow, 2003).

Tissue biopsy is considered the gold standard for wound culture. It provides information on the causative pathogens within the tissue; however, it is invasive and disrupts wound bed healing. Swab cultures are not as invasive but can be inconclusive and unreliable, especially in chronic wounds (Fleck, 2006b). The Levine technique (Levine *et al.*, 1976) (quantitative swab technique) is considered the best technique to obtain a swab culture. It identifies the type and numbers of micro-organisms present and closely approximates quantitative biopsy. The wound should be cleansed first with saline solution as it does not kill organisms. The swab should be taken from the granulation tissue surface avoiding debris and exudate. It is preferable that swabs should be taken following debridement of the wound. Use an alginate or rayon-tipped applicator, moisten the swab in sterile saline and twirl the applicator with sufficient pressure over a 1 cm² surface area of the wound. A zig-zag pattern can be used for wounds larger than 5 cm² (Schultz *et al.*, 2003).

Semi-quantitative swab techniques involve the debridement of the wound bed and cleansing with saline solution. A swab is taken by rolling the swab across the wound bed; it is then inoculated onto a standard media and streaked into four quadrants (Schultz *et al.*, 2003). The greater the quantity of bacteria on the original swab the more quadrants will display bacterial growth (O'Meara *et al.*, 2006).

Each specimen should be labelled clearly with the name, date and site from where the specimen was taken. Additional information regarding the type of wound, the position of the wound, clinical signs of infection and the presence of necrosis and associated malodour will assist the microbiologist (Bowler *et al.*, 2001). Caution must be taken with laboratory results due to the possibility of a false negative result. Microbiological results should be considered in combination with clinical signs and symptoms and general health status. Patients with systemic signs of sepsis should undergo blood cultures.

Does Mary's wound require a culture? Which technique would be appropriate? Give a rationale for your choice.

4.7.3 | Infections by Wound Types

It has been recognized that wounds of varying aetiologies may present with different clinical signs and symptoms. Cutting *et al.* (2005) developed a set of criteria of clinical signs for six different wound types using a Delphi process involving a leading worldwide expert group. These signs and symptoms are not validated as yet, but they provide a more specific set of criteria for infections in different wound types than the commonly used CSSC (Table 4.3). These extensive criteria provide guidance for the advanced wound practitioner. Cellulitis, malodour, delayed wound healing, wound deterioration or breakdown and an increase in exudate were clinical indicators common to all wounds (Cutting *et al.*, 2005).

Table 4.5 presents the four common lower limb wound types. The table provides colour coding in order of importance for signposts of clinical signs which may lead to infection. Clinical signs in the light blue area are important, blue very important and dark blue diagnostic of infection. The more clinical signs that present the more likely that infection is present.

4.7.4 | Masking of Signs and Symptoms

Some signs of wound infection may be "masked" or diminished in certain wound types due to comorbidities of systemic pathologies. In venous leg ulcers, the presence of lipodermatosclerosis and haemosiderin staining can mask features such as erythema. In arterial leg ulcers infection may present as bluish–purple discoloration of soft tissue due to the increased metabolic demands of infection and reduced blood flow to the skin. Diabetic foot ulcers are of the greatest concern as the criteria of infection may not be clear-cut; people with diabetes may not show a typical inflammatory response to infection, i.e. pain, erythema and oedema (Cutting and White, 2005). Pain may not be present due to the loss of protective pain sensation in the presence of neuropathy (Wu and Armstrong, 2005). A wound infection in an immunocompromised or suppressed individual may not show the usual local host–bacteria reaction due to the lack of an immune system response. Also the use of immunosuppressive drugs, such as corticosteroids or cytotoxic drugs, can mask all signs of localized wound infection.

4.7.5 | Differential Diagnosis

The diagnosis of infection in a wound can be complicated by the presence of non-infectious conditions that produce an inflammatory response. It is important for the wound care practitioner to note that an inflammatory reaction can occur as part of the normal physiological response to wound healing and to differentiate between inflammatory and infective wounds. The most common non-infective inflammatory conditions are:

- Allergic contact dermatitis. This is an allergic inflammatory reaction of the skin caused by direct contact with an irritating substance. It appears as inflammation with redness, itching and may have skin blistering at the site of contact with the irritant. Figure 4.6 shows an allergic response to zinc bandaging, the clear demarcation of redness at the foot and below the knee indicates the contact area of the bandage.

	Diabetic foot ulcer	Arterial leg ulcers	Venous ulcers	Pressure ulcers
Diagnostic — Diagnostic clinical indicators of infection	Cellulitis Lymphangitis Phlegmon Purulent Exudate Pus/abscess	Cellulitis Pus/abscess	Cellulitis	Cellulitis
Very important — Subtle clinical indicators of infection	Crepitus in the joint Erythema Fluctuation Increase in exudate level Induration Localized pain in a normally asensate foot Malodour Probes to the bone Unexpected pain/tenderness	Change in colour/viscosity of exudate Change in wound bed colour Crepitus Deterioration of wound Dry necrosis turning wet Increase in local skin temperature Lymphangitis Malodour Necrosis – new or spreading	Delayed healing despite appropriate compression therapy Increase in local skin temperature Increase in ulcer pain/change in nature of pain Newly formed ulcers within inflamed margins of pre-existing ulcers Wound bed extension with inflamed margins	Change in nature of pain Crepitus Increase in exudate volume Pus Serous exudate with inflammation Spreading erythema Viable tissues become sloughy Warmth in surrounding tissues Wound stops healing despite relevant measures

(continued)

Table 4.5

Infections by wound type (adapted from Cutting *et al.*, 2005)

	Diabetic foot ulcer	Arterial leg ulcers	Venous ulcers	Pressure ulcers
Important Signposts of pending infection (critical colonization)	Blue–black discoloration and haemorrhage(halo)	Erythema	Discoloration, e.g. dull, dark brick red	Enlarging wound despite pressure relief
	Bone or tendon becomes exposed at base of ulcer	Erythema in peri-ulcer tissue – persists with leg elevation	Friable granulation tissue that bleeds easily	Erythema
	Delayed/arrested wound healing despite offloading and debridement	Fluctuation	Increase in exudate viscosity	Friable granulation tissue that bleeds easily
	Deterioration of the wound	Increase in exudate volume	Increase in exudate volume	Malodour
	Friable granulation tissue that bleeds easily	Increase in size in a previously healing ulcer	Malodour	Oedema
	Local oedema	Increased pain	New onset dusky wound hue	
	Sinuses develop in ulcer	Ulcer breakdown	Sudden appearance/increase in amount of slough	
	Spreading necrosis/gangrene		Sudden appearance of necrotic black spots	
	Ulcer base changes from healthy pink to yellow or grey		Ulcer enlargement	

Table 4.5
(Continued)

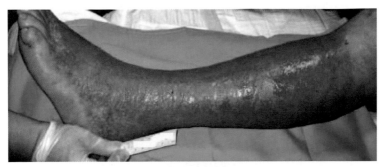

Figure 4.6
Contact dermatitis

- Erythematous maceration. This is a chronic proinflammatory exudate irritation of the peri-wound skin (Figure 4.7). Note the presence of the shiny surface which indicates serous exudate.
- Proinflammatory hypoxic changes related to pressure injury usually located over a pressure point (post-occlusive reactive hyperaemic response). The dominant metabolic process is undetermined and it is fundamentally believed to be either an oxygen deficit or metabolic release from anoxic tissue (Michel and Gillott, 1990). Figure 4.8 is a stage 1 pressure ulcer of the heel: note the dark discoloration which indicates a hypoxic state.
- Vasculitic wounds. This is a skin manifestation of an inflammatory systemic condition which affects the cutaneous blood vessels (very painful, sloughy based wounds with a reddish/purple hue surrounding the wound) (Sibbald *et al.*, 2003). Examples are rheumatoid arthritis, lupus erythematosus, scleroderma, polyarteritis nodosa and calciphylaxis (see Figure 4.9 for an example of a vasculitic wound).
- Pyoderma gangrenosum. This is a skin disease that causes tissue to become necrotic, causing deep wounds that usually occur on the legs. The wounds usually first appear as papules or blisters that progress to larger painful wounds that become necrotic (Sibbald *et al.*, 2003). They are characterized by raised irregular rolled borders and central purulent ulceration (see Figure 4.10).

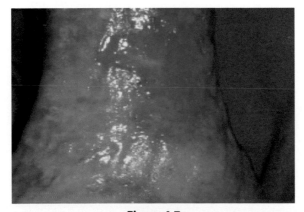

Figure 4.7
Erythematous maceration

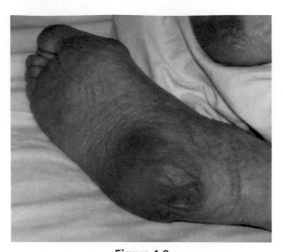

Figure 4.8
Proinflammatory hypoxic changes. (reproduced with kind permission of G. Sussman, Wound Foundation Australia, Monash University)

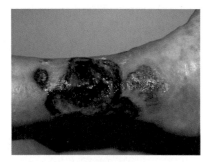

Figure 4.9
Vasculitic wound (reproduced with kind permission of G. Sussman, Wound Foundation Australia, Monash University)

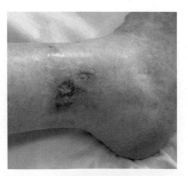

Figure 4.10
Pyoderma gangrenosum (reproduced with kind permission of G. Sussman, Wound Foundation Australia, Monash University)

4.8 | Management of Wound Infection

Generally, once a wound infection has been clinically diagnosed and is felt to have active infection invading beyond the level that can be managed with local wound therapy, appropriate systemic antibiotics should be prescribed (Dow *et al.*, 1999). The wound practitioner may also consider the addition of topical antimicrobials in conjunction with systemic antibiotics.

It must be noted that systemic antibiotics should be used only for specific indications as they may not always be appropriate for all wound infections and to minimize the risk of developing drug resistance (Frank *et al.*, 2005). Guidelines for the treatment of pressure ulcers recommend that systemic antibiotics may not be required for pressure ulcers that exhibit only clinical signs of local infection; this may also be applied to a wider variety of chronic wound types that present with similar microbial flora (Bowler *et al.*, 2001). Furthermore, systemic antibiotics may be ineffective or contraindicated in patients with certain pathologies such as insufficient arterial supply.

The European Wound Management Association (EWMA) has produced a Position Document, *Management of Wound Infection* (Vowden and Cooper, 2006), featuring a detailed algorithm for treatment of wound infection which should be considered by the practitioner (Figure 4.11). The position document suggests that systemic antibiotics should be considered for stage 3 and stage 4 infections. The entire position document is available for download at www.ewma.org.

4.8.1 | Wound Bed Preparation

One of the key principles of wound bed preparation in minimizing or managing wound infection is to reduce the bacterial burden. Excess exudate, slough and necrotic tissue provide a reservoir for bacteria, extend the inflammatory phase and impairs epithelialization. The most important intervention for reducing the level of bacteria is to remove all devitalized tissue. This may be achieved either by topical wound cleansing or debridement (Templeton, 2004).

Topical wound cleansing is usually sufficient in wounds that have simple colonization or contamination and can be accomplished by the use of surface-active agents to remove exudate and dressing adhesive residues and cleansing of the peri-wound (Warriner and Burrell, 2005). Removal of necrotic tissue or slough, which occurs in critically colonized or local infected wounds, should be undertaken with aggressive debridement and the use of topical antimicrobials (Warriner and Burrell, 2005). Debridement can be achieved by either sharp or surgical debridement, high-pressure irrigation debridement, topical negative pressure or even maggot therapy (Ryan, 2007). The type of debridement is dependent on individual circumstances, including the level of colonization and the type of devitalized tissue.

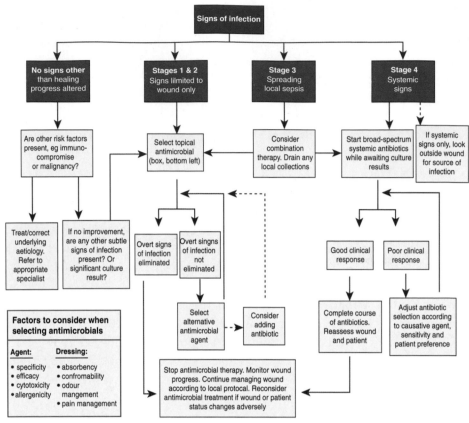

Figure 4.11
Algorithm for managing wound infection (reproduced with permission from Vowden, P. and Cooper, R.A. An integrated approach to managing wound infection, in European Wound Management Association (EWMA) Position Document, 2006, *Management of Wound Infection*, MEP Ltd, London, pp. 2–6)

4.8.2 | Topical Antimicrobials Used in Wound Care

The careful use of topical antimicrobial agents and dressings in the management of critically colonized wounds can lessen the need for systemic antibiotics by topically reducing the bacterial load (bioburden) present at the wound surface (see Table 4.6). The goal of wound care is to restore the bacterial balance of the wound through adequate cleansing and wound hygiene, debridement of devitalized tissue, utilizing topical antimicrobial dressings, and increasing the frequency of dressing changes if required. If a wound is clinically infected, systemic antibiotics and debridement are vital; topical antimicrobials should not be solely relied upon.

It must be noted that there are three categories of antimicrobials used in wound care:

1. Antiseptic
2. Antibiotic: topical or systemic
3. Disinfectant, equipment only

Level of microbial burden	Primary treatment	Adjunct treatment
Nonhealing wound	Antiseptics	
Critical colonization	Topical antiseptics	
Local infection	Systemic antibiotics	Topical antiseptics
Spreading infection	Systemic antibiotics	Topical antiseptics

Table 4.6
A guide to antimicrobial management of wound bioburden (adapted from Sibbald *et al.*, 2003)

The use of these antiseptics and antibiotics in wound bioburden are outlined in Table 4.6.

The types of topical antimicrobial agents commonly used in wound care include traditional antiseptic agents at low dose concentrations, modern antiseptic preparations and a small number of topical antibiotics. An understanding of the different types of topical antimicrobials and their use in wound care is important. Outlines of these are provided in Table 4.7.

Type	Dressing vehicle
Cytotoxicity, pain and allogenicity. Will it harm the patient?	What else does the dressing need to do for the local wound bed? • Debridement • Absorbency • Conformability • Odour management • Pain management
Efficacy. How well does it kill micro-organisms?	Does the topical antimicrobial agent release into the wound bed?
Specificity. What type of micro-organisms are killed?	
Cost-effectiveness. Has there been independent research to show value for money?	

Table 4.7
Factors to consider when choosing antimicrobial agents (adapted from Vowden and Cooper, 2006)

Antiseptics

These are non-selective agents used to kill or inhibit micro-organism growth on skin and living tissues (Healy and Freedman, 2006). More traditional formulations of antiseptics (see Table 4.8) have significant limitations. They can be toxic to both microbial cells and host cells, though this is dependent upon concentrations and time of exposure; in lower concentrations and for shorter periods of time the antiseptic can retain its antimicrobial activity without damaging host cells (White *et al.*, 2001). A short duration of micro-organism kill action requires frequent (and often painful) dressing changes, which in turn reduces the wound bed temperature, adding to a delay in wound healing. The inert dressings used with traditional antiseptics often cause too dry or too wet conditions, which lead to an inability to manage exudate and again adds to a delay in wound healing (see Table 4.8: ionic silver and cadexomer iodine).

Antibiotics

These are defined as drugs that are able to selectively kill or inhibit the growth of bacteria (Healy and Freedman, 2006). Microbes have proven to be very skilful in developing resistance to the extensive antibiotic formulary available today. Systemic antibiotics are to be used when a wound is clinically infected.

Topical antibiotics are no longer advised for use in wound care due to antibiotic resistance and sensitivities that occur in individuals. Also ensuring adequate concentrations of the antibiotic penetration into the tissue in the presence of increased exudate from the infected wound is difficult (e.g. Mupirocin for *Staphylococcus aureus* infections and Metronidazole gel for fungating wounds).

Disinfectants

These are nonselective agents used to kill or suppress the growth of micro-organisms on inanimate objects (Scanlon, 2005). The use of disinfectants in wound care is limited to activities such as cleansing of dressing trolleys and other equipment (e.g. sodium hypochlorite, alcohol 70%).

Silver Products

Silver products should only be used in adequately assessed wounds that are failing to heal with standard treatment, particularly where microbial burden (critical colonization/stage 2 of the clinical stages of infection) (Vowden and Cooper, 2006) appears to be delaying healing (Woodward, 2005). Silver has been shown to denature microbial proteins, impairing their ability to ingest and process food substances and reducing their metabolism and growth. For antimicrobial effectiveness, silver concentrations require either large amounts of silver to be applied regularly or the use of formulations that release enough silver over prolonged periods of time (Woodward, 2005). Recent literature notes that the ideal wound fluid concentration of silver for greatest antimicrobial efficacy should be levels of between 20 and 60 µg/mL (Demling and DeSanti, 2001; Burrell 2005). However, this is debatable as the amount of silver necessary to be bactericidal in the wound environment varies as it is dependent on the type of bacteria present, medium of the dressing and the mode of action (Templeton, 2005). Some dressings release the silver in the wound and some partly release the silver in the dressing (Sussman, 2005). Silver has also been shown to affect microbial DNA.

Type	Advantage	Disadvantage	Usefulness
		Traditional Preparations	
Cetrimide	Effective against most Gram positive and negative micro-organisms. Good detergent action	Can cause hypersensitivity. Even very low concentrations can inhibit fibroblast growth. High toxicity to human tissue	Emulsifying and detergent properties assist when cleaning wounds. Consider where wound healing is not the focus
Chlorhexidine	Active against Gram positive and negative micro-organisms	Skin sensitivity reported. Presence of blood and organic material can decrease its activity	Small effect on human tissue
Povidone iodine (PVI)	Bactericidal effect at 1%. Very broad activity. Active against bacteria, spores, fungi and viruses. Effective against biofilms.	Local irritation and sensitivity may occur. Cannot apply to individuals with thyroid dysfunction, pregnant/lactating women	Useful as a 3–5 minute wound soak at 1% concentration for direct surface contact kill

Table 4.8

Commonly used topical antiseptics (traditional and modern) (McDonnell and Russell, 1999; Carville, 2005; Templeton, 2005)

(continued)

Type	Advantage	Disadvantage	Usefulness
		Modern Preparations	
Silver–ionic silver	20–50 µg/mL concentration required for micro-organism kill effect. Delivery and dressing dependent	Can develop sensitivity	Anti-inflammatory. Useful in chronically inflamed wounds
Cadexomer iodine	Bacteriocidal effect at 0.1%. As for PVI	As for PVI	Pro-inflammatory. Useful in recalcitrant wounds
Medical grade honey or Manuka honey	Broad spectrum bactericidal effect due to the slow release of hydrogen peroxide. Anti-inflammatory. Stimulatory effect on granulation tissue	May cause stinging. May require frequent (daily dressings) dependent upon dressing vehicle	High glucose level is stimulatory to macrophages and lymphocytes. Deodorizing effect
Tea tree oil	New preparations looking at prolonged activity	Toxic to human tissue at high concentrations	Anti-inflammatory properties can assist healing chronic wounds.

Table 4.8
(*Continued*)

Topical antiseptic agents will, however, only reduce wound surface bacterial levels with no reduction in deeper tissue (Sibbald *et al.*, 2001). This superficial effect may be enough to tip the balance and the efficacy of the antimicrobial product should also be merited by its effect on wound healing (Woodward, 2005).

> **?** **What management plan would you choose for Mary? What topical antimicrobial would you choose? What secondary dressings would you use? Give a rationale for your choice.**

4.9 | Summary of Treatment Options and Patient Care Trajectory

4.9.1 | Patient Assessment

Every individual with a wound requires a tailored wound assessment and management plan. The major aetiology of Mary's wound was determined by review of her medical history, physical examination and Doppler studies, which supported the diagnosis of venous hypertension with an element of arterial insufficiency (ankle brachial pressure index (ABPI) 0.8). The goal of care was healing. When reviewing the wound bed preparation model the wound bed required debridement and assessment for wound infection.

Although she is taking six hourly paracetamol that may mask a febrile episode, Mary reports that she is feeling well, her appetite is good and she exhibits no systemic signs of infection. Mary's haemoglobin is 10.1 mmol/L and her serum albumin is 32 mmol/L. Her blood glucose levels are within normal limits. She has lost weight recently; thus a referral to a dietician to review her nutritional intake to support wound healing is vital.

The wound pain is similar to the wound pain Mary previously experienced prior to commencing compression. She reports wound pain reducing when her lower leg is elevated. It is likely that the increase in wound pain is due to lack of compression and oedema formation rather than bacterial bioburden, though this cannot be ruled out.

4.9.2 | Wound Assessment

On review of Mary's wound assessment the practitioner noted that she had increased purulent exudate, an increase in wound base slough, malodour, wound-related pain, peri-wound erythema and no progress in wound healing. The practitioner must consider why compression was ceased by the carer. In this case the carer thought that Mary would have less pain if compression was removed.

However, Mary's ankle and calf circumferences increased in size with subsequent oedema due to lack of compression, which may have been a contributory factor to increased pain.

Mary has five signs of bacterial bioburden (please review the wound infection criteria tables). The wound practitioner may consider this wound to have signposts of infection.

4.9.3 | Treatment Options

Treatment options include:

1. Recommencement of judicious (light) compression as tolerated to control oedema.
2. Encouraging ankle flexion–extension exercises to increase venous return.
3. Taking a wound swab for culture and specificity. Appropriate antibiotics active against the causative organisms should be commenced.
4. Reviewing and assessing analgesia needs.
5. Wound cleansing and debridement of devitalized tissue.
6. Considering commencing suitable topical antimicrobial dressing. If this is not possible more frequent wound cleansing and dressing regimen in conjunction with close monitoring of wound status is pertinent.
7. Minimizing cross-infection.
8. Implementation of appropriate exudate management dressings and peri-wound skin protection.
9. Dietitian review for investigation of weight loss and wound healing supplement.
10. Optimizing and monitoring glycaemic control.
11. Individual education regarding the importance of maintaining judicious compression therapy.
12. Constructing a management plan that details expected progress so that any delays or changes in the wound can be detected early.
13. Communication of wound management strategies with Mary, carer and local doctor.

4.9.4 | Prevention of Wound Infection

"Prevention is better than a cure." An emphasis on standard precaution principles and wound infection risk-minimizing strategies, such as adequate hand washing, ensuring clean storage areas for dressings and ensuring equipment has been disinfected, are all important methods to reduce the risk of wound infection. If an individual experiences repeat wound infections, a review of who is doing the dressings, how they are doing the dressing, how equipment and dressing supplies are being handled and a full assessment of factors supporting the host immune system and local wound environment must be considered.

The support of the host immune system is a part of wound infection prevention. Poor nutrition causes delays in wound healing and increases the risk of wound infection. Malnutrition can arise because of insufficient nutrient intake, systemic disorders, drug intolerances or chemotherapy. In malnourished individuals there is competition for limited nutrients. A nutritionally balanced diet is essential for tissue repair and regeneration (Carville, 2005).

A poor psychological state, such as stress, anxiety and depression, reduces the efficiency of the individual's immune system, which retards healing. A positive attitude by both the patient and the practitioner can help promote wound healing (Carville, 2005). Some considerations to include in risk minimization of wound infections and support of a healthy immune system are as follows:

1. Reduce stressors: ensure a balance of sleep and exercise, smoking cessation strategies and limiting alcohol intake.
2. Ensure adequate nutritional intake to support the immune function with adequate hydration, protein and fruit and vegetable intake. Consider nutritional supplementation and dietician review.
3. Ensure psychosocial support is being received.

A decision as to whether aseptic or clean technique should be undertaken when attending a wound dressing is dependent upon individual client assessment. The focus always should be upon risk minimization.

In any disease process it is always better to aim for prevention rather than trying to cure the condition. Wound infection is no different; the wound practitioner's focus and that of clinical researchers will need to develop further in this area as more antibiotic-resistant strains of virulent micro-organisms develop and threaten lives.

4.10 | Conclusion

Wound infection is a complex interaction between the host, the invading organism and the wound environment. All wounds are contaminated; as the number of bacteria increases the wound can progress from the harmless contaminated state to colonization to critical colonization to infection. Infection occurs when the host's tissue defences cannot overcome the invasion of micro-organisms. This delays the healing process and places the patient at risk, leading to poor patient outcomes.

It is important for the wound practitioner to assess wounds for clinical signs and symptoms of inflammation and infection, and to recognize the subtle clinical changes in the inflammatory response of wound healing to identify and treat the early signs of infection.

This chapter has presented frameworks of clinical signs and symptoms of infection, outlined the clinical indicators for diagnosing bacterial bioburden and provided an overview on the management of wound infection.

References

Ayton, M. (1985) Wound care: wounds that won't heal. *Nursing Times*, **81**(46), s16–s9.

Bennett, G. Dealey, C. and Posnett, J. (2004) The cost of pressure ulcers in the UK. *Age Ageing*, **33**(3), 230–5.

Bowler, P.G., Duerden, B.I. and Armstrong, D.G. (2001) Wound microbiology and associated approaches to wound management. *Clinical Microbiology Reviews*, **14**, 244–69.

Burrell, R. (2005) A scientific perspective on the use of topical silver preparations. *Ostomy Wound Management*, **49**(5A), Suppl., 19–24.

Carville, K. (2005) *Wound Care Manual*, Silver Chain Nursing Association.

Collier, M. (2004) Recognition and managment of wound infections. *World wide wounds.* (online), Available at: `http://www.worldwidewounds.com/2004/january/Collier/Management-of-Wound-infection.html` , Last accessed 2 july 2007.

Cooper, R.A. (2005) Understanding wound infection, In *Identifying Criteria for Wound Infection*, European Wound Managment Association (EWMA) Position Document, MEP Ltd, London.

Crow, S. (1998) Asepsis: back to basics. *Urologic Nursing*, **18**(1), 42–6.

Cutting, K. and White, R.J. (2005) Criteria for identifying wound infection – revisited. *Ostomy Wound Management*, **51**(1), 28–34.

Cutting, K.F., White, R.J., Mahoney, P. and Harding, K.G. (2005) Clinical identification of wound infection: a Delphi approach, In *identifying Criteria for Wound Infection,* European Wound Management Association (EWMA) Position Document, MEP Ltd, London, pp. 6–9.

Davies, P. (2004) Back to basics of wound care: why nurses should question their practice. *Professional Nurse*, **20**(2), 29–31.

Demling, R. and DeSanti, L. (2001) Effects of silver on wound management. *Wounds*, **13**(1), Suppl. A, 4–15.

Dow, G. (2003) Bacterial swabs and the chronic wound: when, how and what do they mean. *Ostomy Wound Management*, **49**(5A), 8–13.

Dow, G., Browne, A. (1999) Infection in chronic wounds: controversies in diagnosis and treatment. *Ostomy Wound Management*, **45**(8), 23–40.

Dumpis, U., Balode, A., Vigante, D., *et al.* (2003) Prevalence of nosocomial infections in two Latvian hospitals. *European Surveillance*, **8**(3), 73–8.

Emmerson, A.M., Enstone, J.E., Griffin, M., Kelsey, M.C. and Smyth, E.T. (1996) The Second National Prevalence Survey of infection in hospitals – overview of the results. *Journal of Hospital Infection*, **32**(3), 175–90.

Eron, L.J., Lipsky, B.A., Low, D.E., Nathwani, D., Tice, A.D. and Volturo, G.E. (2003) Managing skin and soft tissue infections: expert panel recommendations on key decision points. *Journal of Antimicrobial Chemotherapy*, **52**, Suppl. S1, i3–i17.

Fleck, C. (2006a) Fighting infection in chronic wounds FAQs. *Advances in Skin and Wound Care*, **19**(4), 184–8.

Fleck, C. (2006b) Identifying infection in chronic wounds FAQs. *Advances in Skin and Wound Care*, **19**(1), 20–1.

Frank, C.A., Bayoumi, I. and Westendo, C. (2005) Approach to infected skin ulcers. *Canadian Family Physician*, **51**(10), 1352–9.

Gardner, S.E., Frantz, R.,A., Bradley, N. and Doebbeling, M.D. (2001) The validity of clinical signs and symptoms used to identify localized chronic wound infection. *Wound Repair and Regeneration*, **9**(3), 178–86.

Healy, B. and Freedman, A. (2006) Infections. practice: ABC of wound healing. *British Medical Journal*, **332**(7545), 838–41.

Heinen, M.M., van Achterberg, T., Scholte op Reimer, W., van de Kerkhof, P.C.M. and de Laat, E. (2004) Venous leg ulcer patients: a review of the literature on lifestyle and pain-related interventions. *Journal of Clinical Nursing*, **13**, 355–66.

International Committee on Wound Management (ICWM) (1995) An overview of an economic model of cost-effective care. *Advances in Wound Care*, **8**(5), 46.

Johnson, A.P., Pearson, A. and Duckworth, G. (2005) Surveillance and epidemiology of MRSA bacteraemia in the UK. *Journal of Antimicrobial Chemotherapy*, **56**(3), 455–62.

Kingsley, A. (2001) A proactive approach to wound infection. *Nursing Standard*, **15**(30), 50–6.

Kingsley, A. (2003) The wound infection continuum and its application to clinical practice. *Ostomy Wound Management*, **49**(7A), 1–7.

Kingsley, A., White, R.J. and Gray, D. (2004) The wound infection continuum: a revised perspective. *Applied Wound Managment Supplement. Wounds UK*, **1**(1), 13–8.

Levine, N.S., Lindberg, R.B., Mason, A.D. and Pruitt, B.A. (1976) The quantitative swab culture and smear: a quick and simple method for determining the number of viable bacteria on open wounds. *Journal of Trauma*, **16** , 89–94.

McDonnell, G. and Russell, A.D. (1999) Antispetics and disinfectants: activity, action and resistance. *Clinical Microbiology Reviews*, **12**(1), 147–79.

Michel, C.C. and Gillott, H. (1990) Microvascular mechanisms in stasis and ischaemia, in *Pressure Sores, Clinical Practice and Scietific Approach* (ed. D.L. Bader), Macmillan Press, London, pp. 153–64.

Morris, C.D., Sepkowitz, K., Fonshell, C., *et al.* (2003) Prospective identification of risk factors for wound infection after lower extremity oncologic surgery. *Annals of Surgical Oncology*, **10**, 778–82.

Mosby (1983) *Mosby's Medical and Nursing Dictionary*, C.V. Mosby, St Louis, Missouri.

Nelson, E.A., O'Meara, S., Golder, S., Dalton, J., Craig, D. and Iglesias, I. (2006) Systematic review of antimicrobial treatments for diabetic foot ulcers. *Diabetes Medicine*, **23**(4), 348–59.

Nosocomial Infection National Surveillance Serive (NINSS) (2002) *Surveillance of Surgical Site Infection in English Hospitals: A National Surveillance and Quality Improvement Programme*, Public Health Laboratory Service.

O'Meara, S., Nelson, E.A., *et al.* (2006). Systemic review of methods to diagnose infection in foot ulcers in diabetes. *Diabetic Medicine*, **23**, 341–347.

Percival, S. and Bowler, P. (2004) Understanding the effects of bacterial communities and biofilms on wound healing. *World wide wounds* (online), Available at: http://www.worldwidewounds.com/2004/january/Collier/Management-of-Wound-infections.html, accessed 2 July 2007.

Persoon, A., Heinen, M.M., van der Vieuten, C.J.M., de Rooij, M.J., van de Kerkhof, P.C.M. and van Achterberg, T. (2004) Leg ulcers: a review of their impact on daily life. *Journal of Clinical Nursing*, **13**, 341–54.

Plowman, R. (2000) The socioeconomic burden of hospital acquired infection. *European Surveillance*, **5**(4), 49–50.

Ryan, T.J. (2007) Infection following soft tissue injury: its role in wound healing. *Current Opinion in Infectious Diseases*, **20**(2), 124–28.

Scanlon, E. (2005) Wound infection and colonisation. *Nursing Standard*, **19**(24), 57–67.

Schultz, G., Sibbald, G., Falanga, V., *et al.* (2003) Wound bed preparation: a systemic approach to wound management. *Wound Repair and Regeneration*, **11**(s1), S1–S28.

Sibbald, R. and Orsted, H. (2004) Letters to the Editor: five levels of the bacterial chronic wound relationship. *International Wound Journal*, **1**(2), 142–3.

Sibbald, R., Browne, A.C., Coutts, P. and Queen, P. (2001) Screening evaluation of an ionized nanocrystalline silver dressings in chronic wound care. *Ostomy Wound Management*, **47**(10), 38–43.

Sibbald, R., Orsted, H.L., Schultz, G.S., Coutts, P. and Keast, D. (2003) Preparing the wound bed: focus on infection and inflammation. *Ostomy Wound Management*, **49**(11), 24–51.

Sibbald, R., Woo, K. and Ayello, E.A. (2006) Increased bacterial burden and infection: the story of NERDS and STONES. *Advances in Skin and Wound Care*, **19**(8), 447–61.

Sussman, G. (2005) The Australian silver product tour. *Primary Intention. The Australian Journal of Wound Managment*, **13**(4), S23–S25.

Templeton, S. (2004) Using a foam silver dressing to promote healing of a mixed aetiology leg ulcer. *Primary Intention. The Australian Journal of Wound Managment*, **12**(3), 115–120.

Templeton, S. (2005) Management of chronic wounds: the role of silver-containing dressings. *Primary Intention. The Australian Journal of Wound Managment*, **13**(40), 170–9.

Trengrove, N., Stacey, M., McGechie, D. and Mata, S. (1996) Qualitative bacteriology and leg ulcer healing. *Journal of Wound Care*, **5**(6), 277–80.

Vowden, P. and Cooper R.A. (2006) An integrated approach to managing wound infection, in *Management of Wound Infection*, European Wound Management Infection (EWMA) Position Document, MEP Ltd, London, pp. 2–6.

Warriner, R. and Burrell, R. (2005) Infection and the chronic wound: a focus on silver. *Advances in Skin and Wound Care*, **18**, Suppl. 1, 2–12.

White, R.J. (2003) The wound infection continuum, in *Trends in Wound Care UK* (ed. R.J. White), Quay Books.

White, R.J., Cooper, R., Kingsley, A. (2001) Wound colonization and infection: the role of topical antimicrobials. *British Journal of Nursing*, **10**(9), 563–78.

Woodward, M. (2005) Silver dressings in wound healing: what is the evidence? *Primary Intention. The Australian Journal of Wound Managment*, **13**(4), 153–60.

Wu, S. and Armstrong, D.G. (2005) Risk assessment of the diabetic foot and wound. *International Wound Journal*, **2**(1), 17–24.

Zgonis, T. and Roukis, T.S. (2005) A systematic approach to diabetic foot infections. *Advances in Therapy*, **22**(3), 244–62.

Adrienne Taylor

Chapter 5

Leg Ulcers

5.1 | Introduction

Chronic ulceration of the leg is a miserable, painful and socially isolating condition that incurs considerable expense to the National Health Service (NHS). Graham *et al.* (2003), following their systematic review of the literature, found that although estimates vary venous ulcers are thought to affect at least 1% of the elderly population, with women at greater risk than men in the United Kingdom. Briggs and Closs (2003) reviewed the incidence of leg ulcers and found that in the Western world 0.11–0.18% of the general population have an open ulcer and that approximately 1–2% of the population will suffer a leg ulcer at some point in their life.

Chronic venous insufficiency affects a large proportion of individuals, and with the ageing population, its prevalence is bound to increase. In a study of 474 patients presenting with symptoms of chronic venous insufficiency, age was identified as a major factor for increasing severity of venous disease (Capitao *et al.*, 1995). In fact, Margolis *et al.* (2002) found that in people over 65 women were at greater risk than men in the UK; furthermore, MacKenzie *et al.* (2003) identified that a significant number of patients developed their first venous leg ulcer prior to age 50.

Leg ulcers can take a long time to heal and the recurrence of leg ulceration is a significant problem for many (Morison and Moffatt, 2004). Moffatt (2001) argues that leg ulcers which are venous in origin (70%) are most commonly encountered, followed by arterial ulcers (15–20%). She continues that, less commonly, leg ulcers may be caused by conditions such as rheumatoid arthritis, other vasculitis disorders and malignancy. An ulcer that develops as a result of a combination of diseases is referred to as being of mixed aetiology, which makes management more complex (Morison and Moffatt, 2004).

Many leg ulcer patients have complex needs and it is important that the multiprofessional team is involved in the assessment, planning, implementation and evaluation of their care needs. Bowskill (2001) argues that the healing of a leg ulcer can take a considerable amount of time and the recurrence rate is still high even with intervention. Therefore, patients must be involved in their care and have clear instructions on how and when to report problems.

Studies of point and period prevalence of open ulceration report levels between 1.1 and 1.8 per thousand (Callam *et al.*, 1985; Cornwall *et al.*, 1986; Freak *et al.*, 1995), which is equivalent in the UK to between 55 000 and 90 000 patients requiring treatment at any one time. Bosanquet (1992) estimated the annual cost of managing an open leg ulcer to be £1067 while Freak *et al.* (1995) calculated the annual cost in 1995 to be £2356. Similarly, Carr *et al.* (1999) estimated, the cost of treatment of legulcers to be between £1200 and £1400. Few leg ulcer studies have incorporated an analysis of their cost effectiveness and most evidence on this related to one particular four-layer system.

Bosanquet (1992) suggests that failing to use the most cost-effective treatment, thereby creating inefficient services and wasting NHS resources, could amount to a loss of between £350 000 and £1.08 million annually in a typical health authority. Given these findings, Taylor *et al.* (1998a) concluded that the successful management of leg ulcers depended on correct aetiological diagnosis, a high standard of wound management, compression bandaging for venous ulcers, early diagnosis and treatment of infection and allergic complication, and long-term supervision of healed ulcers to minimize recurrence.

The economic and health care burden associated with leg ulceration is vast; however, the personal burden for the affected individual must also be addressed. Franks and Moffatt (2006) stated that practitioners who treat patients with leg ulceration believe there is a significant deficit in health-related quality of life for those living with leg ulceration.

This chapter will discuss the assessment, aetiology and management of leg ulcers and will focus on national guidelines, current best evidence and the need for a holistic and multiprofessional approach to leg ulcer care.

5.2 | Case Scenario

Case Scenario 5

Annie is an 80-year-old lady who lives alone. She had been visited by the district nursing service for the management of a painful leg ulcer which she has had for approximately six months. She is in a lot of pain and according to the district nurses is not compliant with treatment. Her appetite is poor, she has recently lost weight and looks malnourished.

On presentation she appears tired and is still in her nightclothes mid-morning; she informs you she does not bother to dress any more. Her only contact with the outside world is with the district nurses. She has oedema of the right leg accompanied by low-grade cellulitis. She has ulceration over the medial malleolus area of her right leg (see Figure 5.1). Her ankle brachial pressure index (ABPI) was 0.9 and she had clinical evidence of venous hypertension. She had lipodermatosclerosis and varicosities of the lower limb.

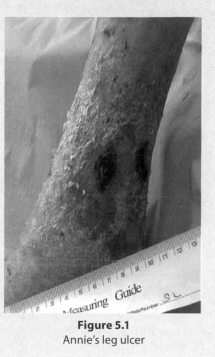

Figure 5.1
Annie's leg ulcer

?   **Ensuring you consider the holistic assessment of the patient, not just the leg ulcer, answer the following questions using the information provided throughout the chapter:**

1. **What are the possible causes of Annie's leg ulcer?**

2. **What is the aetiology of this ulcer?**

3. **What factors may delay healing in this case?**

4. **What are the most appropriate management strategies in this case?**

5. **Are there any correctable risk factors that will speed healing and prevent the risk of recurrence?**

The information provided within the following sections should enable you to answer the five questions posed above. The answers to the case will be further considered towards the end of the chapter.

5.3 | Definition of a Leg Ulcer

Leg ulcers are generally defined as areas of loss of skin/tissue below the knee on the leg or on the foot that take greater than 4 weeks to heal (Scottish Intercollegiate Guidelines Network, 1998).

5.4 | Common Causes of Ulceration of the Lower Limb

According to Morison (2006) there are a number of pathological conditions associated with leg ulceration in the lower limb:

- Chronic venous insufficiency, often associated with incompetent valves in the deep and perforating veins, which results in reflux of venous blood and consequently venous hypertension
- Arterial insufficiency of the lower limit
- Combined chronic venous and arterial insufficiency

Hofman (2000) and Morison (2006) also identify less common causes of leg ulceration:

- Neuropathy, e.g. associated with diabetes mellitus
- Vasculitis, e.g. associated with rheumatoid arthritis, which is further explored in Chapter 9, and other autoimmune disorders such as lupus erythematous
- Malignancy, e.g. basal cell carcinoma and squamous cell carcinoma
- Lymphoedema
- Infection, e.g. leprosy, tuberculosis and tropical ulcers
- Blood disorders, e.g. sickle cell disease and thalassaemia
- Metabolic disorders, e.g. diabetes mellitus
- Iatrogenic, e.g. tight bandaging or hosiery

5.5 | Problems Associated with Leg Ulcers

Chronic leg ulceration is distributed equally across all socioeconomic classes, although the prognosis is less favourable among patients from socioeconomic classes IV and V (Registrar General Classification, 2007). Indeed, Moffatt *et al.* (1992) identified that a higher proportion of the lower social class, unmarried people and those living in rented accommodation more often developed ulceration compared with the general population.

The impact on quality of life associated with leg ulceration can be described as follows (Morison, 2006):

- Pain and discomfort (dependency on analgesics)
- Side effects from medication
- Reduced mobility

- Unpleasant odour
- Social isolation and despair
- Unemployment

Walshe (1995) and Rich and McLachalan (2003) identified that issues, such as high pain levels, poor sleep quality, depression and restricted activities affected the health-related quality of life of patients with leg ulceration. Indeed, Moffatt and Oldroyd (1994) identified a significant reduction in levels of anxiety, depression, pain and interference with daily and social activities in patients whose leg ulcer healed.

5.6 | The Aetiology of Leg Ulcers

? **Consider the anatomy of the venous system of the lower limb to aid you in understanding the causes of leg ulceration.**

Veins in the lower leg carry blood back to the heart. The capillaries that provide the skin with oxygen and nutrients drain into the superficial veins. Small vessels called perforators join the deep and superficial systems. On movement of the leg, contraction of the calf muscle occurs, which squeezes the veins thus forcing the blood up towards the heart. The one-way valves within the veins stop the blood flowing down the veins again when the muscle relaxes (Tortora and Grabowski, 2000).
There are three systems of veins:

- Deep
- Superficial
- Perforating

5.6.1 | Theories of Venous Ulceration

Faulty valves within veins will allow reverse blood flow causing accumulative damage to other valves. Superficial venous hypertension occurs due to valvular incompetence in the perforating veins between the superficial and deep venous systems. Thus, the calf muscle pump during exercise and gravity in the dependent position at rest both force blood at high pressure into the superficial system. This leads to the leakage of red cells, fluid and protein from the distended capillaries. The leaked fibrin forms a cuff around the capillaries, which acts as a barrier to the exchange of oxygen and nutrients to the tissues, with resulting breakdown of the overlying skin and superficial tissues (Vowden and Vowden, 2001). The calf perforator incompetence may be visible or palpable. Gaiter pigmentation, scarring, oedema and inflammation are common. Venous ulcers are almost always in the medial or lateral gaiter area of the lower leg (an area between the mid-calf to approximately

2–3 cm below the malleoli). However, it is possible to have venous ulceration on the dorsum of the foot. If an ulcer is not in the classical medial ankle position, other causative factors are more likely and should be explored.

5.6.2 | Venous Disease

The recognition that leg ulcers occurred in association with venous disease goes back to the era of the ancient Greeks when Hippocrates described "varicose ulcers" (Adams, 1949). According to Vowden and Vowden (1998), the majority of leg ulcers are venous in origin and caused by venous hypertension, although it is important to undertake a holistic assessment prior to treatment commencing. Moffatt (1998) argues that while vascular disease is the most common cause for leg ulceration, the circulation cannot be viewed in isolation; it is important that an overall assessment of the patient is undertaken. Disorders, such as rheumatoid arthritis, ulcerative colitis, Crohn's disease and haematological conditions, such as sickle cell disease and thalassaemia can also lead to leg ulceration.

Venous return from the leg is dependent of the venous calf pump and active leg muscles. Venous insufficiency is caused by damage to the valves in the deep veins and the perforator veins joining the deep and superficial veins of the leg (e.g. by a blood clot in the deep veins, known medically as deep vein thrombosis (DVT)), leading to venous hypertension. Figure 5.2 shows swelling localized to the calf post-DVT.

Studies undertaken by Hopkins et al. (1983) found that the skin beneath an ulcer has a high blood flow and a poor oxygen extraction. Additionally transcutaneous oxygen flux is reduced in the

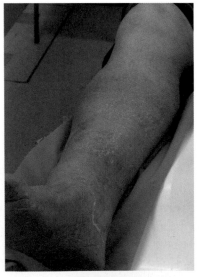

Figure 5.2
Calf swelling post-DVT

patient's skin with lipodermatosclerosis. Lipodermatosclerosis is thickening, induration, pigmentation and inflammation of the skin of the gaiter "regions" or ulcer bearing area (Hopkins *et al.*, 1983), as seen in Annie's case (Figure 5.1).

Recognized factors for venous ulceration

Anderson (2006) describes the following factors:

- Patients with venous ulceration have abnormally raised venous pressure during walking and exercise.
- There is some local abnormality in the calf skin leading to the changes of lipodermatosclerosis.
- Valves within the leg veins become damaged and are less able to prevent the backflow of blood.
- The calf muscle may not be strong enough to assist venous return.
- The venous blood volume increases in the lower leg veins, resulting in a pooling of blood in the veins.
- The walls of the veins in the lower leg stretch, allowing fluid, including proteins and erythrocytes, to leak out into the tissues.
- There is evidence of lymphoedema.
- Venous congestion and hypertension means that nutrients do not get to the tissues and skin, which results in dry skin and often eczema.
- The fluid in the leg is at risk of infection and the skin and tissue are at high risk of trauma.

Other risk factors for venous ulceration include occupation (prolonged periods of standing or sitting), history of DVT and previous trauma (e.g. pre-tibial laceration).

The actual mechanism of venous ulceration is unclear. In many cases local trauma on previously damaged skin leads to a break in the epithelium. Ulceration then progresses because of a failure of the tissues to heal. Almost all leg ulcers are heavily colonized with bacteria. The effects bacteria have on wound healing in leg ulcers is unknown. Browse and Burnard (1982) suggest that venous and capillary hypertension increase permeability and produce tissue oedema and perivascular deposition of fibrin, which creates a barrier to diffusion around the capillaries and results in necrosis (necrosis is caused by lack of oxygen to the tissues).

5.6.3 | Arterial Disease

Arterial disease due to atherosclerosis, can cause occlusion of the vessels as atheroma adhere to the arterial wall, narrowing the vessel lumen, which results in arterial insufficiency to the lower limits which can cause tissue ischaemia, necrosis, and the formation of a deep punched-out ulcer. The toes and feet may be involved with loss of distal pulses, cold skin, nail dystrophy, loss of hair, pallor of the foot on elevation of the limb and marked reactive hyperaemia on lowering again. A history of ischaemic rest pain is more common in the more severe cases and lesser degrees of ischaemia are usually associated with intermittent claudication (pain in the calf muscle which comes on when walking or exercising and is relieved by rest) (Callam *et al.*, 1987a).

Signs and symptoms of arterial problems are highlighted in Chapter 3, but to summarize, Morison (2006) identifies the following symptoms:

- Intermittent claudication
- Ischaemic rest pain

and signs, many of which are suggestive but not specific to ischaemic disease:

- Coldness of the foot
- Poor tissue perfusion
- Atrophic, shiny skin
- Loss of hair on the leg
- Muscle wasting in the calf or thigh
- Trophic changes in the nails
- Gangrene of toes
- Abnormal or absent foot pulses

Clinical signs and symptoms of acute arterial occlusion in the lower limb are:

- Pain of sudden onset and severe intensity
- Pallor
- Paraesthesia
- Pulselessness
- Paralysis
- Perishing cold (polar)

It is important to distinguish between venous, arterial and mixed aetiology ulceration as the management and treatment are very different. Inappropriate treatment can result in damage or lead to amputation of the limb.

Risk factors for arterial disease

The risk of arterial disease increases with age (Callam *et al.*, 1987a). Other factors such as a history of smoking, hypertension, cardiac disease, diabetes and cerebrovascular disease are major contributory factors. When assessing Annie it is important that you ask her if there is any family history of arterial disease and peripheral arterial disease. You will also need to assess Annie for any of the following signs: hairless, shiny legs, a pale poorly perfused leg or any evidence that her leg pales on elevation. It is advisable to check for any signs of diabetes as this may lead to arterial disease (Scott, 2005). If Annie presents with peripheral arterial disease or diabetes it is imperative that a podiatrist is involved in Annie's care. Both are significant preceding factors in lower extremity amputation. Studies have demonstrated the positive impact of podiatry in the care of these patients, with amputation rates significantly reduced in those who receive regular podiatric care (Van Gils *et al.*, 1999; Plank *et al.*, 2003).

During your assessment with Annie you should identify with her if she has any pain on walking and, if so, how far can she walk before the pain is felt, as this is indicative of claudication. If the distance is reducing over time the underlying disease, atherosclerosis, may be worsening. You will need to refer her to her GP or the vascular team for further investigation.

Careful assessment for underlying arterial disease is mandatory for patients with chronic leg ulcers before patients are treated with high-compression bandages.

5.6.4 | Rheumatoid Arthritis

Ulceration of the lower limb occurs with greater frequency in patients with rheumatoid arthritis than in the general population, although the incidence of ulceration in rheumatoid disease is poorly researched. If there is a clear history of rheumatoid arthritis or scleroderma, there should be no difficulty with diagnosis (rheumatoid arthritis is almost always associated with sero-positive rheumatoid factor). Rheumatoid ulcers are usually broad and shallow (Negus, 1991), are frequently multiple and may present on the lateral or posterior aspect of the lower leg. They can, however, appear in the malleoli regions and mimic venous ulceration, usually without surrounding lipoder-matosclerosis.

Diagnosis can be difficult when patients present with evidence of venous incompetence without physical evidence of rheumatoid arthritis. It may not be recognized as a complicating factor until the patient fails to respond to treatment for venous ulceration. In some patients examination of the joints of the hands (Figure 5.3), enquiring regarding previous surgery (Figure 5.4) and examination

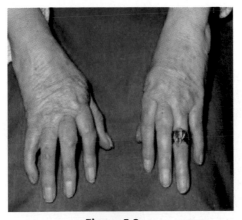

Figure 5.3
Typical changes in the hand with RA

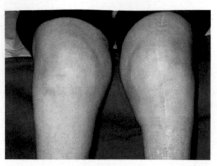

Figure 5.4
Previous surgical site scar of total knee replacement

of the feet will reveal signs of rheumatoid disease. However, specific screening will provide a precise diagnosis. The treatment for rheumatoid arthritis is often disease-modifying antirheumatic drugs or steroids; both can delay wound healing and increase infection risk, making this group of patients very difficult to treat. Chapter 9 specifically discusses rheumatoid ulceration in the lower limb.

Vasculitis (inflammation of the blood vessels) is common to rheumatoid disease and may affect the vascular tree at any level, but typically affects the lower leg and feet. Vasculitic ulcers do not normally mimic venous ulceration; specific investigations will provide a precise diagnosis. Medical supervision from a rheumatologist or dermatologist should be sought. Please refer to Chapter 9 for a more comprehensive guide to vasculitis and rheumatoid ulcers.

> **?** **What factors do you need to include in your assessment of Annie to identify the underlying aetiology of the leg ulcer?**

5.7 | Leg Ulcer Assessment

All patients with a leg ulcer must undergo a full holistic assessment before any treatment is instigated. Although vascular disease in one form or another is the most common cause for leg ulceration, the circulation cannot be viewed in isolation. It is important that a full overall assessment includes the holistic requirement of care planning. This will include information relating to the patient, the skin, the circulation, the limb and the ulcer. This should be combined with additional information derived from investigations (Vowden and Vowden, 2001).

The assessment should be able to address the following questions:

- What is the aetiology of this ulcer?
- What factors may delay healing?

- What is the most appropriate treatment?
- Are there any correctable risk factors that will speed healing and reduce the risk of occurrence?
- What are the patient's feelings regarding the ulcer and how is this affecting the quality of life?

Assessment should include investigations such as blood pressure, height, weight and urinalysis. Blood pressure is taken to monitor cardiovascular disease, weight is measured at the baseline to monitor weight loss if the patient is obese and urinalysis is undertaken to detect any undiagnosed diabetes mellitus. The need for additional blood and biochemical investigations will depend on the patient's clinical history and local protocols. Measurement of ABPI is essential to rule out arterial insufficiency in the ulcerated limb (Royal College of Nursing, 2006, Section 1.8).

If considered to be appropriate, blood tests should be taken to exclude anaemia, diabetes, and renal and hepatic failure. Screening for autoantibodies, including rheumatoid factor, may be indicated if a vasculitic or previously undiagnosed rheumatoid arthritis is suspected (Gibson, 1995).

5.7.1 | The Patient

The management of chronic leg ulcers will often be influenced by the patient's comorbidity, e.g. cardiac failure, and other causes of limb swelling such as renal disease, lymphoedema and osteomyelitis. It is important that the cause of the ulcer is ascertained and if possible treated to prevent reoccurrence. Mekkes *et al.* (2003) state that although most leg ulcers are caused by venous insufficiency (45–60%), arterial insufficiency (10–20%) or both (10–15%), more uncommon underlying disorders may be involved and should not be discounted, especially if the ulcer is unresponsive to conventional treatment.

Annie will be able to provide you with a history that will assist you to identify the underlying aetiology of her ulcer. A detailed history should include information on existing medical conditions, including risk factors for venous disease such as multiple pregnancies, previous limb trauma and history of DVT. As with all wounds, it is advisable to examine the nutritional status of the patient. This should be undertaken using a validated nutritional assessment scale and referral made to the dietician as appropriate.

5.7.2 | The Leg

The shape of the leg

Patients present with legs of all shapes and sizes, e.g. large, slim, straight, champagne bottle shaped, as illustrated in Figure 5.5, or oedematous due to underlying disease processes. The shape of the leg will have implications if compression bandaging is indicated. For example, it is very difficult to try to apply graduated compression to a champagne bottle shaped leg, as seen in Figure 5.5.

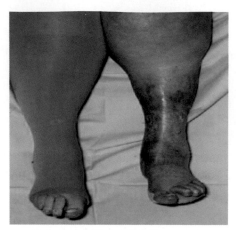

Figure 5.5
Champagne bottle shaped limbs

Measurement of both legs can be useful to detect any alteration in limb size. A great deal of skill is required to build up the narrow part of the limb with wadding bandage. Additionally a very thin leg will be susceptible to tissue damage.

The skin

A lot can be learned by observation of the patient's skin. For example, the colour of the skin can indicate underlying disease processes. Patients with venous disease often have brown staining (lipodermatosclerosis), signs of atrophie blanche, peratolytic plaques and/or varicose eczema, which may be itchy. Patients with very pale cold skin often have underlying arterial disease. Observation of the condition of the skin is an important aspect when planning the patient's management. Evidence of previous ulceration may be apparent. If the skin is red with associated pain and excessive exudate the patient may have an underlying cellulitis. Chapter 3 offers a greater insight into skin changes associated with vascular disease.

Foot pulses

The palpation of foot pulses is primarily used for assessing peripheral vascular disease. All four foot pulses should be palpated: peroneal, anterior tibial, posterior tibial and dorsalis pedis pulses. Figure 5.6 illustrates palpation of the latter two. Examination reveals weak or absent foot pulses if peripheral arterial disease is present (Epstein *et al.*, 1992). The practitioner must be aware that during palpation if oedema is present it may be difficult to palpate the pulses effectively. Moffatt and O'Hare (1995) warn that reliance on palpation can be an unreliable predictor of arterial disease; therefore the use of Doppler ultrasound and the ankle brachial pressure index (ABPI) are useful clinical adjuncts. Doppler ultrasound provides audible signals that enable clinicians to determine the presence or absence of arterial disease (Figure 5.7). The Doppler ultrasound is now commonly used to establish an ABPI measurement and is a safe and reliable method of monitoring arterial disease (Marshall, 2004).

The ABPI (ankle brachial pressure index) is a simple ratio between the blood pressure in the arm and the distal calf. With the patient lying down, the anterior tibial, dorsalis pedis, posterior tibial and

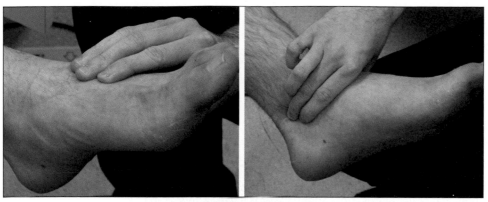

Figure 5.6
Palpation of dorsalis pedis pulse (left) and posterior tibial pulse (right)

peroneal arteries are isolated at the foot and the pressure required to occlude the vessel is measured with a blood pressure cuff around the leg, just above the ankle (*it is important with large limbs that a large thigh cuff is used*). The probe should be held at an angle of 45–60 degrees towards the skin and must be used with ultrasound gel. Systolic pressure at all four pulses should be recorded as

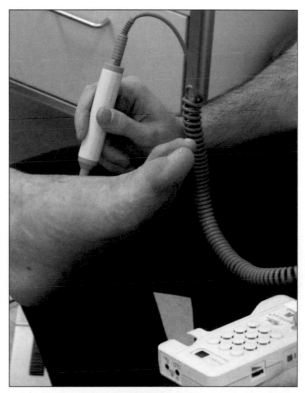

Figure 5.7
Droppler Ultrasound

well as brachial systolic pressure in both arms. The ABPI ratio is calculated by dividing the highest systolic pressure obtained from the foot pulses by the highest brachial systolic pressure as seen in the equation below:

$$ABPI = \frac{\text{highest ankle pressure}}{\text{highest arm pressure}}$$

In the absence of arterial disease the ABPI should be 1.0–1.3 as blood pressure may be a little higher at the foot because of gravity. Progressively more severe arterial disease reduces this, but the ABPI may be significantly reduced with no symptoms if the patient has good collateral vessels or rarely exercises. As a general guide, patients complain of calf cramps on exercise when the ABPI falls below 0.85 and are at risk of spontaneous arterial ulceration or rest pain when the ABPI is below 0.3 (Taylor and Smyth, 2001). Table 5.1 offers a guide to interpreting ABPI ratios.

In some patients, typically those with diabetes or chronic renal failure, the ABPI may be artificially high (greater than 1.3) because of arterial calcification, which reduces compressibility (Grasty, 1999). This type of patient should be referred to specialist clinics for further vascular investigation. Vowden and Vowden (2001) highlight common problems and errors that may arise:

- The cuff is repeatedly inflated for long periods. This can cause the ankle pressure to fall.
- The pulse is irregular or the cuff is deflated too rapidly. The true systolic pressure may be missed.
- If vessels are calcified, common in diabetes, or if the legs are large, fatty or oedematous, the cuff size is inappropriate, or the legs are elevated or dependent the result may be inaccurate.

Vowden and Vowden (2001) suggest Doppler ultrasound as a valuable tool in leg ulcer assessment, when used by skilled practitioners, but they advise caution when interpreting results. They argue

- ABPI normally >1.0–1.3

- ABPI < 0.9 indicates some arterial disease

- ABPI < 0.8 not suitable for compression

- ABPI > 0.4 and < 0.9 can be associated with claudication so this type of patient should be referred for further assessment

- ABPI < 0.4 indicates severe arterial disease and may be associated with gangrene, ischaemic ulceration or rest pain and warrants urgent referral for a vascular opinion

Table 5.1
Interpretation of ABPI values

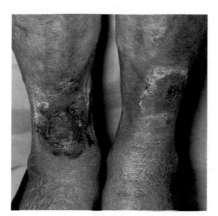

Figure 5.8
Arterial leg ulcers on the anterior aspect of the legs

that nurses can place undue reliance on an ABPI of 0.8 in their decision making, rather than regarding it as only one aspect of information relating to what is a multifaceted assessment. The ABPI should be used in conjunction with all other aspects of the structured and systematic assessment, to determine the aetiology of the ulcer.

The ulcer(s)

The location of the ulceration often is a clue to the aetiology. For example, venous ulcers are almost always in the medial/lateral gaiter areas of the lower limb. Occasionally they can present elsewhere. Ischaemic ulceration tends to be on the foot or anterior aspect of the lower limb, as seen in Figure 5.8, but also can present elsewhere.

? **Annie has presented with an ulcer on her medial malleolus, as seen in Figure 5.1. What do you suspect is the aetiology of the wound?**

The history regarding the development and the duration of the ulcer is very important. Venous ulcers tend to develop more slowly and are usually shallow with irregular borders. Ischaemic ulcers are frequently punched out and develop more rapidly. Ulcers with an unusual appearance (rolled edges) or with a history of bleeding should be referred for tissue biopsy to rule out malignant change.

The ulcer appearance should be examined. Venous ulcers tend to be colonized with bacteria, but this does not usually affect the healing process. Most venous ulcers will heal with compression bandaging. However, ulcers with offensive odour and clinical signs of infection should be swabbed and treated with appropriate antibiotics. Many venous ulcers present with a clean base. Ulcers with a fixed sloughy base will require wound debridement. There are many methods of wound debridement; local guidelines and formularies will provide information on wound care products recommended locally.

If sharp debridement is indicated this should only be undertaken by a skilled practitioner who has undergone training. Specialist podiatrists may be able to offer training packages for nurses.

All ulcers should be measured and the wound bed described as part of the assessment process. Assessment should include pain assessment, nutritional status and photographs where possible (please refer to your local guidelines regarding consent).

5.7.3 | Assessment of Wound Pain

Annie has stated that she is in a lot of pain from her ulcer and therefore it is important to assess the site and severity of the pain. Assessment of wound pain in patients with leg ulcers is difficult for practitioners because pain is personal and influenced by many complex factors. Hollinworth (2000) found nurses did not perceive patients' wound pain correctly, were disinclined to administer sufficient analgesics to adequately relieve pain and did not have accurate information about the pharmacology of analgesic drugs. Singer *et al.* (1999)confirmed that there was poor correlation between individual patients and practitioner pain scores and suggested that practitioners may not always be good judges of their patient's pain during painful procedures.

Methods for assessing wound pain include verbal and visual assessment together with monitoring physiological and behavioural changes such as increased pulse rate, perspiration, restlessness and moaning. Wound pain assessment tools are an essential part of the holistic wound care assessment process. Simple tools appear to have the most relevance to wound care.

As a practitioner you should assess Annie's pain using a pain assessment scale and record the response in her notes. The verbal rating score is recognized as a tool that is generally good to use with older people as it is less complicated that other tools (Jensen and Karoly, 1992). It is important that consistency in the use of tools is maintained to allow effective comparison of the scores. Dobson (2000) considers the "sociocultural" dimension of pain which describes the impact of a long-standing painful wound on the patient and her family and social network. It is important that you discuss Annie's feeling of loneliness and make provision for her to integrate with others, with her consent. Discussions with Annie should include whether she would like to attend a day care centre where she will be able to meet other people on a regular basis. It is important to identify whether any analgesics have previously been prescribed for annie, whether she takes the recommended dose and when they were last reviewed. Annie's analgesic may require review to ensure that she receives the correct type and amount to control her pain. The World Health Organization (1996) has developed an analgesic ladder as a useful guideline for titrating the strength and dose of analgesia to the level of pain. It is recommended that the type of analgesic used should have a short time-to-peak effect, be easily titrated to changing requirements and cause minimal side effects. The final choice of drug will be dictated by Annie's history, severity of pain and clinical setting (Heafield, 1999). Referral to her GP and the community chronic pain team will be beneficial to the assessment and management of Annie's pain.

5.8 | Treat the Surrounding Skin

The skin needs to be kept clean and in a healthy condition. All patients should have their legs washed, as per local guidelines, between bandage changes. Pay particular attention to the feet and in between the toes. Observe the conditions of the toenails and assess for callus or corns and, if necessary, refer the patient to a podiatrist to promote foot health. Following assessment skin may require treating with an emollient; please refer to your local guidelines. Additionally patients with unmanageable skin conditions, such as varicose eczema, may need to be reviewed by a dermatologist.

5.9 | Management of Leg Ulcers

Treatment directed at the leg will largely depend on the aetiology of the ulcer: accurate diagnosis is therefore the primary objective when a patient presents with leg ulceration. Noninvasive tests including the ABPI and a comprehensive history take will assist in diagnosis and inform management planning.

5.9.1 | Types of Leg Ulceration

Marston and Vowden (2003) placed leg ulceration into five categories:

- Uncomplicated venous ulceration
- Complicated venous ulceration
- Mixed arterial and venous ulceration
- Arterial ulceration
- Other causes, e.g. malignancy

Management strategies will differ for each category of leg ulceration.

Uncomplicated venous ulceration
Marston and Vowden (2003) defined uncomplicated venous ulceration as an ulcer occurring due to venous disease, without the presence of other medical diseases and in a limb with an ABPI ratio of >0.8.

The concept of compression for the management of uncomplicated venous leg ulcers is well established. Moffatt (2003) suggests that few other interventions can claim such drastic improvements in care, with patients reporting an improvement in pain, mobility and quality of life as their ulcer heals due to compression therapy. Given this, it is not surprising that graduated compression, as

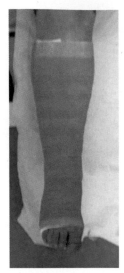

Figure 5.9
Graduated Compression: four-layer compression bandage

illustrated in Figure 5.9, has become recognized as the single most important conservative form of treatment for the management of venous ulcers (Partsch, 2003). Moffatt (1992) suggests that graduated compression has been shown to:

- Reduce the distension of the superficial veins and reverse venous hypertension
- Improve venous return to the heart by improving the blood flow velocity in the deep veins
- Reduce oedema, which in turn reduces the pressure difference between the capillaries and the tissues
- Enhance the clearance of sodium from the subcutaneous tissue of the foot from patients with a history of deep vein thrombosis
- Improve the healing rate of chronic venous ulcers
- Reduce the symptoms of venous disease by preventing excessive venous distension

It is well established that graduated compression (i.e. compression that delivers the highest pressure at the ankle and gaiter area and progressively diminishes as it ascends the leg) controls or reverses venous insufficiency.

Complicated venous ulceration
Marston and Vowden (2003) define complicated venous ulceration as an ulcer occurring due to venous disease with other confounding medical disease that could prevent the use of high compression and/or presents on a limb with an ABPI ratio <0.8. In these patients alternative forms of compression may be considered.

However, compression is not appropriate for all leg ulcers. Patients with arterial disease with an ABPI less than 0.8 may be harmed by graduated compression, as may people with diabetes, in which the ABPI may be unreliable because of arterial calcification. Neuropathy may confer an additional risk.

First layer: wadding, which will act as an absorbency layer to absorb exudates, protect the bony prominences and help to redistribute pressure

Second layer: light support bandage will provide a smooth surface, conserving the elastic energy of the compression layer

Third layer: high elastic compression layer will provide sustained compression for up to one week

Fourth layer: a lightweight cohesive bandage which will maintain the bandages in place for up to a week; this bandage also provides compression

Table 5.3
Four-layer bandaging

Drug Tariff and is based on Stemmner's calculation that 40 mmHg is required to reverse venous hypertension (Stemner *et al.*, 1980).

All compression layers of bandage, as detailed below, are applied at mid-stretch and are classed as long-stretch bandages. The action of the calf muscle pump will allow the bandages to expand. Short-stretch bandages are inelastic and applied at full stretch. These bandages provide a low resting pressure which increases to high pressure during activity. These bandages need to be applied on a more regular basis and require a great deal of skill in the application.

When assessing the patient for compression therapy it is important that patients with acute infection, acute deep vein thrombosis, fragile or damaged skin are *not* treated with compression. Specialist referral and advice must be sought for the diabetic patient as there is a risk of microvascular disease. Patient education is paramount when compression is applied and the patient must understand that should they suffer any pain, irritation, change in the colour of the feet/toes or tightness under the compression they must seek urgent advice.

5.9.4 | Bandaging Skills

Nurses need specific training on how to apply compression bandages. Involvement on a regular basis is recommended in order to acquire and maintain good bandaging skills. It is important that bandages are applied evenly, both in respect to tension and overlap to prevent skin damage. Bandages applied incorrectly will not provide graduated compression and may delay wound healing. This may contribute to the patient losing confidence in the treatment, thus affecting compliance. Taylor *et al.* (1998b) identified only that 50% of nurses demonstrated good bandaging skills; however, this improved to 81% with the use of a sub-bandage pressure monitor. Venous ulcers are mainly dealt with in the community setting by district nurses who are involved regularly in order to maintain skills. Problems tend to arise in secondary care where nurses are not involved on a regular basis.

Remember that all patients must have a Doppler assessment prior to application of compression bandaging. Arterial perfusion should also be reviewed on a regular basis for those receiving compression therapies. Marston and Vowden (2003) stress the need to closely monitor arterial perfusion, particularly in the elderly, in whom arterial disease is prevalent and can develop rapidly.

5.10 | Managing the Wound

Consideration needs to be given to the physiological, psychological and social aspect of care relating to the management of patients with leg ulcers. The aims of treatment are (Moffatt *et al.*, 1992):

- To provide a wound environment that promotes healthy granulation tissue
- To prevent secondary infection
- To prevent further damage to the ulcer or surrounding skin
- To control odour
- To control pain and provide a socially and psychologically acceptable form of treatment for the patient
- To treat the underlying cause
- To reduce the risk of recurrence once the ulcer has healed

All ulcers should be measured and evaluated at the initial assessment. Trace a round the wound edges with an acetate pen on to acetate or measure the length and width of the ulcer. It is important to describe the ulcer bed and note whether there are any signs of infection. In the absence of clinical signs of infection (e.g. cellulitis) there is no indication for routine bacterial swabbing venous ulcers (Hanson *et al.*, 1995). All ulcers will be colonized by micro-organisms at some point, and colonization in itself is not associated with delayed healing (Trengrove *et al.*, 1996). The value of antimicrobial dressings in the management of leg ulcers is not clear due to a current lack of evidence.

The vast majority of venous ulcers will heal with adequate compression bandaging. The use of a simple nonadherent dressing is usually sufficient. There are many products on the market that are available for use under compression bandaging. It is important for practitioners to adhere to their local formulary. Increased exudate levels can cause problems with the frequency of bandage changes. Compression can be left on for up to seven days; this will depend on the patient and problems related to the wound. It is acceptable to use foams or low-adherent contact materials under compression if required.

Most venous ulcers will heal spontaneously with compression bandaging; however, practitioners should measure wounds on a regular basis (every four weeks). Ulcers that fail to reduce in size by 50% by 12 weeks should be reassessed. There are many reasons why ulcers fail to heal. The incidence of malignancy in leg ulceration is reported to be less than 1% of the total population.

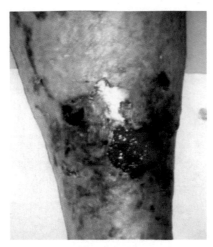

Figure 5.10
Squamous cell carcinoma

Taylor (2003) reported a higher malignancy rate of 6% in 193 patients reporting to a community-based leg ulcer service. This study highlighted the need for nurses to be aware of the need for tissue biopsy in patients where there is diagnostic uncertainty. Figures 5.10 and 5.11 illustrate malignant skin changes on the leg.

5.10.1 | Factors Affecting Healing

Although most venous ulcers will respond to management with compression bandaging and heal within a reasonable period of time, there are cohorts of chronic nonhealing ulcers that fail to respond to treatment. It is important to examine and re-examine the underlying aetiology: are there underlying disease processes or local factors that are affecting wound healing? For example, does the patient have a low-grade infection that has not been addressed?

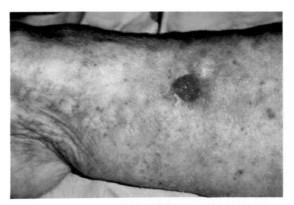

Figure 5.11
Basal cell carcinoma on the leg

Moffatt (2003) states that the majority of venous leg ulcers will heal with the application of high-compression bandaging and a nonadherent dressing. However, they argue that the challenge for effective wound bed preparation is the early detection of those ulcers unlikely to heal by simple compression therapy alone, and for which additional therapeutic interventions may accelerate or facilitate healing. Harper *et al.* (1995) and Moffatt *et al.* (1992) state that there is currently no internationally agreed standard healing rates of uncomplicated venous ulcers: reported healing progress at 12 weeks ranges from 30% to over 75%. Although a number of risk factors for delayed healing are recognized, there are many possible reasons why healing rates vary so widely. However, the percentage of wound reduction during the first three to four weeks of treatment can be used to predict subsequent healing, with a 44% reduction in the initial area at week 3 correctly predicting healing in 77% of cases (Flanagan, 2003).

5.11 | Lymphoedema

One significant pathology that can give rise to complex leg ulceration is lymphoedema. The lymphatic system consists of a vast network of lymph vessels and over 700 lymph nodes. It has an important role in maintaining tissue fluid balance, transporting fats and proteins and supporting the immune response. Swelling develops when part of the lymphatic system fails as a result of an intrinsic problem with the lymph vessels or nodes (primary lymphoedema) or secondary damage within the system as a result of surgery, radiotherapy trauma or infection (secondary lymphoedema). This produces a protein-rich lymphoedema associated with characteristic skin thickening and a positive Stemmer's sign: the inability to pinch a fold of skin on the second toe (Williams, 2006). Primary lymphoedema of the leg may be the result of an absence of collector lymphatic vessels or lymph node fibrosis. Bilateral swelling is more often associated with obliteration of distal lymphatics and is most commonly seen in females.

The primary management aim in a patient with lymphoedema is to reduce swelling and relieve pain. According to Casley-Smith *et al.* (1998), the four main treatment approaches include:

- Skin care: daily washing and the application of an emollient cream and any other appropriate skin care treatments
- Manual lymphatic drainage (MLD) massage: helps redirect the fluid away from the oedematous areas and enhances the removal of protein from the tissues
- Exercises: walking and swimming
- Compression therapy: is long-term therapy and should be used in conjunction with other treatments

Williams (2006) recommends that a comprehensive assessment of the patient should be undertaken, identifying the following:

- Is this lymphoedema and what is the cause(s) of the swelling?
- How extensive is the swelling and does it include the trunk, breast or genital areas?
- What is the limb volume? Is shape distortion present and does the limb fit the size ranges for standard garments?

- What skin and tissue changes are present?
- What other problems or contributing factors are present, such as obesity, immobility, cardiac disease or active cancer?
- What is the impact of lymphoedema on the person and what factors may influence the outcome of treatment?

Further recommendations include limb volume measurement by a practitioner who is experienced in the method. This can be used to compare swollen and unswollen limbs through calculating the excess limb volume. Assessment of arterial status should be undertaken, including the use of Doppler ultrasound to measure the ankle brachial pressure index (ABPI). However, this may present difficulties if the limb is very swollen and fibrotic. Specialist advice should be sought if the ABPI is <0.8 or >1.3.

5.11.1 | Multiprofessional Approach

A multiprofessional approach to the care of the patient with lymphoedema is important. The patient should be assessed by a lymphoedema specialist initially and appropriate referrals made to other members of the team. These members may include the following professionals:

- Lymphoedema nurses
- Diabetic specialist nurses
- Tissue viability specialist podiatrists
- Vascular nurse specialists
- Vascular medical team
- Pain management team
- Tissue viability specialist nurses
- Dieticians

5.12 | Criteria for Specialist Referral

The Royal College of Nursing (RCN) (2006) recommend that specialist medical referral may be appropriate for:

- Treatment for underlying medical problems
- Ulcers of nonvenous aetiology (rheumatoid, diabetes related, arterial mixed aetiology)
- Suspected malignancy
- Diagnostic uncertainty
- Reduced ABPI (e.g. <0.8 for routine vascular referral; <0.5 for urgent vascular referral) (however, these may vary according to local protocols)
- Increased ABPI (e.g. >1.0) (however, these may vary according to local protocols)
- Rapid deterioration of ulcers
- Newly diagnosed diabetes mellitus
- Signs of contact dermatitis (spreading eczema, increased itch)

- Cellulitis
- Healed ulcers (with a view to venous surgery)
- Ulcers that have not received adequate treatment and have not improved after three months
- Recurring ulceration
- Ischaemic foot
- Infected foot
- Pain management

The RCN (2006) cite a randomized controlled trial undertaken by Vandongen & Stacey (2000) who reported that wearing class III compression stockings significantly reduced ulcer recurrence at six months, compared with not wearing compression stockings. Furthermore, the RCN (2006, 15.1) state that the use of compression stockings reduces venous ulcer recurrence rates and is cost-effective. Patients should be encouraged to wear class III compression, if this is not contraindicated and they can tolerate it; otherwise the highest level of compression they will tolerate.

The author would like to point out that in clinical practice elderly patients, and even many younger patients, are unable to comply with class III compression hosiery. They are very difficult to apply and you run the risk of non-compliance.

5.13 | Healed Ulcers

Chronic leg ulcers almost always recur unless a strategy for prevention is maintained. Prevention strategies include the use of graduated compression hosiery or surgery, but not all patients are suitable for surgery or will consider surgery if this is available to them.

5.13.1 | Compression Hosiery

Compression hosiery can be recommended for patients with no signs of arterial disease and have an ABPI of 0.8 and above (Grasty, 1999). Most stocking companies provide tape measures and measuring guides to ensure correct measurement.

Classification of compression hosiery
Compression hosiery available on the Drug Tariff is British standard (it should be noted that European standards of compression are higher):

Class I provides 14–17 mmHg at the ankle, giving light support.
Class II provides 18–24 mmHg, providing medium support for the prevention of recurrence.
Class III provides 25–33 mmHg at the ankle for strong support.

Compression stockings can be difficult to apply and some patients will also, for various reasons, have problems with wearing them. Class I stockings may be a more acceptable choice for these patients.

? Examine the photograph of Annie's wound (Figure 5.1). Using the information and illustrations provided develop a management plan for her care.

5.14 | Case Scenario Revisited

1. **What is the history of leg ulceration in this patient (first or recurrent episode trauma, etc.)?**
   This is Annie's first episode of ulceration. The ulcer is described as chronic as it has been present for a duration of 6 months.

2. **What is the aetiology of this ulcer?**
   The ulcer presents on the medial aspect of her leg; this anatomical location is highly indicative of a wound of venous aetiology. In addition, on observation of the limb, lipodermatosclerosis and mild oedema were visible, both clinical signs associated with venous dysfunction. A vascular assessment, including ABPI, supported this finding. Annie's ABPI result was 0.9, indicating some arterial disease, but the underlying aetiology of the wound in this case was venous disease.

3. **What factors may delay healing in this case?**
   The fact that Annie has venous disease and some arterial disease suggests that healing could be delayed in this case. In addition, the presence of infection, poor compliance to treatment and poor nutritional status could all contribute to the chronicity of Annie's ulcer.

4. **What are the most appropriate management strategies in this case?**
   As Annie's ABPI value was 0.9 she is appropriate for graduated compression bandaging – the gold standard treatment in the management of venous leg ulceration. In addition, local wound bed preparation and management of infection is essential to optimize healing.

5. **Are there any correctable risk factors that will speed healing and prevent the risk of recurrence?**
   A wound swab identified that Annie had a *Staphylococcus aureus* wound infection that required treatment with systemic antibiotics. Due to her low morale and feeling of despair it was decided to bring her to the local leg ulcer clinic to mix with other patients. She was prescribed oral antibiotics by her GP. She commenced treatment with multilayer compression bandaging. She enjoyed attending the leg ulcer clinic weekly. Her appetite and appearance improved dramatically and she was completely healed within 16 weeks. When her ulcer healed she was provided with class II compression hosiery and regularly attended the healed ulcer clinic.

5.15 | Conclusion

Leg ulcers can pose a significant clinical, financial and personal burden to all affected. The clinician is often faced with the complexities associated with managing leg ulceration of various aetiologies and ensuring appropriate treatment strategies are adopted dependent on cause, best practice and patient requirements. This chapter has explored best practice in leg ulcer care, based on evidence and clinical guidelines, while encouraging a holistic approach to patient care.

> **?** **Reflection**
>
> **Take time to reflect upon your learning from this chapter. Ask yourself:**
>
> 1. **What knowledge did I possess prior to reading this chapter?**
>
> 2. **How has my knowledge developed?**
>
> 3. **How will I implement this into my future practice?**

References

Adams, E.F (1949) *The Genuine Works of Hippocrates*, Sydenham Press, London.

Anderson, I. (2006) Aetiology, assessment and management of leg ulcers. *Wound Essentials*, **1**, 21–37.

Bosanquet, N. (1992) Costs of venous ulcers: from maintenance therapy to investment programmes. *Phlebology*, **1**, Suppl., 44–6.

Bowskill, D. (2001) Compression hosiery in venous insufficiency: a nurse-led field. *Journal of Community Nursing*, **6**(7), 356–62.

Briggs, M. and Closs, S.J. (2003) The prevalence of leg ulceration: a review of the literature. *EWMA Journal*, **3**(2), 14–20.

Browse, N.L. and Burnand, K.G. (1982) The cause of venous ulceration. *Lancet*, **2**(8292), 243–5.

Callam, M.J., Ruckley, C.V., Harper, D.R. and Dale, J.J. (1985) Chronic ulceration of the leg: extent of the problem and provision of care. *British Medical Journal*, **290**, 1855–6.

Callam, M.J., Harper, D.R., Dale, J.J. and Ruckley, C.V. (1987a) Arterial disease in chronic leg ulceration: an underestimated hazard? Lothian and Forth Valley leg ulcer study. *British Medical Journal* (*Clinical Research Edition*), **294** (6577), 929–31.

Callam, M.J., Harper, D.R., Dale, J.J. and Ruckley, C.V. (1987b) Chronic ulcer of the leg clinical history. *British Medical Journal* (*Clinical Research Edition*), **294** (6584), 1389–91.

Capitao, M.L., Menezes, J.D. and Oliveria, G.A. (1995) Clinical predictors of the severity of chronic venous insufficiency of the lower limbs: a multivariate analysis. *Phlebology*, **10**, 155–9.

Carr, L., Philips, Z., and Posnett, J. (1999) Comparative cost-effectiveness of four layer bandaging in the treatment of venous ulceration. *Journal of Wound Care*, **8**(5), 243–8.

Casley-Smith, J.R., Boris, M., Weindorf, S. *et al.* (1998) Treatment for lymphoedema of the arm – the Casley–Smith method: a non-invasive method produces continued reduction. *Cancer*, **15**(83), (12 Suppl. American), 2843–60.

Cornwall, J.V., Dore, C.J., and Lewis, J.D. (1986) Leg ulcers: epidemiology and aetiology. *British Journal Surgery*, **73**, 693–6.

Cullum, N.A., Nelson, E.A., Fletcher, A.W. and Sheldon, T.A. (2001) Compression for venous leg ulcers (Cochrane Review), The Cochrane Library, Oxford, update software (2).

Dobson, F. (2000) The art of pain management. *Professional Nurse*, **15**(12), 786–90.

Epstein, O., Perkin, G.D., de Bono, D.P. *et al.* (1992) *Clinical Examination*, Mosby, London.

Flanagan, M. (2003) Wound measurement: can it help us to monitor progression to healing? *Journal of Wound Care*, **12**(5), 189–94.

Franks, P.J. and Moffatt, M. (2006) Do clinical and social factors predict quality of life in leg ulcertation? *The International Journal of Lower Extremity Wounds*, **5**(4), 236–43.

Freak, L., Simon, D., Kensella, A., McCollum, C., Walsh, J., and Lane, C. (1995) Leg ulcer care: an audit of cost-effectiveness. *Health Trends*, **27**, 133–6.

Gibson, B. (1995) The nursing assessment of patients with leg ulcer, in *Leg Ulcers: Nursing Management*, (eds N. Cullum and B. Roe), Scutari, Harrow.

Graham, I.D., Harrison, M.B., Nelson, E.A., Lorimer, K. and Fisher, A. (2003) Prevalence of lower-limb ulceration: a systematic review of prevalence studies. *Advanced Skin Wound Care*, **16**, 305–16.

Grasty, M.S. (1999) Use of the hand held Doppler to detect peripheral vascular disease. *The Diabetic Foot*, **2**(1), 18–21.

Hanson, C., Hoborn, J., Moller, A. *et al.* (1995) The microbial flora in venous leg ulcers without clinical signs of infection. Repeated culture using a validated standardised microbiological technique. *Acta Dem Venereol*, **75**, 24–30.

Harper, D.R., Nelson, E.A., Gibson, B. *et al.* (1995) A prospective randomised trial of Class 2 and Class 3 elastic compression in the prevention of venous ulceration. *Phlebology*, Suppl. 1, 872–3.

Heafield, H. (1999) The management of procedural pain. *Professional Nurse*, **15**(2), 127–9.

Hofman, D. (2000) Management of leg ulcers. Quick reference guide. *Nursing Standard*, **14**(29), Suppl.

Hollinworth, H. (2000) *Pain and Wound Care*, Educational Leaflet, Wound Care Society, London.

Hopkins, N.F.G., Spinks, T.J., Rhodes, C.G. *et al.* (1983) Position emission tomography in venous ulceration and liposclerosis; a study of regional tissue function. *British Medical Journal*, **296**, 333.

Jensen, M.P., and Karoly, P. (1992) Self report scales and procedures for assessing pain in adults, in *Handbook of Pain Assessment*, (eds D. Turk and R. Melzack), Guilford Press, New York, pp. 135–52.

MacKenzie, R., Brown, D., Allan, P., Bradbury, A. and Ruckley, C. V. (2003) A comparison of patients who developed venous leg ulceration before and after their 50th birthday. *European Journal of Vascular and Endovascular Surgery*, **26**(2), 176–8.

Margolis, D.J., Bilker, W., Santanna, J. and Baumgarten, M. (2002) Venous leg ulcer: incidence and prevalence in the elderly. *Journal of Academic Dermatology*, **46**(3), 381–6.

Marshall, C. (2004) The ankle: brachial pressure index. A critical appraisal. *British Journal of Podiatry*, **7**(4), 93–5.

Marston, W. and Vowden, K. (2003) Compression therapy: a guide to safe practice, in Position Document, Understanding Compression Therapy, European Wound Management Association (EWMA) Medical Education Partnerships Ltd, pp. 11–7.

Mekkes, J., Loots, M., Van der Wal, A. *et al.* (2003) Causes, investigation and treatment of leg ulceration. *British Journal of Dermatology*, **148**(3), 388–401.

Moffatt, C.J. (1992) Compression bandaging the state of the art. *Journal of Wound Care*, **1**(1), 45–50.

Moffatt, C. (1998) Issues in the assessment of leg ulcers. *Journal of Wound Care*, **7**(9), 469–73.

Moffatt, C. (2001) Leg ulcers, in *Vascular Disease: Nursing and Management* (ed. S. Murray), Whurr, London, pp. 200–37.

Moffatt, C. (2003) Understanding compression therapy, in Position Document Understanding Compression Therapy, European Wound Management Association (EWMA), Medical Education Partnerships Ltd, p. 1.

Moffatt, C. and O'Hare, L. (1995) Ankle pulses are not sufficient to detect impaired arterial circulation in patients with leg ulcers. *Journal of Wound Care*, **4**(3), 134–8.

Moffatt, C.J. and Oldroyd, M.I. (1994) A pioneering service to the community. *Professional Nurse*, **9**(7), 486–90.

Moffatt, C.J., Franks. P.J., Oldroyd, M. *et al.* (1992) Community clinics for leg ulcers and impact on healing. *British Medical Journal*, **305**(6866), 1389–92.

Morison, M. (2006) *Leg Ulcers: An Educational Booklet* (sponsored by Smith and Nephew), Wounds UK Publishing, Aberdeen.

Morison, M.J., and Moffatt, C. (2004) Leg ulcers, in *Chronic Wound Care: A Problem Based Learning Approach* (eds M.J. Morison, L.G. Ovington and K. Wilkie) Mosby, Edinburgh, pp. 164–76.

Negus, D. (1991) *A Practical Approach to Leg Ulcers*, Butterworth-Heinneman Ltd, Oxford, pp. 97–8.

Nelzen, O., Bergqvist, D., Lindhagen, A. *et al.* (1994) Venous and non-venous leg ulcers; clinical history and appearance in a population study. *British Journal of Surgery*, **81**, 182–7.

Partsch, H. (2003) Understanding the pathophysiological effects of compression, in Position Document Understanding Compression Therapy European Wound Management Association (EWMA) Medical Education Partnerships Ltd, pp. 2–4.

Plank, J., Haas, W., Rakovac, I. *et al.* (2003) Evaluation of the impact of chiropodist care in the secondary prevention of foot ulcerations in diabetic subjects. *Diabetes Care*, **26**(6), 1691–5.

Registrar General Classification (2007) The National Statistics Socio-economic Classification (online), Available at: http://www.statistics.gov.uk/methods_quality/ns_sec/default.asp, Last accessed 15 February 2007.

Rich, A. and McLachalan, I. (2003) How living with a leg ulcer affects people's daily life: a nurse led study. *Journal of Wound Care*, **12**, 51–4.

Royal College of Nursing (RCN) (2006) *Clinical Practice Guidelines. The Nursing Management of Patients with Venous Leg Ulcers. Recommendations*, RCN, London.

Scott, A.R. (2005) Risk factors, in *Vascular Complications of Diabetes*, (eds R. Donnelly and E.S. Horton) 2nd edn, Blackwell Publishing, London and Oxford, pp. 60–8.

Scottish Intercollegiate Guidelines Network (SIGN) (1998) The care of patients with chronic leg ulcer: A National Clinical Guideline, Available at: http://www.sign.ac.uk/pdf/sign26.pdf, Last accessed 15 February 2007.

Singer, A.J., Richman, P.B., Kowalska, A. *et al.* (1999) Comparison of patient and practitioner assessments of pain from commonly performed emergency department procedures. *Annals of Emergency Medicine*, **33**(6), 562–58.

Stemner, R., Marescaux, J. and Furderer, C. (1980) Compression therapy for the lower extremities particularly with compression stockings. *Hautarzt*, **31**, 355–65.

Taylor, A. (2003). Leg ulcer management and the diagnosis of malignant ulceration. *Nurse2Nurse*, **3**(3), 49–50.

Taylor, A. and Smyth, V.J. (2001) A multidisciplinary approach to leg ulcer management in primary care. *British Journal of Community Nursing*, **6**(9), Profore Suppl., 12–6.

Taylor, A.D., Taylor, R.J. and Marcuson, R.W. (1998a) Prospective comparison of healing rates and therapy costs for conventional and four-layer high-compression bandaging treatments of venous leg ulcers. *Phlebology*, **13**, 20–4.

Taylor, A.D., Taylor, R.J. and Said, S.S.S. (1998b) Using a bandage pressure monitor as an aid in improving bandaging skills. *Journal of Wound Care*, **7**(3), 131–3.

Tortora, G.J. and Grabowski, S.R. (2000) *Principles of Anatomy and Physiology*, John Wiley and Sons, Ltd, Chichester.

Trengrove, N.J., Stacey, M.C., McGechie, D.F., Stingemore, N.F., and Mata, S. (1996) Qualitative bacteriology and leg ulcer healing. *Journal of Wound Care*, **5**, 97–100.

Van Gils, C.C., Wheeler, L.A. and Mellstrom, M. (1999) Amputation prevention by vascular surgery and podiatry collaboration in high-risk diabetic and non-diabetic patients: The Operation Desert Experience. *Diabetes Care*, **22**(5), 678–83.

Vowden, K. and Vowden, P. (1998) Venous leg ulcers Part 2: assessment. *Professional Nurse*, **13**(9), 633–8.

Vowden, P. and Vowden, K. (2001) Investigation in the management of lower limb ulceration. *British Journal of Community Nursing*, **6**(9), 4–11.

Walshe, C. (1995) Living with a venous ulcer: a descriptive study of patient's experiences. *Journal of Advanced Nursing*, **22**, 1092–100.

Williams, A.F. (2006) A clinical audit of Actico cohesive short stretch bandages. *Journal of Community Nursing*, **20**(2), 4–10.

World Health Organization (1996) *Cancer Pain Relief*, 2nd edn, WHO, Geneva.

Jacqui Fletcher

Chapter 6

Surgical Wounds

6.1 | Introduction

Surgical wounds vary in size and complexity but are increasingly presenting greater management challenges as patients live longer with more complex underlying disease processes. Changes in health care delivery mean patients requiring minor procedures frequently have their surgery in a community setting and those who undergo surgery as inpatients are being discharged much earlier due to pressure on hospital beds (Dowsett, 2002). Increasingly, patients who would previously have been deemed unsuitable for surgery because of high mortality are now being operated on because of advanced technologies, but alongside this comes an almost inevitable rise in complications. Patients are often sicker, and with more complex underlying pathologies their potential to heal in a straightforward way, as outlined in Chapter 2, is reduced. In addition, the growing number of patients with obesity and malnutrition compounds these problems (Harrison, 2006). Therefore, clinicians need to ensure that the best environment possible for healing is sought.

The aim of this chapter is to consider assessment and management strategies, based on best evidence, to promote healing in lower extremity surgical wounds.

6.2 | Case Scenario

Case Scenario 6

Consider the following case scenario. Raymond is a 41-year-old man with learning disabilities; he was admitted to the orthopaedic unit with a hot, red, swollen great toe on the left foot. On examination there was a break in the skin which was discharging a creamy white granular substance (see Figure 6.1).

Although the area was clearly painful, Raymond was adamant that it was "OK" as long as he took the tablets (nonsteroidal anti-inflammatories) given to him regularly by the nurse. He had no past medical history of note and was otherwise fit and well. He was accompanied by his frail elderly parents and also a care assistant from the home in which he had lived for the past five years.

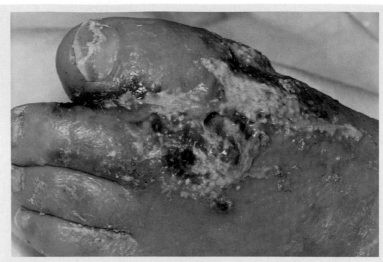

Figure 6.1
Raymond's left foot on admission

Following discussion with the care home staff it became evident that the toe had been inflamed for some days and the footwear he had been wearing had caused additional pressure on the area. Despite their best efforts to persuade him otherwise Raymond had insisted on wearing his trainers as they had been a birthday present; when they had tried to remove them he became extremely distressed. Although care home staff had applied dressings to the wound he regularly removed them.

On investigation his blood tests revealed a normal CRP (C reactive protein, a marker of infection) but a slightly raised serum uric acid level and analysis of the discharge from the wound confirmed the presence of gout. Raymond was taken to theatre for incision and drainage and returned with an open wound which was clean and granulating (see figure 6.2).

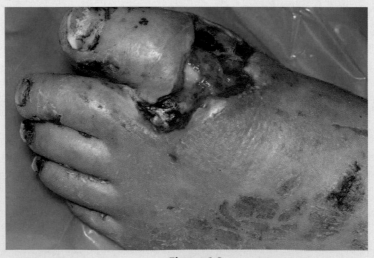

Figure 6.2
Raymond's left foot post-debridement

> **Consider the following questions:**
>
> 1. **What particular factors may need to be considered in Raymond's post-operative care? Consider especially the need to keep pressure off the area and also the need to prevent infection.**
>
> 2. **When selecting dressings for this wound what would be the main objectives of treatment?**
>
> 3. **Why was this wound not suitable for primary closure?**
>
> 4. **What factors may delay healing in this wound?**

The information provided within the following sections should enable you to answer the four questions posed above. The answers to the case will be further considered towards the end of the chapter.

6.3 | Surgical Wounds – Defining the Problem

Defining how many people undergo surgery of the lower limb is difficult as the clinical coding system used in the UK is not sufficiently sophisticated to discriminate between patient diagnoses, e.g. between sites of amputations. Table 6.1 presents a summary of some of the most relevant statistics presented for 2004/2005 (Hospital Episode Statistics (HES), 2006).

Diagnostic code	Completed patient episodes	Bed days used
Arteries and veins	176 872	892 611
Other arteries	8 715	44 779
Varicose veins of the leg	37 896	22 558
Veins and other blood vessels	106 963	385 842
Reconstruction of hand or foot	2 579	9 611
Other bones and joints	612 383	3 358 477
Amputation	14 984	251 359

Table 6.1
Statistics for frequency of operations (HES, 2006)

The most common reasons for surgery of the lower limb include peripheral arterial disease, orthopaedic surgery and amputation. Patients requiring surgery of the lower limb are usually cared for in specialist vascular or orthopaedic units. There are a large number of surgical interventions of the lower limb for other miscellaneous reasons, as highlighted in the case study above. Excision and drainage of wounds, grafting of ulcers or burns, repair of minor orthopaedic trauma, excision of varicose veins, etc., may be cared for on a variety of surgical areas.

6.3.1 | Peripheral Arterial Disease (PAD)

PAD (or PAOD, peripheral arterial occlusive disease) encompasses a large series of disorders affecting arterial beds exclusive of the coronary arteries. There is a high (up to 29% of the population) prevalence of lower extremity PAD across Europe, America and Asia; this occurrence rate increases with advancing age and exposure to atherosclerosis risk factors (Hirsch *et al.*, 2005). When considering the possibility of surgery thought must be given to the extent of the arterial disease, acuity of ischaemia and feasibility of restoring blood flow. It should be considered that the mortality rates associated with this type of surgery, even in appropriately selected candidates, may be up to 6%, but more importantly for major amputation of the lower limb there is a 30-day mortality risk of 4–30% with a 20–37% risk of significant morbidity such as myocardial infarction (MI), stroke or infection (Hirsch *et al.*, 2005). In addition, the long-term prognosis for the patient must be considered. In one study of infrainguinal bypass with a reversed saphenous vein for critical limb ischaemia (Chung *et al.*, 2006) 25% of patients did not achieve healing at 1 year, 19% had lost ambulatory function and 5% had lost independent living status. The wound healing for these patients was prolonged and they had many episodes of complications including infections.

A Cochrane review identified that although surgical bypass of an occluded arterial segment is the mainstay of treatment for patients with critical limb ischaemia there is little clear evidence to support this in preference to percutaneous transluminal angioplasty (PTA). In the six trials reviewed there were no clear differences between bypass surgery and PTA. Mortality and amputation rates did not differ significantly, although primary patency was significantly higher in the bypass group after 12 months (but not after four years). Compared with thrombolysis, amputation rates were significantly lower in the bypass group but mortality rates did not differ (Leng *et al.*, 2000).

Revascularization surgery is beneficial in enhancing the quality of life for patients with PAD as it removes the pain associated with critical ischaemia or severe claudication. An ankle brachial pressure index (ABPI), a test used to quantify the vascular status of the lower limb, of 0.5 or less is considered significant enough to require surgical intervention. Revascularization surgery results are usually good with long-term (three years and over) patency rates being approximately 80% for a vein graft to a proximal artery and 55% for an expanded polytetrafluoroethlene graft to a distal vessel (Herbert, 1997).

Cause of lower limb amputation	Percentage
Dysvascularity	75
Neoplasia	2
Neurological disorder	2
Infection	7
Trauma	9
Other	3
No cause provided	2
The dysvascularity group can broken down as follows:	
Diabetes mellitus	42
Nondiabetic arteriosclerosis	29
Patients for whom no additional detail was available	24
Other dysvascularity	5

Table 6.2
Conditions that contribute to lower limb amputation (reproduced from National Amputee Statistical Database, *National Amputee Statistical Database Annual Report*, NASDB, Edinburgh, 2005)

6.3.2 | Orthopaedics/Amputations

Amputations of the lower limb occur for a variety of reasons, the most common being PAD and diabetes mellitus. The lower limb amputee population in the UK is thought to be around 52 000 (National Amputee Statistical Database, 2005). The UK Prosthetics Service Annual Report for 2004/2005 (2005) suggests that 75 % of patients referred for prostheses had undergone amputation because of dysvascularity (see Table 6.2). Nine out of ten amputations were performed at either the transtibial (52 %) or the transfemoral (38 %) level and 70 % of lower limb amputees referred to prosthetics centres were male.

Figure 6.3 shows common levels of lower limb amputation. These are as follows (Harker, 2006):

- Above knee
- Through knee

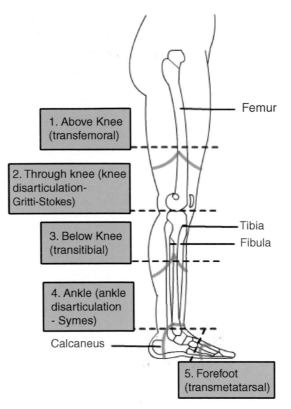

Figure 6.3
Common levels of lower extremity amputations

- Below knee. Two types of skin flap can be used. The posterior myocutaneous flap is well vascularized and contains muscle and skin and is designed to compensate for the poorly vascularized anterior skin flap. If a skew flap is used the join of the flap is oblique; thus the tibial crest is covered by the gastrocnemius muscle and blood supply to the flap is preserved.
- Ankle
- Forefoot

Amputations may be managed as open wound or closed via a flap; this depends upon the amount of salvageable skin available to flap and the extent of any infection. Where there has been deep-seated infection with bone involvement the amputation is frequently left open to facilitate any necessary further debridement.

Amputations result in a whole range of specific considerations for both the clinician and patient, perhaps the uppermost of which is the possibility of further loss of limb and reduction in mobility and independence. For most patients their prognosis depends very much on the reason for amputation in the first place, as some of the main causes are progressive disease processes, e.g. PAD. This progression may be ameliorated by successful preventative care and management of underlying symptoms. Patients requiring amputation require considerable psychological support as the loss of a body part may be equated to a bereavement. For most patients, reaching the decision to undergo amputation is complex and difficult and where possible they should be given sufficient time to assimilate information and understand the future consequences. Rybarczyk *et al.* (2004) suggest that consideration should be given to post-amputation depression and anxiety, body image, feelings of vulnerability, social support changes, grief, pre-amputation psychological issues and phantom limb pain and sensations. They state that psychological assessment and referrals for treatment should be included as part of the routine care provided to individuals with amputations, irrespective of the length of time that has passed since the amputation.

6.3.3 | Amputations Related to PAD

For many patients with critical limb ischaemia amputation may be the only option or certainly the best option in terms of improved quality of life. Revascularization may have been attempted and, successful or not, considered a reasonable option because of the extent of the underlying disease. The aim of amputation is to relieve pain, remove dead or severely ischaemic (see Figure 6.4) or infected tissue whilst maintaining function and quality of life.

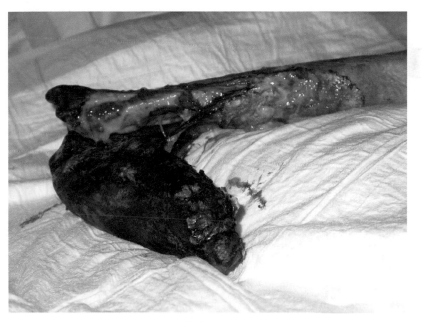

Figure 6.4
Severe ischaemia in the lower limb

As patients with lower extremity PAD frequently have widespread arterial disease and additional cardiovascular, respiratory and neurological disease, there is a high level of perioperative morbidity and mortality associated with amputation (Potterton and Galland, 2002). Due to the underlying cause of amputation and the progression of arterial disease, nearly a third of patients who have single limb amputation will progress to bilateral amputation within three years and approximately 50 % die within five years (Herbert, 1997).

6.3.4 | Amputation Related to Osteomyelitis

Forefoot amputation is a common sequalae of osteomyelitis, and is also frequently a precursor to major leg amputation. Berceli *et al.* (2006) in their study of 204 patients identified that, despite repeated operative debridement and apparently successful wound healing, many patients developed recurrent infections, which led to major amputation at a rapid rate regardless of their initial treatment approach.

6.3.5 | Amputations Related to Burns

Although amputation following burn surgery is not common it can reduce mortality in the management of severely burned extremities. The causation which results in amputation is most likely to be flame injury, usually from road traffic accidents or high-voltage electrical injury. In one study of 1858 patients there were 34 amputations in 27 patients, 9 immediate amputations with 25 delayed. The survival rate in these patients was 89 % and the presence of pre-existing psychiatric disease significantly impaired rehabilitation of some patients (Kennedy *et al.*, 2006). Amputation in this patient group frequently results in complications; Parrett *et al.* (2006) identified increased hospital stay (mean 76 days) and high rates of cellulitis, deep vein thrombosis and bacteraemia in the 18 % of their patients who required amputation following fourth degree burns.

6.3.6 | Amputation Related to Combined Vascular/Orthopaedic Wounds

Complex extremity trauma involving both arterial and skeletal injuries is rare, comprising only 0.2 % of all military and civilian traumas and only 0.5 %–1.7 % of all extremity fractures and dislocations. Combined arterial and skeletal extremity trauma imparts a substantially higher risk of limb loss and limb morbidity than isolated skeletal and arterial injuries. Even the most experienced trauma centres (where less than 5 % of limbs are lost following either arterial or skeletal trauma) report amputation rates approaching 70 %. Limb loss most commonly is attributed to delay in diagnosis and revascularization in most published series of this unique trauma. Major nerve damage, extensive soft tissue injury which disrupts collaterals and prevents adequate vessel coverage, infection and compartment syndrome are other reasons for such a high rate of loss of these severely compromised limbs (Frykberg, 2005).

6.4 | Patient Assessment

6.4.1 | Pre-operative Assessment

Vascular review

Assessment of any patient who is to undergo surgery of the lower limb should include a thorough review of the arterial status of the limb, as the blood supply to the limb will probably be the primary determinant of the ability to heal. Hirsch *et al.* (2005) suggest that there are key components to vascular physical examination:

- Measurement of blood pressure in both arms and notation of any interarm asymmetry
- Palpation of the carotid pulses and notation of the carotid upstroke and amplitude and presence of bruits.
- Auscultation of the abdomen and flank for bruits.
- Palpation of the abdomen and notation of the presence of aortic pulsation.
- Palpation of the pulses at the brachial, radial, ulnar, femoral, popliteal, dorsalis pedis and posterior tibial sites.
- Auscultation of both femoral arteries for the presence of bruits.
- Pulse intensity should be assessed and recorded numerically as follows: 0, absent; 1, diminished; 2, normal; 3, bounding.
- The shoes and socks should be removed, the feet inspected, the colour, temperature and integrity of the skin and intertrigineous areas evaluated and the presence of ulceration recorded.
- Additional findings suggestive of severe PAD, including distal hair loss, trophic skin changes and hypertrophic nails should be sought and recorded.

It is not always possible to manually palpate pulses; using a hand-held Doppler instrument is a more efficient way of determining the presence or absence of a pulse.

If there is any suggestion of abnormality in arterial flow Doppler studies, it is beneficial to identify the ABPI and patients may be referred for a colour duplex scan for a more detailed review of the vasculature. Angiography is the most definitive investigation to establish the position and extent of the blockage in the vessels (Herbert, 1997). Other investigations that may be considered include:

- Toe brachial pressure indices
- Segmental pressure examination (to determine the approximate level of the disease)
- Pulse volume recording
- Continuous wave Doppler ultrasound (Hirsch *et al.*, 2005)
- Blood tests, full blood count, creatinine, urea and electrolytes, lipid levels, group and cross-matching (usually for at least 4–6 units) and coagulation tests (including screening for anti-thrombin III, as a deficiency may lead to post-operative arterial thrombus formation) (Herbert, 1997)

The limb should be inspected for oedema, skin changes, colour, and movement and mobility. These may indicate poor perfusion or additional underlying disease processes such as congestive cardiac failure (Stubbing and Chesworth, 2001).

Fontaine			Rutherford		
Stage	Clinical	Grade	Category		Clinical
I	Asymptomatic	0	0		Asymptomatic
IIa	Mild claudication	I	1		Mild claudication
IIb	Moderate–severe claudication	I	2		Moderate claudication
		I	3		Severe claudication
III	Ischaemic rest pain	II	4		Ischaemic rest pain
		III	5		Minor tissue loss
IV	Ulceration or gangrene	IV	6		Ulceration or gangrene

Table 6.3
Classification of PAD: Fontaine's staging and Rutherford's categories (Dormandy and Rutherford, 2000)

The severity of any PAD is usually classified according to either Fontaine's stages or Rutherford's categories (see Table 6.3).

6.4.2 | Post-operative Assessment

Post-operative assessment criteria depend on the cause of the wound/surgery, but would usually include:

- Wound assessment
- Assessment of infection
- Assessment of circulation
- Pain assessment (which may address phantom limb pain)
- Health promotion activities

Wound assessment

For closed surgical wounds a simple assessment chart that records the presence of erythema, exudate, oedema and the presence of haematoma is sufficient. Additional categories found in many comprehensive wound assessment tools, such as the size of the wound and percentage of tissue type present, are not necessary and render the chart long and not user friendly. The example shown in Table 6.4 illustrates a chart suitable for closed wounds healing in a straightforward way. Should complications such as infection or dehiscence occur a more comprehensive wound assessment chart would be needed.

Patient details: Site of wound: Type of closure: Sutures yes / no How many? .... Clips yes / no: How many? .... Paper strips yes / no: How many?			
Date			
Exudate Heavy/moderate/light Clear/blood stained Watery/mixed/thick			
Erythema of surrounding skin Around stitches only Extending beyond stitches			
Oedema None/minimal/moderate/severe			
Haematoma Severe/moderate/none			
Pain at wound site Yes/no			
Frequency of pain Continuous/intermittent/procedural			
Pain score 0–10			
Odour None/normal/unusual			
Infection Suspected/swab sent			
Signature			

Table 6.4
Assessment of closed surgical wounds

If the wound is open, either because it has been left to heal by secondary intention or has dehisced due to infection or other patient-related factors, a more detailed assessment will be required. There are a variety of assessment frameworks that can be used to assist in this process, e.g. the TIME framework which looks at tissue, infection/inflammation, moisture levels and epithelial edge advancement (Fletcher, 2005). More detailed measurement is required to determine wound progress or deterioration and a visual record of the wound is required; this can be a line drawing but a tracing or a photograph is preferable. Digitized tracing equipment is now available that allows easy tracking of changes in wound dimensions and tissue types (Gethin and Cowman, 2006).

Assessment of infection

By definition, surgical wounds are usually created in a clean environment so the risk of infection should be low, but this depends very much on the type of surgery. Costs associated with surgical site infection (SSI) are high for both the NHS and the patient, with increased length of stay and pain intensity reducing the quality of life for the patient. Surveillance of orthopaedic infections became compulsory in 2004 and infection rates for other specialities will follow (Donaldson and Mullally, 2003). Currently infection rates in orthopaedic implant patients are believed to be between 1 and 15 % depending on the data-collection method used (Reilly *et al.*, 2005). Data collected on inpatients does not always reflect the true infection rate, as with faster discharge many patients do not develop the signs and symptoms of infection until after they are discharged. Reilly *et al.* (2005) studied infection rates post-discharge and identified a higher rate of infection post-discharge than as an inpatient. Therefore, it is important that good wound assessment is continued into the community setting and where possible patients' assessments charts transferred with them to allow the community team to highlight changes quickly. Identification of real rates of infection which include those identified post-discharge has advantages for both patients and staff. A post-discharge surveillance study across all surgical specialities with feedback to ward staff and surgeons was able to demonstrate cost savings of between £347 and £491 by producing a significant reduction in the rates of infection within four years (Wilson *et al.*, 2006).

The risk of wound infection is increased by many different factors, e.g. pre-operative hair removal or the type of marker pen used to mark the skin. Tanner *et al.* (2006) completed a systematic review of the literature on hair removal and concluded that there was no difference in surgical site infection rates between those patients who had hair removal and those that did not. They suggest that if hair removal is required, e.g. to give better access to the site or reduce trauma on dressing change, then both clipping and depilatory cream give better results than using a razor. Wilson and Tate (2006) suggest that there is a theoretical risk of cross-infection of methicillin-resistant *Staphylococcus aureus* (MRSA) from the use of skin markers, with one type of pen producing MRSA cultures for up to three weeks. Increased length of pre-operative stay in hospital also increases the rate of infection (Cruse and Foord, 1973) and the patient's ability to fight infection is crucial, so their general health and any medication they are taking should be considered. The material used for wound closure also affects the risk of infection, with wounds closed by tapes having the greatest resistance to infection as the material does not pass through the skin; stapled wounds have a lower rate of infection than sutured (Gotrup, 1999). Individual patient-related factors, as in the initial case study, where the patient removed the dressing and touched the wound, also increase the risk of infection considerably.

The most widely recognized definition of SSI splits infection into three groups: superficial, deep and organ space (Horan *et al.*, 1992). The straightforward signs and symptoms of heat, redness, pain and immobility do not always manifest, particularly in patients with other disease processes or on drug therapy that may mask these signs. Therefore, additional more subtle criteria for identifying wound infection have been suggested (Cutting *et al.*, 2005):

- Delayed healing (compared with the normal rate for site/condition)
- Discoloration
- Friable granulation tissue that bleeds easily
- Unexpected pain/tenderness
- Pocketing at the base of the wound
- Bridging of epithelium or soft tissue
- Abnormal smell
- Wound breakdown

Melling *et al.* (2005) suggest some basic recommendations for the early recognition of SSI. These cover general issues and practice points (see Table 6.5).

General Issues	Practice points
It is important to recognize when the normal inflammatory process becomes abnormal and when this is due to infection	Any redness/inflammation around the wound lasting several days should be a cause for concern, particularly if the inflamed skin is warmer than the surrounding area and painful to touch
The level of suspicion should be raised if more than one indicator of infection is present	Pain that begins or increases around the wound area in conjunction with other signs of Inflammation/erythema several days after surgery is of concern
The presence of pus in whatever form is an immediate indicator of infection, although this may be difficult to identify	Any discharge from the wound 48 hours after surgery requires further investigation. Offensive smelling discharge is a clearer indication of infection. Discharge due to infection is most common around 5–10 days post surgery
When wounds simply fail to heal or where there are disturbances to the normal healing process further investigation is required	Reasons other than infection for disturbances in the wound healing process should be excluded prior to a diagnosis of infection (e.g. poor suturing, etc.)
To define infection use validated tools (e.g. Centres for Disease Control and Prevention definition)	Consistent application of a scoring system is required

Table 6.5
Early recognition of surgical site infection

Assessment of circulation

Assessment of peripheral circulation should continue post-operatively and simple test, such as capillary refill time, should be performed to the digits to determine the level of capillary perfusion. If the patient has a good cardiac output and digital perfusion the refill time should be less than 3 seconds, a refill time of more than 5 seconds is considered abnormal and indicative of poor peripheral perfusion (Stubbing and Chesworth, 2001).

Pain assessment

According to the Commission on the Provision of Surgical Services (1990) failure to relieve pain is morally and ethically unacceptable. A thorough pain assessment should be carried out to determine the type, nature and intensity of the pain:

- Type of Pain. The type of pain is usually described as continuous, intermittent or procedural.
- Nature of pain. This describes the characteristics of the pain, whether it is sharp and stabbing, dull, aching, etc. This description can sometimes help to determine the cause of the pain.
- Intensity of pain. There are a variety of scales used for assessing intensity, including numerical and verbal scales, visual scales and pain diaries, where a continuous pain rating is required.

Unresolved pain negatively affects wound healing and quality of life. The World Union of Wound Healing Societies (WUWHS) (2004) consensus document on pain suggests that practitioners:

- Assume that all wounds are painful.
- Over time wounds may become more painful.
- Accept that the skin surrounding the wound can become sensitive and painful.
- Accept that for some patients the lightest touch or simply moving air across the wound can be excruciatingly painful.
- Know when to refer for specialist assessment.

Patients who have undergone amputation may also experience phantom limb pain. Edwards and Wallbridge (2002) suggest that almost all (55–85 %) amputees will experience these sensations, usually within a few days of surgery, although it may be later. This pain is very real and should be treated appropriately; patients will often describe it as shooting, burning, throbbing or stabbing in nature and located in the distal part of the missing limb. Phantom pain should be distinguished from stump pain and other less common causes of pain such as osteomyelitis, ischaemia and bony spurs.

6.5 | Health Promotion Activities

In order to achieve the best healing outcome and prevent recurrence of the disease it is important to address the risk factors that may have led the patient to require surgery in the first place. Many of the changes required of these patients reflect *The Health of the Nation* (Department of Health, 1992) targets for coronary heart disease/strokes/blood pressure, diet, nutrition and smoking and so are very familiar to most patients as they have been widely discussed in the national news and media.

This does not mean that they are easy to achieve. For most patients they are being asked to make considerable modifications to their lifestyle and many will need professional help and guidance to do this. The role of the multiprofessional team cannot be overemphasized in supporting patients at this stressful time. It cannot be assumed that an increase in knowledge will result in a change in lifestyle; behavioural change is also influenced by personal, psychological and social variables. Timing of information giving and provision of support are crucial in affecting change. It must also be acknowledged that not all risk factors can be reduced or removed. Ockenden (2001) suggests that there are risk factors which are modifiable and those which are not (see table 6.6 below).

6.6 | Wound Management

Wounds closed by primary intention are generally believed not to require covering after 48 hours, the role of the primary dressing being primarily to stem bleeding and provide mechanical and bacterial protection for the newly formed tissues (Aindow and Butcher, 2005). These wounds are frequently dressed with fabric-based self-adhesive post-operative dressings, which have several disadvantages:

- They are not transparent and therefore the wound cannot be assessed without removing the dressing.
- Although they form an effective bacterial barrier when dry, once they come into contact with fluid a moist pathway for transmission of bacteria into or out of the wound is set up.
- They have limited capacity to stretch when *in situ*. This can lead to blistering if there is localized oedema around the wound.

Modifiable risk factors	Nonmodifiable risk factors
Cigarette smoking	Age
Low-density lipoprotein cholesterol	Gender
Physical inactivity	Family history
Obesity	
Diabetes mellitus	
Hypertension	
Homocysteine (raised levels)	
Thrombogenic factors	

Table 6.6
Modifiable and nonmodifiable risks for the development of atherosclerosis

The products that appear to give the best management of surgical wounds are those that combine a film backing (which is stretchy, flexible and waterproof) with a central fabric pad that will absorb the minimal amount of exudate expected from a healing surgical wound. Although the pad obscures the wound, the film allows visualization of the peri-wound area so that redness, etc., can quickly be observed (Aindow and Butcher, 2005).

Wounds healing by secondary intention, such as those in the case study, should be managed according to the presenting symptoms, e.g. high level of exudate, malodour and necrotic tissue. A systematic review of dressings and topical agents for surgical wounds healing by secondary intention (Vermeulen *et al.*, 2005) suggests that there is little strong evidence to support the choice of any one dressing over another. They suggest, however, that foam is preferable to gauze in terms of pain control, patient satisfaction and reduction in nursing time. It would appear that there is, however, sufficient evidence to support the use of modern wound dressings that maintain a moist environment over the use of gauze (Jones, 2006).

6.7 | Complications of Surgery

Deep vein thrombosis (DVT) is an eminently preventable complication of surgery. Simple interventions, such as regular physical activity and elevation of the legs without calf compression, will reduce the risks of DVT, particularly in combination with correctly fitting compression hosiery (Vowden and Vowden, 1997). For patients who have had lower limb surgery, undertaking these preventative activities may appear daunting and some may believe that it may increase the level of pain experienced; therefore appropriate support and education is required.

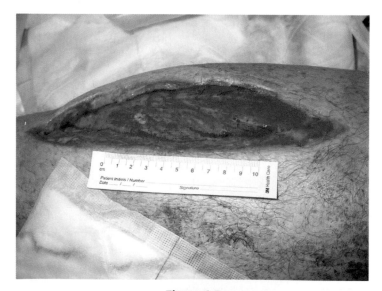

Figure 6.5
Fasciotomy wound

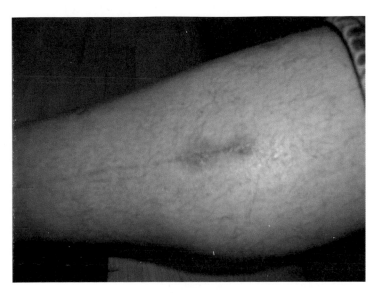

Figure 6.6
Calf wound six months post-operation

6.7.1 | Compartment Syndrome

Compartment syndrome is a very serious complication of acute limb ischaemia. There may be excessive swelling within the fascia, putting extreme pressure on the muscle, bone, nerves, arteries and veins. Urgent surgical intervention is necessary and the patient will require a fasciotomy (opening of the fascial compartment with incisions to both sides of the calf; see Figure 6.5). Patients may require skin grafting following fasciotomy if the wound edges cannot be apposed.

Careful monitoring of calf measurement, sensation and pedal pulses is necessary to avoid missing this condition (Herbert, 1997). Figure 6.6 shows that a calf wound six months post-surgery is still inflamed and painful.

6.8 | Case Scenario Revisited

Consider the initial questions posed:

1. **What particular factors may need to be considered in Raymond's post-operative care? Consider especially the need to keep pressure off the area and also the need to prevent infection.**
   Because of Raymond's learning difficulties he has difficulty processing and retaining information. Therefore, he will need close supervision and constant reminding of what is expected of him. It is worth talking to his carers from the home to find out how they help

him to deal with information. The footwear has been a particular problem in exacerbating the damage and a way of managing this to prevent further pressure damage needs to be considered, remembering that there will be additional bulk from the dressing on his foot. In terms of preventing infection, again referring back to the history from the care staff, Raymond frequently removed dressings that they applied so care will need to be taken to find either a dressing that is difficult to tamper with (e.g. putting additional layers of bandaging in place but remembering the potential for extra bulk in the footwear) or to find ways of minimizing cross-infection.

2. **When selecting dressings for this wound what would be the main objectives of treatment?**

   The long-term objective is to encourage the wound to heal without complications. Short-term objectives would include prevention of infection, management of exudate, management of any pain and prevention of additional pressure. Broader objectives would include management of the underlying problem, gout and a focus on patient education to perhaps include working with the care staff and his parents to give them a better understanding of the problem so that should this occur again he would be referred earlier for treatment.

3. **Why was this wound not suitable for primary closure?**

   The amount of tissue removed meant that it was not possible to appose the skin edges without causing undue tension. Additionally, the wound was still exuding the uric crystals and these needed a point of free egress from the wound.

4. **What factors may delay healing in this wound?**

   The main factor that may cause a problem is Raymond removing the dressings. This renders him vulnerable to infection. He has no other underlying medical problems that may delay healing and as he is very mobile he is encouraging blood flow to the area.

6.9 | Conclusion

There are a huge variety of surgical wounds that may be regularly seen on the lower limb. These can heal by primary or secondary intention. The healing trajectory of these wounds relates greatly to the underlying cause or disease that gave rise to the surgery in the first instance. Infection (SSI) is a major problem in many of these wounds, which may be poorly vascularized and oxygenated. Therefore, every precaution must be taken both pre- and post-operatively to prevent this occurring. As with all surgical wounds, controlling pain is an important consideration both in terms of patient comfort but also in encouraging patients to return to activity that may be helpful in preventing complications such as deep vein thrombosis. An understanding of the underlying disease process is essential in planning appropriate patient focused post-operative care.

Reflection

Take time to reflect upon your learning from this chapter. Ask yourself:

1. **What knowledge did I possess prior to reading this chapter?**

2. **How has my knowledge developed?**

References

Aindow, D. and Butcher, M. (2005) Films or fabric: is it time to re-appraise postoperative dressings? *British Journal of Nursing*, **14**(19), Suppl., S15–S20.

Berceli, S.A., Brown, J.E., Irwin, P.B. and Ozaki, C.K. (2006) Clinical outcomes after closed, staged and open forefoot amputations. *Journal of Vascular Surgery*, **44**(2), 347–51.

Chung, J., Bartelson, B.B., Hiatt, W.R. *et al.* (2006) Wound healing and functional outcomes after infrainguinal bypass with reversed saphenous vein for critical limb ischemia. *Journal of Vascular Surgery*, **43**(6), 1183–90.

Commission on the Provision of Surgical Services (1990). *Report of the Working Party on Pain after Surgery*, Royal College of Surgeons of England and The College Anaesthetists, London.

Cruse, P.J.E. and Foord, R. (1973) A five-year prospective study of 23,649 surgical wounds. *Archives of Surgery*, **107**, 206–10.

Cutting, K., White, R.J., Maloney, P. and Harding, K.G. (2005) Clinical identification of wound infection: a Delphi approach, in *Identifying Criteria for Wound Infection*, European Wound Management Association Position Document, MEP Ltd, London.

Department of Health (1992) *The Health of the Nation: A Strategy for Health in England*, Department of Health, London.

Donaldson, L. and Mullally, S. (2003) *Surveillance of Healthcare Associated Infections*, Department of Health, London.

Dormandy, J.A. and Rutherford, R.B. (2000) Management of peripheral arterial disease (PAD). TASC Working Group. TransAtlantic Inter-society Consensus (TASC). *Journal of Vascular Surgery*, **31** (1, pt 2), S1–S296.

Dowsett, C. (2002) The management of surgical wounds in a community setting. *Wound Care*, **June**, 33–8.

Edwards, N. and Wallbridge, A. (2002) The chronic pain clinic, in *Pathways of Care in Vascular Surgery* (eds J.D. Beard and S. Murray), Tfm Publishing Limited, Shrewsbury.

Fletcher, J. (2005) Wound bed preparation and the TIME principals. *Nursing Standard*, **20**(12), 57–65.

Frykberg, E.R. (2005) http://www.trauma.org/vascular/vascskeletal.html.

Gethin, G. and Cowman, S. (2006) Wound measurement comparing the use of acetate tracings and Visitrak digital planimetry. *Journal of Clinical Nursing*, **15**(4), 422–7.

Gottrup, F. (1999) Wound closure techniques. *Journal of Wound Care*, **8**(8), 397–400.

Harker, J. (2006) Wound healing complications associated with lower limb amputation, available at: http://www.worldwidewounds.com/2006/september/Harker/Wound-Healing-Complications-Limb-Amputation.html, Last accessed 14 November 2006.

Harrison, M. (2006) Discussion on wound care in the 21st century. *British Journal of Nursing*, **15**(19) Suppl., S12–S16.

Herbert, L. (1997) *Caring for the Vascular Patient*, Churchill Livingstone, Edinburgh.

Hirsch, A.T., Haskal, Z.J., Hertzer, N.R. *et al.* (2005) *Practice Guidelines for the Management of Patients with Peripheral Arterial Disease (Lower Extremity, Renal, Mesenteric, and Abdominal Aortic)*, A Collaborative Report from the American Association for Vascular Surgery/Society for Vascular Surgery,* Society for Cardiovascular Angiography and Interventions, Society for Vascular Medicine and Biology, Society of Interventional Radiology, and the ACC/AHA Task Force on Practice Guidelines (Writing Committee to Develop Guidelines for the Management of Patients with Peripheral Arterial Disease): Endorsed by the American Association of Cardiovascular and Pulmonary Rehabilitation, National Heart, Lung, and Blood Institute, Society for Vascular Nursing, TransAtlantic Inter-Society Consensus and Vascular Disease Foundation. *Circulation*, March 2006, **113**, e463–e654, Available at: http://circ.ahajournals.org/cgi/reprint/113/11/e463?maxtoshow=&HITS=10&hits=10&RESULTFORMAT=&fulltext=vascular+guidelines&searchid=1&FIRSTINDEX=0&resourcetype=HWCIT, Last accessed 14 November 2006.

Horan, T.C., Gaynes, R.P., Martone, W.J. *et al.* (1992) CDC definitions of nosocomial surgical site infections 1992. A modification of CDC definitions of surgical wound infections. *Infection Control and Hospital Epidemiology*, **13**, 606–8.

Hospital Episode Statistics (HES) (2006) Main operations summary 2004/2005, available at: http://www.hesonline.nhs.uk/Ease/servlet/AttachmentRetriever?site_id=1937&file_name=d:\efmfiles\1937\Accessing\DataTables\Operations\summary\MainOps.pdf&short_name=MainOps.pdf&u_id=5710, Last accessed 14 November 2006.

Jones, V.J. (2006) The use of gauze: will it ever change? *International Wound Journal*, **3**(2), 79–86.

Kennedy, P.J., Young, W.M., Deva, A.K. and Haertsch, P.A. (2006) Burns and amputations: a 24 year experience. *Journal of Burn Care Research*, **27**, 183–8.

Leng, G.C., Davis, M. and Baker, D. (2000) Bypass surgery for chronic lower limb ischaemia (Cochrane Review). *The Cochrane Database of Systematic Reviews*, Issue 3, Article No. CD002000, DOI:10.1002/14651858.CD002000.

Melling, A., Hollander, D.A. and Gottrup, F. (2005) Identifying surgical site infection in wounds healing by primary intention, in *Identifying Criteria for Wound Infection*, European Wound Management Association Position Document, MEP Ltd, London.

National Amputee Statistical Database (NASDAB) (2005) *National Amputee Statistical Database Annual Report 2004/2005*. NASDAB, Edinburgh, Available from URL: http://www.nasdab.co.uk, Last accessed 14 November 2006.

Ockenden, L.J. (2001) Aetiology and pathology of vascular disease, in *Vascular Disease. Nursing and Management* (ed. S. Murray), Whurr Publishers, London.

Parrett, B.M., Pomahac, B., Demling, R.H. and Orgill, D.P. (2006) Fourth degree burns to the lower extremity with exposed tendon and bone: a ten year experience. *Journal of Burn Care Research*, **27**(1) 34–9.

Potterton, J.A. and Galland, R.B. (2002) Lower limb amputation and rehabilitation, in *Pathways of Care in Vascular Surgery* (eds J.D. Beard and S. Murray), Tfm Publishing Limited, Shrewsbury.

Reilly, J., Noone, A., Clift, A., Cochrane, L., Johnston, L., Rowley, D.I., Philips, G. and Sullivan, F. (2005) A study of telephone screening and direct observation of surgical wound infections after discharge from hospital. *Journal of Bone and Joint Surgery (British)*, **87-B**, 997–9.

Rybarczyk, B., Edwards, R. and Behel, J. (2004) Diversity in adjustment to a leg amputation: case illustrations of common themes. *Disability Rehabilitation*, **26**(14–15), 944–53.

Stubbing, N. and Chesworth, J. (2001) Assessment of patients with vascular disease, in *Vascular Disease. Nursing and Management* (ed. S. Murray), Whurr Publishers, London.

Tanner, J., Woodings, D. and Moncaster, K. (2006) Preoperative hair removal to reduce surgical site infection. *Cochrane Database of Systematic Reviews*, 19 July 2006, Issue 3, CD004122.

UK Prosthetics Service (2005) *The Amputee Statistical Database for the United Kingdom Annual Report 2004/2005*, available at: http://www.nasdab.co.uk/pdf.pl?file=nasdab/news2004-05_annual_report.pdf. Last accessed 20 August 2007.

Vermeulen, H., Ubbink, D.T., Goosens, A., deVos, R. and Legemate, D.A. (2005) Systematic review of dressings and topical agents for surgical wounds healing by secondary intention. *British Journal of Surgery*, **92**, 665–72.

Vowden, K. and Vowden, P. (1997) Vascular assessment in compression therapy. *Professional Nurse*, April, **12**(7Suppl.), S3–S6.

Wilson, A.P.R., Hodgson, B., Lui, M., et al. (2006) Reduction in wound infection rates by wound surveillance with post discharge follow up and feedback. *British Journal of Surgery*, **93**, 620–38.

Wilson, J. and Tate, D. (2006) Can pre-operative skin marking transfer methicillin-resistant *Staphylococcus aureus* between patients? *Journal of Bone and Joint Surgery (British)*, **88-B**(4), 541–2.

World Union of Wound Healing Societies (2004) *Principles of Best Practice: Minimising Pain at Wound Dressing Related Procedures. A Consensus Document*, MEP Ltd, London, Downloadable from http://www.molnlycke.net//Files/Tendra/Paris/consensus%20final%20for%20press.pdf, Last accessed 14 November 2006.

Karen Ousey and Caroline McIntosh

Chapter 7

Pressure Ulcers

7.1 | Pressure Ulcers: An Introduction to the Problem

The prevention and management of pressure ulcers poses a significant challenge to health care providers. The economic implications for the National Health Service are considerable, with estimated costs amounting to £1.4–2.1 billion annually (Bennett *et al.*, 2004). This monetary figure does not, however, take into account the indirect costs to the patient living with a pressure ulcer in terms of pain experienced, anguish suffered and reduced quality of life. Health care professionals play a pivotal role in the prevention and management of pressure ulcers. The ability to detect those vulnerable to pressure ulcers is challenging for health care providers, but early identification of risk factors can prevent extensive tissue damage and adverse patient outcomes. Likewise, timely management based on best evidence can significantly improve the likelihood of wound healing.

This chapter will discuss the common causes of pressure ulcers; the prevention, assessment and management of pressure ulcers; the use of appropriate pressure redistributing devices; wound dressings; national guidelines; accountability issues; and the role of the multiprofessional team in pressure ulcer management. Emphasis will be placed on the care of lower extremity pressure ulcers, where nurses and podiatrists are most likely to be involved in the shared care of individuals at risk of or suffering from pressure ulceration.

7.2 | Case Scenario

Case Scenario 7

Consider the image and information provided for this case scenario. All information provided is based on a case seen in a secondary care setting.

Jack is a 62-year-old gentleman who was brought to the Accident and Emergency Department by paramedics, after being found by a stranger, passed out drunk on the street. Jack has no fixed abode and no family. He has been admitted to a medical ward following referral from the Accident and Emergency Department. On observation he is thin, frail and looks unkempt.

During the assessment it is noted that his clothes are in a dirty state and his footwear is ill-fitting. When he removes his shoes and socks there is an unpleasant odour arising from the right heel area and on examination a pressure ulcer is discovered (Figure 7.1). He states that his heel has been painful for the past ten days but he thought it would get better. He is not registered with a general practitioner and has limited access to health and social care services.

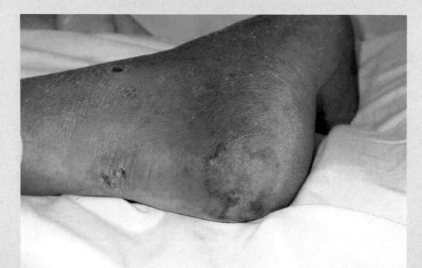

Figure 7.1
Pressure ulcer on the right heel (image reproduced with kind permission of Jacqui Fletcher)

What do I need to know?
Before continuing consider the following questions:

1. **What factors may have contributed to Jack's pressure ulcer?**

2. **What interventions could you now commence that would improve his general condition?**

3. **What are the causes of pressure ulcer development?**

4. **How can you prevent further deterioration of his skin?**

5. **Which members of the multiprofessional team need to be involved in his care?**

6. **Are there any national policies that you need to access to ensure his care will be evidence based?**

The information provided within the following sections should enable you to answer the six questions posed above. Answers will be considered towards the end of the chapter.

7.3 | National Policy Documents

There are a number of national policy documents in existence that aim to ensure practitioners can meet the benchmark standards in pressure ulcer care. For example, the National Institute for Health and Clinical Excellence (NICE) (2005) published clinical guidance on the management of pressure ulcers in primary and secondary care in England and Wales, while the Clinical Resource Efficiency Support Team (CREST) (1998) and the NHS Quality Improvement Scotland (NHS QIS) (2005a, 2005b) introduced guidelines and best practice statements for use in Northern Ireland and Scotland respectively (Beldon, 2006). In order to achieve optimum standards in pressure area care assessment and management, strategies must be underpinned by evidence from research. This chapter incorporates guidance from published national policy documents.

7.4 | Financial Cost of Pressure Ulcers

The financial costs associated with the treatment of pressure ulcers have become a concern for all involved, with Collier (1999) estimating the cost of treatment to be £40 000 for a grade IV pressure ulcer. More recently Bennett *et al.* (2004) described the cost to treat a pressure ulcer as ranging from £1064 to £10 551 depending upon its severity. The Department of Health (DH) (1992) recognized the significant costs of pressure ulcers and set targets to reduce the prevalence by between 5% and 10%, as detailed in *The Health of the Nation* document (1992). Yet Reid and Morison (1994) reviewed the literature pertaining to the prevalence of pressure ulcers and concluded the rate lay between 6% and 14%, while more recent reports claims this figure continues to be much higher than this; a prevalence of 21.9% was reported in the UK in 2001 (Clark *et al.*, 2004) and according to Bennett *et al.* (2004) approximately 412 000 individuals will develop a pressure ulcer annually in the UK. Therefore, the need for education for all professionals involved in pressure area care and the ability to utilize the available resources in an effective and efficient manner remains central in any plan to achieve optimum patient outcomes.

7.5 | Pressure Damage

Pressure damage may be referred to as a "bed sore", "pressure sore", "decubitus ulcer" and "pressure ulcer", all of which refer to the same problem encountered by many patients and are all caused by the same common denominator, that of sustained pressure (Farley, 2002). Courtenay (2002) defined a pressure ulcer as an area of damage caused by prolonged or excessive soft tissue pressure. Furthermore, the European Pressure Ulcer Advisory Panel (EPUAP) (1999) defined a pressure ulcer as an area of localized damage to the skin and underlying tissue caused by pressure, shear or friction, or a combination of these.

7.5.1 | Causes of Pressure Ulcers

Pressure, shear and friction, as illustrated in Figure 7.2, are major contributory factors that lead to skin damage. It is pertinent therefore to define the three common causative factors in pressure ulcer development.

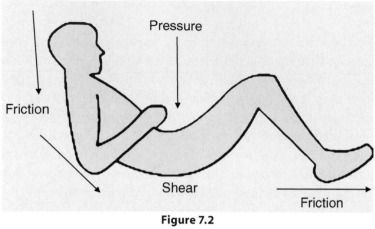

Figure 7.2
Causes of pressure ulcers

Pressure

Pressure can be described as a force exerted perpendicularly to the tissue. Pressure ulcers often develop as a result of external pressure, which in turn results in an occlusion of blood vessels and endothelial damage to the arterioles and microcirculation. Prolonged pressure on an area of tissue can cause ulceration or can delay wound healing in an already established ulcer for a number of reasons. Wysocki (1999) suggests pressure ulcers are pressure-induced ischaemic–reperfusion injuries. Prolonged pressure causes a reduced perfusion to the skin; when the pressure is released reperfusion occurs, causing an ischaemic–reperfusion injury. It is thought that hypoxia (lack of oxygen) associated with ischaemia triggers a cascade of events that results in loss of cell membrane integrity and apoptosis (cell death) and ultimately tissue necrosis.

Shear

Shear is a force exerted parallel to the tissue. According to Flanagan and Fletcher (2003), shear is an internal force caused when adjacent surfaces slide across each other, resulting in twisting and tearing of the underlying blood vessels, and leads to tissue ischemia and localized tissue death.

Friction

Friction is the force caused when two touching surfaces move in opposite directions and may result in superficial scuffing or abrasion of the skin (Flanagan and Fletcher, 2003). Friction can also result in superficial damage through the stripping of the epidermis and may be exacerbated by the presence of moisture, increasing the probability of pressure ulcer development when accompanied by pressure and/or shearing forces (Dealey, 1997; Defloor, 1999).

The combination of shear and friction is particularly damaging to the integrity of skin. It is therefore important that when moving and handling individuals they are not "dragged" along a surface. All members of the multiprofessional team must be educated and trained in correct moving and handling techniques and employ these on every occasion. The use of appropriate aids to move and handle an individual must be used. If they are unavailable then the manager of the health care setting must be made aware of this.

7.5.2 | Risk Areas for Pressure Ulcer Development

As external pressure is a major causative factor of pressure damage it follows that areas of skin where pressure is sustained over bony prominences are at greatest risk of tissue breakdown. Figure 7.3 highlights anatomical sites vulnerable to pressure damage. In the lower limb the heel is a vulnerable site for pressure damage as there is little subcutaneous tissue to protect the underlying bone, as seen in Jack's case.

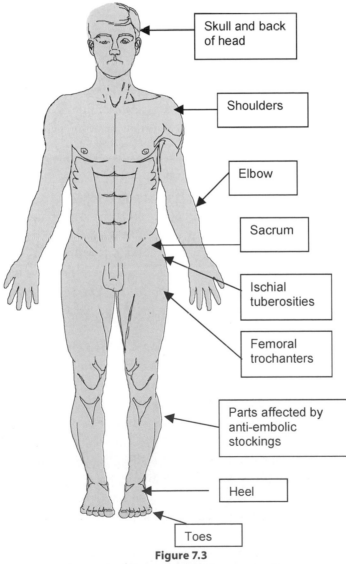

Figure 7.3
Anatomical sites vulnerable to pressure ulcers

In the lower extremities, ill-fitting footwear or foot deformities resulting in high pressures during gait should be considered as a potential causative factor leading to skin damage due to prolonged or sustained pressure, friction and shearing forces. Individuals who are considered to be at greater risk of pressure damage, e.g. people with diabetes, should be instructed on the importance of wearing correctly fitting footwear. If foot deformities exist and/or there is damage to the foot or heel then referral to, and involvement of, podiatrists and orthotists is vital.

7.5.3 | Other Factors Affecting Pressure Ulcer Development

A number of other factors can contribute to pressure ulcer development and should be explored as part of a comprehensive assessment.

Mobility/immobility

Reduced mobility is a major factor in pressure ulcer development. An immobile patient is unable to move their own position or weight sufficiently enough to relieve pressure. This must be taken into account when positioning individuals who spend substantial amounts of time in a chair or wheelchair, ensuring that their feet are fully supported to prevent pressure ulcers developing.

Malnutrition

The European Pressure Ulcer Advisory Panel's (EPUAP) (2006) *Nutritional Guidelines for Pressure Ulcer Prevention and Treatment* recommends that recording the patient's weight should follow a specified protocol, where the individual is weighed ideally at the same time of day using the same scales with an appropriate weight range (up to 350 kg). Before weighing the patient any outdoor clothes and shoes should be removed. If possible, all weight measurements should be made by a single recorder. In addition to weight measurement, waist circumference is a reliable marker for intra-abdominal fat mass. The waist measurement should be carried out at a specific location halfway between the superior iliac crest and the rib cage, in the mid-axillary line.

Nutritional assessment may also include nutritional intake over the past one, three or seven days; this information may be gathered using a 24 hour recall, self or carer reported food intake records or through the involvement of a dietician, where available. It is important to consider why the intake of food and fluids is at the reported level. It may be pertinent to explore the patient's ability to shop for food and prepare meals, as well as enquiring regarding any available assistance, particularly for elderly patients.

The patient's nutritional intake and requirements should be assessed using a recognized nutritional screening tool (British Association for Parental and Enteral Nutrition, 2005). The chosen tool will largely depend upon local policy and guidelines. Patients suffering from nutritional deficit will require referral to a dietician as soon as possible following admission.

Biochemical measurements such as serum albumin, haemoglobin and potassium may be helpful when considering nutritional status, although these indicators may provide more information on chronic rather than acute depletion of specific nutrients. In general, it is unlikely that biochemical measurements will provide more information than other indicators such as undesired weight loss.

? **As Jack has no fixed abode and limited access to health and social care there are a number of issues to address. Jack has no means of preparing food and has limited finances, so as a result he often chooses to substitute alcohol for food. He also experiences difficulty chewing food as a result of ill-fitting dentures and regularly suffers from painful mouth ulcers.**

1. **What can be done to overcome these issues?**

2. **Which professionals should be involved in Jack's care?**

Medical history

It Is essential that health professionals involved in pressure ulcer care undertake a comprehensive medical history. Numerous factors can increase the likelihood of pressure ulcer occurrence and can impact negatively on the healing process in the presence of active ulceration, some of which are explored below.

Sensory impairment

Patients with sensory impairment will be vulnerable to localized pressure. Certain illnesses and conditions, such as diabetes mellitus, stroke and spinal cord injury, can result in sensory neuropathy (loss of sensation). Individuals who have lost protective pain sensation are unable to feel tissue damage caused from pressure, shear and friction, which can result in episodes of unnoticed trauma/ulceration. Preventative strategies to protect the skin must be implemented. This includes educating the patient on suitable clothing and footwear and changing their position at regular intervals to prevent skin damage.

Diabetes mellitus is a significant risk factor for ulceration in the lower limb. Individuals with diabetes are at an increased risk of sensory neuropathy, a reduced blood supply to the lower limb due to peripheral vascular disease, and are at a greater risk of infection (please refer to Chapter 8). Therefore, any breach in skin integrity from pressure damage can rapidly ulcerate.

Practitioners should be aware that a foot ulcer in a diabetic patient can have devastating outcomes. The Amputee Statistical Database (2005) reports that amputations due to the chronic complications of diabetes accounted for 42% of all lower limb amputations in the UK in 2004–2005. In order to prevent such devastating outcomes the diabetic foot should be inspected regularly for early signs of pressure damage. If early signs of pressure damage are observed strategies should be implemented immediately to minimize pressure and prevent tissue breakdown. Nurses and podiatrists must collaborate to improve standards of care for patients with diabetes who develop pressure ulcers on the lower limb to ensure rapid assessment of neurological, vascular status and foot function. When a pressure ulcer is present on the diabetic foot rapid management strategies, based on best-practice guidelines in diabetes, should be initiated (see Chapter 8).

Peripheral vascular disease

Tissue viability bears a direct correlation to the vascular status of the individual. In the presence of peripheral vascular disease characteristic skin changes will be apparent (see Chapter 3) and ulceration risk is increased.

Whenever an individual presents with a pressure ulcer on the lower limb it is imperative a vascular assessment is undertaken. This will:

- Provide a useful baseline measurement to monitor any future deterioration
- Allow an informed judgement on a likely prognosis for wound healing
- Identify individuals who require referral for further vascular assessment and revascularization

It is important to investigate symptoms associated with arterial disease such as intermittent claudication (pain in the calf or instep when walking), indicative of significant peripheral arterial disease; and ischaemic rest pain (severe pain in the lower limbs at rest), indicative of critical limb ischaemia.

Pulse palpation should be one of the first aspects of a vascular assessment. There are two pulses in the foot that are commonly assessed: dorsalis pedis and posterior tibial pulses. However pulse palpation is not always accurate; e.g. if the limb is oedematous it can be difficult to palpate pulses due to excess fluid. Doppler ultrasound is the most commonly used modality to investigate vascular status in the lower limbs (Vowden, 1999). Doppler examination allows the practitioner to listen to arterial sounds and make a judgement on vascular status by listening to the strength, pitch and phasicity of the pulse; this is particularly beneficial in identifying arterial impairment in patients with necrotic heel ulcers. The ankle brachial pressure index is a further clinical adjunct allowing practitioners to make a more objective measure of vascular status. This involves measuring brachial (arm) systolic pressure and comparing this to ankle systolic pressure to arrive at a ratio (Marshall, 2004). The results of the ratio allow practitioners to establish vascular status and the likelihood of wound healing.

Medication

Certain medication can increase the risk of pressure ulcer formation and/or delayed wound healing. Medication, such as corticosteroids, nonsteroidal anti-inflammatory drugs (NSAIDs) and disease-modifying antirheumatic drugs (DMARDs), can considerably impact on infection rates due to their effect on the immune system (Cooper, 2005). Additionally, drugs such as antiplatelets and anticoagulants can disrupt the clotting cascade, thus disrupting the normal physiology of wound healing. It is essential therefore that a comprehensive patient assessment includes details of current and past prescribed and nonprescribed drugs.

It is apparent that numerous factors can increase the risk of pressure ulcer development. Therefore, the aetiology of pressure ulcers is often multifactorial, requiring multifaceted patient assessment. This is essential to identify potential factors that either increase the risk of pressure damage or may delay wound healing when pressure damage has occurred.

> **Are there any other factors in the case provided that may affect the integrity of Jack's skin?**

7.6 | Preventing Pressure Ulcer Development

Various national policy documents have been developed over a number of years that attempt to reduce the incidence of pressure ulcer development (CREST, 1998; NICE, 2005; NHS QIS, 2005a). These guidelines offer evidence-based recommendations to members of the multiprofessional team for the implementation of preventative strategies. It is essential that all members of the multiprofessional team understand and implement preventative strategies for pressure ulcer formation working together in partnership. NICE (2005) has identified the importance of involving patients, carers and the multiprofessional team in the prevention of pressure ulcers.

Patients and carers should be made aware of the NICE (2005) recommendations and be referred to the version *Information for the Public*. This will encourage patient and carer involvement in shared decision making about the management of pressure ulcers. Additionally, health professionals are advised to respect and incorporate the knowledge and experience of people who have had, or have, a pressure ulcer.

The approach to care should be multiprofessional, involving all those needed in the management of pressure ulcers. Collier (2002) identifies the principles of pressure ulcer development as exemplified in Table 7.1.

7.6.1 | Education

Health promotion and health education are important aspects of the care-giving process. It is vital that patients and their carers are actively involved in the prevention and treatment of pressure ulcers to allow them empowerment and to promote a patient-centred approach to care. Florian and Elad (1998) explain that empowerment assists the individual to develop proactive healthy behaviours for themselves, while Walker (1998) argues that empowerment is a process through which a nurse and client work together to change unhealthy behaviours.

- Assess individual for risk factors

- Ensure regular changes of position and assess each patient on an individual basis

- Maintain skin cleanliness and hygiene

- Prevent mechanical, physical and chemical injury

- Ensure adequate nutrition and hydration

- Promote control of continence

- Ensure good body alignment and positioning

- Use appropriate pressure redistributing systems

- Inspect the skin for any changes at regular intervals

- Promote mental alertness and orientation

- Educate all professionals and carers involved in the patient's skin care routine

Table 7.1
Principles of preventing pressure ulcer development (adapted from Collier, 2002)

7.6.2 | Cultural Issues

The United Kingdom is a multicultural nation and as such the multiprofessional team must understand the varying cultural needs of the population. It may be necessary to employ the skills of an interpreter to convey information. It is worth remembering that relatives may not be the most appropriate people to interpret as they may not understand fully what is being explained. Writing down information will also assist the patient in understanding. However, if written information is provided it should be ensured that literacy skills are of a sufficient standard to enable them to understand.

Included in cultural issues will be the religious beliefs of patients. Certain religions will not allow the patient to eat various foodstuffs and as such dietary requirements need to be established and arrangements made for the patient to achieve the optimal nutrients for their diet to assist in pressure ulcer healing. Similarly, certain religions will undertake periods of fasting and arrangements will need to be in place to ensure that meals are available when the patient is eating. Additionally, it is imperative that practitioners respect religious and cultural preferences to receiving treatment from a member of the opposite gender, particularly when the need arises to expose the lower limbs.

7.7 | Risk Assessment

Risk assessment tools are used to help identify patients who are at risk of developing pressure damage. Nixon and McGough (2001) identified at least 38 alternative risk assessment scales that had been described in the literature, and most of those exist in several variants. All these tools are relatively easy to use but must be accompanied by the relevant training to ensure that practitioners understand the correct assessment technique. Nixon and McGough (2001) warn that there is no evidence that risk assessment scales are better than nurses' clinical judgement in identifying patients at risk and that the predictive value of the risk assessment scales is questionable.

Risk assessment tools developed over the past few decades include:

- Norton Risk Assessment (Norton *et al.*, 1975)
- Waterlow Risk Assessment (Waterlow, 2005)
- Gosnell Risk Assessment (Gosnell, 1973)
- Pressure Sore Prediction Score (Lowthian, 1989)
- Braden Scale (Braden and Bergstrom, 1987)

Risk assessment tools are useful as an aide-memoire and do not replace clinical judgement. The tool used should be in line with local policy. The National Institute for Clinical Excellence (NICE) (2005) recommends that a pressure ulcer risk assessment should be completed within six hours of admission to hospital. In the community setting assessment should be undertaken by the community nurse at the first visit or by the district/practice nurse.

> **As Jack spent four hours in Accident and Emergency ideally his risk assessment should occur within two hours following admission on to the medical ward.**

7.8 | Grading Systems

Once a pressure ulcer has developed it is important to grade its severity. Currently there is no one accepted method of assessing pressure ulcers universally, yet it is important that a grading system is used to promote communication between the multiprofessional team when planning and implementing care interventions. The European Pressure Ulcer advisory Panel (EPUAP) (Table 7.2) classification tool is the choice of the Royal College of Nursing (RCN) (2005) and NICE (2005), as it identifies not only the skin colour change of grade 1 pressure ulcers but also other physiological signs resulting from tissue damage that many other tools ignore, namely the changes in skin temperature and skin texture due to the inflammation process. The classification system is about what the skin/tissue looks like and is not related to patient group/environment/context. These items are part of pressure ulcer risk assessment tools (NICE, 2005; RCN, 2005).

Grade 1	Nonblanching erythema (redness of the tissues that does not blanch (turn white) when pressed) of intact skin, the heralding lesion of skin ulceration
Grade II	Partial thickness skin loss involving epidermis and/or dermis. The ulcer is superficial and presents clinically as an abrasion, blister or shallow crater
Grade III	Full thickness skin loss involving damage or necrosis of subcutaneous tissue that may extend down to, but not through, underlying fascia. The ulcer presents clinically as a deep crater with or without undermining of adjoining tissue
Grade IV	Full thickness skin loss with extensive destruction, tissue necrosis or damage to muscle, bone or supporting structures. Undermining and sinus tracts may be associated with stage IV pressure ulcers

Table 7.2
EPUAP grading system

 Using the EPUAP grading system, what grade is Jack's ulcer?

It is important to recognize that pressure ulcer grading cannot be used in reverse as the ulcer heals. The National Pressure Ulcer Advisory Panel (1998) states this is impossible as the healing wound does not exhibit re-growth of subcutaneous tissue, muscle and fascia; the healing cavity wound produces granulation tissue which eventually becomes scar tissue once the ulcer has healed.

Other, less commonly used, grading systems include:

- Stirling Pressure Sore Severity Scale (Reid and Morison, 1994)
- Torrance Grading System (Torrance, 1983)

The grading system chosen will depend upon local policy. However, it is worth remembering that there are a number of assessment scales available and a patient may be admitted from a unit that uses a different scale. If this should occur it is important that the grade of the ulcer is documented using the scale recommended in the health care setting where the patient is being cared for. No grading system is 100% reliable but they do allow for professionals to assess an ulcer using a predefined set of guidelines. It is worthy to mention that these systems do allow for objectivity and it is therefore important that clinical judgement is used during all assessments.

? **Think about how you would identify a pressure ulcer. What would you be looking for when assessing a patient's skin condition? What information would you document in Jack's notes following your assessment?**

7.9 | Identification of a Pressure Ulcer

Correct identification of a lower extremity pressure ulcer can be ascertained through the use of a grading system. Prior to using a grading system, skin should be inspected for any signs of damage. The assessment of a patient's skin must be documented in the notes and signed each time an assessment is undertaken.

Although some skin damage, e.g. a break in the skin (Figure 7.4), is obvious, other types are less obvious. Health care professionals must be able to recognize the signs of potential skin breakdown prior to a break developing. In fact EPUAP (1999) grade 1 classification includes damage where the skin is not actually broken (Figure 7.5).

When assessing the skin, observation should be made for any signs of:

- Persistent erythema
- Nonblanching erythema

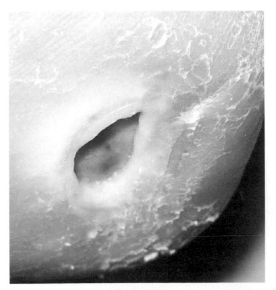

Figure 7.4
Pressure ulcer on the plantar aspect of the heel

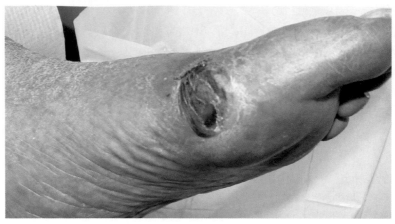

Figure 7.5
Pressure damage on the medial aspect of the first metatarsolphalangeal joint

- Skin discoloration
- Purplish-blue discoloration and localized heat in darkly pigmented skin
- Localized heat
- Localized oedema
- Blisters

7.9.1 │ Assessing the Lower Extremity Wound

Patients with pressure ulcers should receive an initial and ongoing pressure ulcer assessment. When a cause is identified strategies should be implemented to remove/reduce these to encourage healing.

Pressure ulcer assessment should include (NICE, 2005; RCN, 2005):

- Identifying the cause of the pressure ulcer, e.g. ill-fitting footwear
- Position of the ulcer/wound
- Wound dimensions (width, height, surface area, depth)
- Stage or grade
- Appearance and condition of surrounding skin
- Any evidence of skin maceration
- Any signs of neurological deficit
- Any vascular impairment
- Size of the ulcer/wound
- Any odour
- Amount and colour of exudate

- Any pain that the patient may have in relation to the wound
- Any pain that the patient may have in the surrounding areas
- Assessment of the wound bed
- Any signs of clinical infection such as:
  - Localized heat
  - Increased pain (at the wound site or surrounding skin)
  - Increased exudate and discharge
  - Malodour
  - Cellulitis
  - Undermining/tracking

Bacteria often contaminate many pressure ulcers with no clinical signs of multiplication or host reaction; therefore, it is unnecessary to swab these wounds unless signs of infection are apparent. Chronic pressure ulcers are commonly colonized with bacteria. Falanga (2005) attributes this to the fact that these wounds remain open for prolonged periods and are frequently associated with a poor blood supply to the area due to tissue hypoxia from pressure and concomitant disease processes. Cutting *et al.* (2005) published criteria for identifying infection in a number of types of wounds, including pressure ulcers. Chapter 4 provides a comprehensive guide to management of infected wounds.

> **?** **Does Jack's wound display any of the classical signs of infection? Give a rationale for your response.**

7.9.2 | Documenting your Assessment

When assessment of the ulcer is complete all information must be recorded in the patient's notes. Documentation of the wound should include measurements of the wound margins, which may be drawn, traced on acetate or photographed, dependent upon the unit's policy. If the wound is to be photographed it will be necessary to gain the patient's or their relatives' written consent to do so.

The aim of pressure ulcer assessment is to:

- Establish the severity of the pressure ulcer
- Generate a plan of care and treatment
- Evaluate treatment
- Assess for possible complications
- Communicate information regarding the pressure ulcer to all health professionals involved in the care (NICE, 2005)

Write down what information you would document in Jack's notes following your assessment of the ulcer.

When assessing, planning, implementing and evaluating the care of a patient with a pressure ulcer the following should be remembered.

Assessing

Establish the risk status of the patient using the tool advocated by local policy. If there is evidence of pressure damage then grade the damage using the EPUAP (1999) grading tool. Record the results of the assessment in the patient's plan of care and review on an individual basis, identifying the review date clearly.

Planning

Following assessment of the patient develop a plan of care ensuring that relevant members of the multiprofessional team are involved. The plan should include:

- Nutritional assessment and support
- Ordering of and use of pressure redistributing devices
- Referral for appropriate mobility aids
- Referral for pain management strategies
- Appropriate selection of wound dressings
- Discussion with the patient and carers explaining the plan of care and gaining consent for all interventions

Implementation

Following the planning stage, care may be implemented. It is important that all interventions are documented and the patient and/or carers understand the rationale for the care implemented and, where necessary, informed consent is sought.

Evaluation

Evaluation of patient care will need to be undertaken on a regular basis, where the regularity will be on an individual need basis. When evaluating patient care it is important that the multiprofessional team discusses all care interventions and plan how to develop the care based on patient need. All patient evaluations must be documented. Clear explanations of any change in the care plan must be documented clearly and rationales offered for the change in interventions.

7.10 | Pressure Ulcer Management

Effective communication is imperative between members of the multiprofessional team, both verbal and written, when caring for a patient with a lower extremity pressure ulcer, as highlighted in Chapter 1. When an individual develops a pressure ulcer, care needs to be planned and implemented to treat the ulcer and prevent further skin deterioration.

7.10.1 | Choosing a Pressure-Redistributing Device

Effective pressure redistribution is the mainstay of treatment for the prevention of pressure ulcers, facilitating wound healing in established ulcers and prevention of recurrence once pressure ulcers have healed.

Pressure redistribution can be achieved by a number of strategies. These include pressure redistributing devices such as mattresses and pressure-relieving boots, but such devices should not replace basic nursing principles that underpin pressure ulcer prevention and care. Basic principles include regular skin assessment, basic skin care, repositioning of the patient at regular intervals and appropriate manual handling to minimize shear and friction.

NICE (2005) recommend that patients with pressure ulcers should have access to pressure-redistributing support surfaces and strategies, e.g. mattresses and cushions, 24 hours a day. All individuals assessed as having a grade 1–2 pressure ulcer should, as a minimum provision, be placed on a high-specification foam mattress or cushion with pressure-reducing properties combined with very close observation of skin changes, and a documented positioning and repositioning regime. If there is any perceived or actual deterioration of affected areas or further pressure ulcer development, an alternating pressure (replacement or overlay) or sophisticated continuous low-pressure system, e.g. low air loss, air fluidized, air flotation or viscous fluid, should be used. NICE (2005) further recommend that individuals requiring bed rails and alternating pressure overlay mattresses should be placed on a reduced-depth foam mattress to maintain their safety.

Depending on the location of the ulcer, individuals assessed as having grade 3–4 pressure ulcers, including intact eschar, where depth, and therefore grade, cannot be assessed, should, as a minimum provision, be placed on an alternating pressure mattress (replacement or overlay) or sophisticated continuous low-pressure system. If alternating pressure equipment is required, the first choice should be an overlay system, unless other circumstances such as patient weight or patient safety indicate the need for a replacement system (NICE, 2005).

? **When Jack's assessment has been completed, arrangements for pressure-redistributing equipment should be made to prevent further breakdown of the skin. What pressure-distributing device(s) should be used?**

When choosing a piece of equipment Torrance (1983) suggests addressing the following:

- Does the equipment distribute pressure evenly, provide frequent relief of pressure or constant low pressure?
- Does the equipment minimize friction and shearing forces?
- Does the equipment provide a well-ventilated, comfortable surface that does not unduly restrict movement?
- Does the equipment maintain skin at a constant optimal temperature?
- Is the equipment acceptable to the patient?
- Does the equipment allow care interventions and provide a hard surface for resuscitation procedures?
- Is the equipment easily cleaned and maintained?
- Is the equipment easily operated by both carers and patients?
- Does it have height adjustments, tilt facility and sufficient clearance for hoist use?

If the equipment does not fit these characteristics then it may be advisable to choose another product.

> **In Jack's case it is important that pressure is reduced over his heel and foot. The use of a device such as the heel lift suspension boot would be advisable to prevent shear forces and to prevent excessive pressure being applied to the vulnerable and compromised heel area, as seen in Figure 7.6. The boot works by hanging the heel in suspension thus completely relieving pressure on the heel. This can be used in conjunction with pressure-relieving mattresses.**

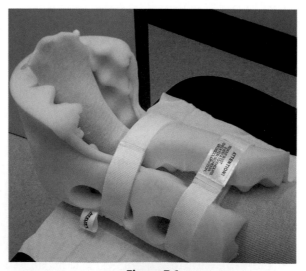

Figure 7.6
Heel lift suspension boot

T	Tissue nonviable or deficient
I	Infection or inflammation
M	Moisture imbalance
E	Edge of wound nonadvancing or undermined

Table 7.3
TIME acronym

While pressure redistribution and the use of pressure redistributing devices is a fundamental aspect of pressure ulcer treatment it is important to recognize that this is only one aspect of care in pressure ulcer management. Optimum wound care is also required to promote wound healing.

7.10.2 | Wound Management

It is important to assess the wound bed to determine the stage of the healing process and identify the most suitable management strategies. The acronym TIME was introduced by an expert working group in 2002 to assist practitioners in assessing the wound bed (Shultz *et al.*, 2003) (Table 7.3)

Tissue management is imperative to encourage wound healing. The presence of necrotic tissue or nonviable tissue, such as slough, as seen in Figure 7.7, is common in chronic wounds.

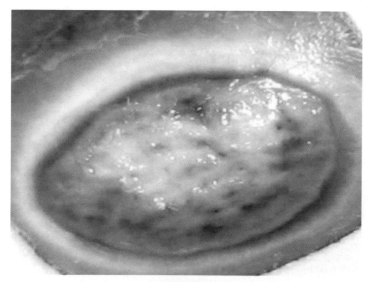

Figure 7.7
Presence of slough in the wound bed

Falanga (2004) suggests that the removal of nonviable tissue from the wound bed (known as wound debridement) is beneficial to the healing process for a number of reasons:

- Removal of nonviable tissue decreases the amount of nonvascularized tissue.
- Wound debridement decreases bacterial burden and cells that impede healing.
- Removal of nonviable tissue promotes an optimum environment for healing.

There are a number of methods of debridement available to the practitioner, namely sharp debridement, enzymatic debridement, autolytic debridement and mechanical debridement.

Sharp debridement is the physical removal of nonviable tissue with a scalpel or tissue scissors. This form of debridement offers the most rapid method of wound debridement and is considered by many as the "gold standard" (Leaper, 2002; König et al., 2005). However McIntosh (2006) highlights a number of factors that must be considered before undertaking this skilled procedure (see Table 7.4).

Less invasive methods of wound debridement include enzymatic debridement, mechanical debridement and autolytic debridement:

Enzymatic debridement can be achieved by the application of manufactured proteolytic enzymes, e.g. streptokinase, or by applying biological products that secrete proteolytic enzymes, e.g. larvae. There is limited evidence to support the use of manufactured proteolytic enzymes such as streptokinase over alternative methods of debridement (Leaper, 2002). Evidence to support the use of larvae therapy is also largely anecdotal but clinical trials are ongoing.

Autolytic debridement occurs, to some extent, naturally in all wounds. The body can exert its own form of debridement by releasing phagocytic cells and proteolytic enzymes to the wound bed,

- The practitioner must consider whether he/she has received sufficient training and is sufficiently skilled to undertake the procedure; if not a referral must be made to a skilled member of the team

- Extreme caution must be exercised on ischaemic wounds to prevent further tissue damage

- Sharp debridement should not be performed on individuals with severe bleeding disorders or those who are severely immunocompromised

- Informed consent from the patient is essential prior to undertaking the procedure

- A pain assessment should be undertaken. Sharp debridement can be painful so pain control may be necessary prior to undertaking the procedure

Table 7.4
Factors to consider before sharp debridement

which act to liquefy and separate necrotic tissue and slough (König et al., 2005). Moist wound dressings facilitate autolytic debridement. This form of debridement poses minimal discomfort to the patient but if there is a large amount of wound debris autolytic debridement may be prolonged, thus delaying the healing process.

Mechanical debridement is the physical removal of wound debris by methods such as wound irrigation and hydrotherapy. This is a relatively slow technique and the risk of cross-infection should be considered.

7.10.3 | Cleansing the Wound

Prior to applying the wound dressing the wound will require assessment of the need for cleansing. If the wound is clean then there is no need to cleanse it, but a variety of reasons exist for cleansing wounds:

- To remove debris from the surface of the wound
- To rehydrate the surface and provide a moist environment
- To clean the surrounding area, thus preventing contamination
- To facilitate assessment of the wound
- If the wound is dirty

A recent Cochrane systematic review concluded that there is currently insufficient evidence to determine the most effective cleansing solution for pressure ulcers, but results indicate that wounds cleansed with saline spray containing aloe vera, silver chloride and decyl glucoside showed improved healing over wounds cleansed with isotonic saline solution (Moore and Cowman, 2005).

7.10.4 | Choosing a Wound Dressing

Winter (1962) demonstrated the concept of a moist healing environment to be the most efficient conditions in which partial thickness wounds heal. The ideal dressing will therefore provide a moist environment, maintain humidity at the wound, remove excess exudate, provide thermal insulation, be impermeable to bacteria, be free from particulate and toxic contaminants, and allow removal without damage to the skin (Turner, 1985; Thomas 1997).

An optimum wound healing environment can be created by using modern dressings, for example:

- Hydrocolloids
- Hydrogels
- Hydrofibers™
- Foams
- Films
- Alginates
- Soft silicones, in preference to basic dressing types, e.g. gauze, paraffin gauze and simple dressing pads.

There are a plethora of dressings available but many health care settings now have a wound care formulary. It is important that these are complied with and practitioners are familiar with the formulary.

> **?** **What type of wound dressing would you choose for Jack? Give a rationale for your choice.**

Types of dressings

Flanagan and Fletcher (2003) identify two main categories that dressing products may be broken into. Passive dressings, they argue, are products that have no direct effect on the wound. These dressings have little absorbency and become saturated quickly, which often leads to leakage and the dressing falling off the wound. In wounds that have a small amount of exudate, the dressing becomes dry and thus becomes painful and traumatic to remove. These dressings may be useful as a secondary dressing.

Alternatively they state that interactive dressings provide the optimum environment at the wound interface. These products may be occlusive or semi-occlusive. They highlight the fact that many manufacturers are now developing dressings that combine the two groups, thus offering the benefits of both categories.

Exudate management

Exudate is vital to wound healing but in excess can prove to be detrimental to the healing process and the surrounding skin. Watret (1997) argues that traditionally exudate has been described in terms of its perceived volume, e.g. as light/low, moderate or heavy. This form of assessment is very subjective and difficult to quantify in the absence of significant investigation, such as the weighing of dressing pre- and post-use.

Vowden and Vowden (2003) suggest that exudate volume should not be viewed in isolation but in conjunction with the viscosity. By considering both of these aspects, they argue that it offers an insight into the underlying condition of the wound and of the patient. They further state that wound exudate volume and viscosity are assessed by:

- Considering the exudate that is retained within the dressing
- The number of dressing changes required in 48 hours
- Visual inspection of the wound

It is important that when caring for an exuding wound the surrounding skin is protected from damage. This may be achieved via the use of barrier products. It is important that the wound dressing chosen to contain the exudate fits the wound, allowing for it to absorb the exudate and preventing any leakage on to undamaged skin. Table 7.5 identifies an example of a dressing selection guide.

Table 7.5

Dressing selection guide.

EXUDATE VOLUME	NECROTIC	SLOUGHY	GRANULATING	EPITHELIALIZING	INFECTED*	ODOROUS
	Characterized by: Dead or devitalized tissue, often black in colour	Characterized by: A yellow covering	Characterized by: A clean, deep pink or red colour	Characterized by: Pink/grey covering over the wound base	Characterized by: Heat, redness, inflammation, pain and/or malocour	Characterized by: Malodour
	Treatment aims: Debride Remove eschar Rehydrate Relieve Pain	Treatment aims: Remove slough Provide a clean base for granulation tissue	Treatment aims: Promote granulation Provide a clean base for epithelializing tissue	Treatment aims: Promote epithelialization Promote wound maturation	Treatment aim: Manage infection	Treatment aim: Control odour
Low Level	Primary Dressing: Hydrogel Hydrocolloid	Primary Dressing: Hydrogel	Primary Dressing: Hydrogel Tulle	Primary Dressing: Tulle	Primary Dressing*: Antimicrobial	Primary Dressing: Hydrogel
	Secondary Dressing: Foam Films	Secondary Dressing: Foam Film	Secondary Dressing: Foam Film	Secondary Dressing: Foam	Secondary Dressing: Foam Film	Secondary Dressing: Activated charcoal dressing

*Assess signs of infection and refer for antibiotics if indicated.

(continued)

EXUDATE VOLUME	NECROTIC	SLOUGHY	GRANULATING	EPITHELIALIZING	INFECTED*	ODOROUS
Medium level	**Primary Dressing:** Alginate Hydrocolloid Hydrofibers™ **Secondary Dressing:** Foam	**Primary Dressing:** Hydrofibers™ **Secondary Dressing:** Foam	**Primary Dressing:** Hydrofibers™ **Secondary Dressing:** Foam	Epithelializing wounds produce minimal exudate	**Primary Dressing:** Hydrogel Hydrofibers™ Antimicrobial **Secondary Dressing:** Foam	**Primary Dressing:** Activated charcoal dressing Hydrofibers™ **Secondary Dressing:** Foam
High Level	Necrotic wounds are often dry so high exudate is unlikely	**Primary Dressing:** Hydrofibers™ **Secondary Dressing:** Foam	**Primary Dressing:** Hydrofibers™ **Secondary Dressing:** Foam	Epithelializing wounds produce minimal exudate	**Primary Dressing:** Hydrofibers™ Antimicrobial **Secondary Dressing:** Foam	**Primary Dressing:** Hydrofibers™ Activated charcoal dressing **Secondary Dressing:** Foam

Table 7.5
(*Continued*)

> **?** **Which members of the multiprofessional team should be included in the care of Jack? What information would you give to Jack to ensure he understands how to care for the pressure ulcer on discharge? What information does Jack require to prevent further skin damage?**

7.11 | Accountability

NICE (2005) guidelines for the assessment and prevention of pressure ulcers stipulate that all health care professionals involved in pressure ulcer risk assessment and prevention should receive relevant training in risk assessment, selection, use and maintenance of pressure-relieving devices and providing education for people vulnerable to pressure ulcers. With the increased number of complaints regarding patient care issues and the rise in litigation, the prevention and treatment of pressure ulcers is a multiprofessional responsibility (Knowlton, 2003).

7.12 | Case Scenario Revisited

Consider the initial questions posed:

1. **What factors may have led him to develop a pressure ulcer?**

   Jack has a number of factors in his history that make him vulnerable to pressure ulcers. Jack has no fixed abode and no family support; he regularly sleeps rough on the streets. Jack struggles with personal hygiene, has limited financial resources, poor clothing and ill-fitting footwear, all of which contribute to poor tissue viability. He also has a history of alcohol abuse. Jack's nutritional status is poor; he was thin and frail on admission to the ward. Jack has had limited access to health and social care, so while he has little in his medical history it is important to recognize that this may be due to a lack of medical diagnoses rather than the fact that Jack does not suffer from any medical pathologies.

2. **What interventions could you now commence that would improve his general condition?**

   An "at-risk" assessment of Jack will need to be undertaken, e.g. using the Waterlow assessment tool, and his pressure ulcer should be graded using the EPUAP guidelines and grading system. Jack will require a nutritional assessment and referral to the dieticians for additional advice and support. To improve nutritional status Jack also requires dental intervention to replace his poorly fitting dentures and reduce mouth ulcer incidence. Advice regarding abstinence of alcohol should also be offered. Jack should have a vascular assessment to inform a prognosis for healing. He will also require adequate pressure relief and therefore will need a pressure redistributing mattress and referral to the podiatrists who will be able to suggest "off-loading" strategies and will liaise with the nursing staff regarding the choice of appropriate wound dressings.

3. **What are the causes of pressure ulcer development?**

   The main cause of pressure ulcer development is pressure. Other causes are shear and friction. In Jack's case ill-fitting footwear has contributed to his pressure ulcer, as has sleeping rough on hard surfaces.

4. **How can you prevent further deterioration of his skin?**

   Pressure will need to removed from Jack's heel to promote healing. Correctly fitting footwear is essential so Jack may benefit from podiatry and orthotist assessment and intervention. While in hospital Jack requires a diet that contains nutrients that will promote wound healing and wound dressings that promote a moist, warm healing environment. Jack will require health promotion and health education to explain how to prevent further breakdown of the skin. As Jack has no fixed abode the involvement of social services, with Jack's permission, is important to arrange appropriate support and care following discharge from hospital.

5. **Which members of the multiprofessional team need to be involved in his care?**

   Members of the multiprofessional team to be involved in Jack's care are:

   - Ward nurses
   - Tissue viability nurses
   - Podiatrists
   - Orthotists and prosthetics
   - Dieticians
   - Physiotherapists
   - Occupational therapists
   - Social workers
   - Medical staff
   - Dentists

6. **Are there any national policy documents that you need to access to ensure his care will be evidence based?**

   The policy documents you will need to access are:

   - NICE (2005)
   - CREST (1998)
   - NHS Quality Improvement Scotland (2005a)
   - DH (1992)

7.13 | Conclusion

Pressure ulcer prevention and management remains a challenging area in tissue viability. This chapter has identified and discussed common causes and accurate identification of pressure ulcers, exploring policy documents that influence the care planning and implementation. The importance of effective skin assessment and the use of the EPUAP guidelines have also been highlighted. Pressure ulcer care requires a multiprofessional approach to promote optimum outcomes. Thus the role of the multi-professional team in caring for Jack and lower limb pressure ulcers has been investigated.

? Reflection

Take time to reflect upon your learning from this chapter. Ask yourself:

1. **What knowledge did I possess prior to reading this chapter?**

2. **How has my knowledge developed?**

3. **How will I implement this into my future practice?**

References

Amputee Statistical Database (2005) (online) Available at: http://www.nasdab.co.uk/, Last accessed November 2006.

Beldon, P. (2006) Pressure ulcers: prevention and management. *Wounds Essentials*, **1**, 68–81.

Bennett, G., Dealey, C. and Posnett, J. (2004) The cost of pressure ulcers in the UK. *Age Ageing*, **33**(3), 230–235.

Braden, B. and Bergstrom, N. (1987) A conceptual schema for the study of the aetiology of pressure sores. *Rehabilitation Nursing*, **12**(1), 8–12.

British Association for Parental and Enteral Nutrition (2005) *Malnutrition Screening Tool*, BAPEN, Redditich, available at: www.bapen.org.uk/uk, Accessed 6 July 2006.

Collier, M. (1999) Pressure ulcer development and principles for prevention, in *Wound Management: Theory and Practice* (eds D. Glover and M. Miller), EMAP, London, pp. 84–95.

Collier, M. (2002) Caring for the patient with a skin or wound care need, in *Watson's Clinical Nursing and Related Sciences* (ed. M. Walsh), Baillière Tindall. Edinburgh, pp. 925–59.

Clark, M., Defloor, T. and Bours, G. (2004) A pilot study of the prevalence of pressure ulcers in European hospitals, in *Pressure Ulcers: Recent Advances in Tissue Viability* (ed. M. Clark), Quay Books, MA Healthcare Ltd, London.

Cooper, R. (2005) Understanding wound infection, in, *Identifying Criteria for Wound Infection* European Wound Management Association (EWMA) Position Document, MEP Ltd, London.

Courtenay, M. (2002) Movement and mobility, in *Foundations of Nursing Practice: Making the Difference* (eds R. Hogston and P.M. Simpson), Palgrave, London, pp. 262–85.

Clinical Resource Efficiency Support Team (CREST) (1998) *Guidelines for the Prevention and Management of Pressure Sores. Recommendations for Practice*, Belfast, Northern Ireland, available at: www.crestni.org.uk/publications/pressure_sores.pdf, Last accessed 8 July 2006.

Cutting, K.F., White, R.J., Mahoney, P. *et al.* (2005) Understanding wound infection, in *Identifying Criteria for Wound Infection*, European Wound Management Association (EWMA) Position Document, MEP Ltd, London, pp. 2–5.

Dealey, C. (1997) *Managing Pressure Sore Prevention*, Quay Books, Mark Allen Publishing Ltd, Salisbury.

Defloor, T. (1999) The risk of pressure sores: a conceptual scheme. *Journal of Clinical Nursing*, **8**, 206–16.

Department of Health (DH) (1992) *The Health of the Nation. A Consultative Document*, HMSO, London.

European Pressure Ulcer Advisory Panel (EPUAP) (1999) Guidelines on treatment of pressure ulcers. *EPUAP Review*, **1,** 7–8.

European Pressure Ulcer Advisory Panel (EPUAP) (2006) *Nutritional Guidelines for Pressure Ulcer Prevention and Treatment*, available at: www.epuap.org/, Accessed 7 July 2006.

Falanga, V. (2004) Wound bed preparation: science applied to practice, in *Wound Bed Preparation in Practice*, European Wound Management Association (EWMA) Position Document, MEP Ltd, London, pp. 2–5.

Falanga, V. (2005) Wound healing and its impairment in the diabetic foot. *The Lancet*, **366**, 1736–43.

Farley, M. (2002) Oh my, the pressure! *Can Operating Room Nursing Journal*. **20**(2), 9–13, 20.

Flanagan, M. and Fletcher, J. (2003) Tissue viability: managing chronic wounds, in *Nursing Adults: The Practice of Caring* (eds C Brooker and M. Nicol), Mosby, London.

Florian, V. and Elad, D. (1998) The impact of mothers' sense of empowerment on the metabolic control of their children with juvenile diabetes. *Journal of Paediatric Psychology*, **23**(4), 239–47.

Gosnell, D.J. (1973) An assessment tool to identify pressure sores. *Nursing Research*, **22**(1), 55–9.

König, M., Vanscheidt, W., Augustin, M. *et al.* (2005) Enzymatic versus autolytic debridement of chronic leg ulcers: a prospective randomised trial. *Journal of Wound Care*, **14**(7), 320–3.

Knowlton, S.P. (2003) The medical record: treatment tool or litigation device? *Advanced Skin Wound Care*, **16**(2), 97.

Leaper, D. (2002) Sharp technique for wound debridement, in *World Wide Wounds* (online), Available at: http://worldwidewounds.com/2002/december/Leaper/Sharp-Debridement.html.

Lowthian, P. (1989) Identifying and protecting patients who get pressure sores. *Nursing Standard*, **4**(4), 26–9.

McIntosh, C. (2006) *Diabetic Foot Ulcers: An Educational Booklet* (sponsored by Smith & Nephew), Wounds UK Publishing, Aberdeen.

Marshall, C. (2004) The ankle: brachial pressure index. A critical appraisal. *British Journal of Podiatry*, **7**(4), 93–5.

Moore, Z.E. and Cowman, S. (2005) Wound cleansing for pressure ulcers, in Cochrane Database Systematic Review 4 CD004983.

National Institute for Clinical Excellence (NICE) (2005) *Pressure Ulcers: The Management of Pressure Ulcers in Primary and Secondary Care: A Clinical Guideline CG029*, National Institute for Clinical Excellence, London.

National Pressure Ulcer Advisory Panel (1998) *Pressure Ulcer Scale for Healing*, available at: www.npuap.org/, Accessed 7 July 2006.

NHS Quality Improvement Scotland (2005a) *Best Practice Statement: The Treatment/Management of Pressure Ulcers*, NHS QIS, Edinburgh.

NHS Quality Improvement Scotland (2005b) *Best Practice Statement: Pressure Ulcers Prevention*, NHS QIS, Edinburgh.

Nixon, J. and McGough, A. (2001) Principles of patient assessment: screening for pressure ulcers and potential risk, in *The Prevention and Treatment of Pressure Ulcers* (ed. M.J. Morison), Mosby, Edinburgh, pp. 55–74.

Norton, D., McLaren, R. and Exton-Smith, A.N. (1975) *An Investigation of Geriatric Nursing Problems in Hospital*, Churchill Livingstone, Edinburgh.

Reid, J. and Morison, M. (1994) Towards consensus: classification of pressure sores. *Journal of Wound Care*, **3**(3), 157–60.

Royal College of Nursing (RCN) (2005) *The Management of Pressure Ulcers in Primary and Secondary Care: A Clinical Practical Guideline*, Royal College of nursing, London, pp. 1–245.

Shultz, G.S., Sibbald, R.G., *et al.* (2003) Wound bed preparation: a systematic approach to wound management. *Wound Repair and Regeneration*, **11**(2), Suppl. 1, S1–S28.

Thomas, S. (1997) A structured approach to the selection of dressings (online), Available at: http://www.worldwidewounds.com/1997/july/Thomas-Guide/Dress-Select.html, Last accessed December 2006.

Torrance, C. (1983) *Pressure Sores: Aetiology, Treatment and Prevention*, Croom Helm, London.

Turner, T.D. (1985) Which dressing and why? in *Wound Care* (ed. S. Westerby), Heinmann Medical Books, London.

Vowden, P. (1999) Doppler ultrasound in the management of the diabetic foot. *The Diabetic Foot*, **2**(1), 16–7.

Vowden, K. and Vowden, P. (2003) Understanding exudate management and the role of exudate in the healing process. *British Journal of Community Nursing*, **6**:(9Suppl.), 4–14.

Walker, R. (1998) Diabetes: reflecting on empowerment. *Nursing Standard* **12**(23): 49–56.

Waterlow, J. (2005) Waterlow score card, Available at: `http://www.judy-waterlow.co.uk/downloads/waterlow` (24 March 2007).

Watret, L. (1997) Know how: management of wound exudate. *Nursing Times*, **93**(30), 38–9.

Winter, G. (1962) Formulation of the scab and the rate of epithelialisation in the skin of the domestic pig. *Nature*, **193**, 293–4.

Wysocki, A.B. (1999) Skin anatomy, physiology and pathophysiology wound care management. *Nursing Clinics of North America*, **34**(4), 777–97.

Caroline McIntosh and Veronica Newton

Chapter 8

Diabetic Foot Ulcers

8.1 | Diabetic Foot Ulcers: the Broader Picture

A person living with diabetes has a 12–25% risk of developing foot ulceration during their lifetime (Cavanagh et al., 2005; Singh et al., 2005). However, the global prevalence of diabetes is predicted to rise from 71 million in 2000 (2.8% prevalence) to 366 million (4.4% prevalence) by 2030 (Wild et al., 2004) and thus the burden of diabetic foot disease is set to escalate. This predicted rise will have a significant impact on diabetes care provision. Diabetic foot ulcers and diabetes-related lower extremity amputations represent a significant financial cost to the National Health Service (Valk et al., 2006). An estimate of costs for diabetes-related ulceration and amputation was £244 million (Shearer et al., 2003). However, personal costs for the individual affected must also be considered in terms of loss of earning, days lost to sickness, restricted activities and anxiety and stress.

It is therefore crucial that systems of care are developed and implemented into clinical practice (Department of Health (DH), 2001). National Institue for Clinical Excellence (NICE) (2004) recommend a risk identification system to identify the at-risk limb, with suggested care pathways dependent on risk status and presenting problems (Table 8.1).

All health care professionals working in diabetes service provision for management of diabetic foot ulcers are recommended within national guidelines (*National Service Framework for Diabetes* (DH, 2001); NICE, 2004) to collect, assimilate and act upon identified clinical risks and complications within tight timeframes to optimize effective care and achieve positive clinical outcomes. Prevention of ulceration remains the optimum management, but this is not always possible. When an individual presents with diabetic foot ulceration NICE (2004) regard this as an emergency situation and stress that the patient should be assessed by a member of the diabetes foot care team within 24 hours. Accurate assessment of diabetic foot ulcers is imperative to identify the underlying cause of the wound, inform management planning and offer a prognosis for wound healing.

Risk status	Review	Recommended assessments/treatment
Low risk (normal sensation, normal foot pulses)	Annual review	• Negotiate and agree a foot management plan with the patient • Patient education
Increased risk (loss of sensation or absent foot pulses or other risk factors)	Review every 3–6 months	• Inspect patient's feet • Determine the need for vascular assessment • Assess footwear • Patient education
High risk (loss of sensation or absent foot pulses plus other risk factors, e.g. skin changes or deformity)	Review every 1–3 months	If required, ensure appropriate provision of: • Footwear and insoles • Skin and nail care • Patient education
Current ulcer	Emergency situation: to be seen by the multiprofessional foot care team within 24 hours	• Urgent assessment and management of the ulceration

Table 8.1
Identifying risk status of the diabetic foot (adapted from NICE, 2004)

This chapter has two broad aims:

1. To suggest and outline wound assessment and wound management models for diabetic foot ulcer management
2. To explore the use of clinical guidelines and the best available evidence to generate a thorough systematic protocol-based approach to the management of diabetic foot ulcers

Within this chapter emphasis is placed on the need for a multiprofessional team approach to the management of patients with diabetic foot ulcers in order to ensure that patients receive integrated health and social care, thus minimizing the impact of foot ulceration and maximizing the quality of life for people with foot ulceration.

8.2 | Case Scenario

Case Scenario 8

Consider the following case scenario. Walter, an 80-year-old man, presents with a new episode of foot ulceration (see Figure 8.1). His wife is in attendance and is concerned about his lack of health care to date. He has a 15-year duration of type 2 diabetes controlled with oral hypoglycaemic therapy, until recently when his diabetologist recommended he commence insulin therapy. He reports his blood glucose levels have been up and down: "typically 5 before lunch but anything up to 20 by the evening". He has a history of (ischaemic) heart disease and hypertension.

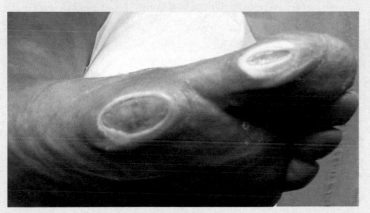

Figure 8.1
Areas of ulceration presenting on the forefoot

His wife informs you that she noticed some blisters (recognized above clinically as two ulcerated areas) on his foot (see Figure 8.1) that are not healing. The family doctor has referred him to you. The patient reports no pain from the wounds. On removal of the soiled dressings you observe a green, purulent exudate.

?   **Consider the following questions prior to reading this chapter:**

1. **What are the possible causes of these ulcers?**

2. **Identify which factors in the patient's history increase the risk of foot ulceration.**

3. **What assessments should be undertaken before implementing a management plan?**

4. **Outline management strategies appropriate for this case.**

5. **Who should be involved in this patient's care?**

The information provided within the following sections should enable you to answer the five questions posed above. The answers to the case will be considered towards the end of the chapter.

8.3 | Causes of Diabetic Foot Ulcers

Current evidence suggests that the normal wound healing physiology, as outlined in Chapter 2, is impaired in individuals with diabetes. Falanga (2005a) attributes this to a number of intrinsic factors:

- Peripheral neuropathy (dysfunction of the nerves in the lower limbs) (see Section 8.4)
- Ischaemia (a reduced blood supply) (see Section 8.4)
- Hyperglycaemia (excess glucose in the blood)

and extrinsic factors such as:

- Wound infection
- Abnormal foot pressures and callus formation

When a patient presents with diabetic foot ulceration a comprehensive assessment is essential to identify causative factors. The next section will consider assessment strategies for diabetic foot ulcers.

8.4 | Wound Assessment Model for Diabetic Foot Ulcers

The following wound assessment model has two recommended stages which should be sequenced as follows:

1. The *"hands off"* stage involves verbal *information gathering* consisting of:

    (a) Aetiology of the wound
    (b) General medical history (management of glycaemic levels)
    (c) Medication (regarding coexisting diseases)
    (d) Nutritional factors
    (e) Social factors

2. The *"hands on"* stage involves semi-quantitative *physical measurement* of:

    (a) Skin
    (b) Foot deformity
    (c) Wound characteristics
    (d) Vascular status
    (e) Neurological status

8.4.1 | "Hands Off" Stage

(a) Aetiology of the wound

Establishing the aetiology of a diabetic foot ulcer is the first stage in achieving a positive outcome in wound management. Effective identification of the aetiological factors in diabetic foot ulceration is a challenge as the origins of these wounds are often multifactorial.

The ALERT assessment framework (McIntosh and Newton, 2005) is recommended to assist the health care practitioner at pre-ulcerative or newly presenting ulcer stage:

Ask the patient. Encourage the patient to vocalize their concerns.
Look at the skin. Scrutinize the surrounding tissues to spot early or established skin changes
Examine for signs of infection.
Review previous treatment and treatment notes
Think about an individualized management plan.

Ischaemia, a reduced arterial blood supply, and peripheral neuropathy, nerve dysfunction, are common long-term complications in diabetes and are both associated with poor glycaemic control and are significant risk factors for diabetic foot ulcers. Peripheral neuropathy can affect many nerve pathways, namely sensory, autonomic and motor pathways. The most common expression of diabetic peripheral neuropathy is polyneuropathy affecting all pathways; hence it is a common cause of foot ulceration in the diabetic patient (Dinh and Veves, 2005).

Edmonds and Foster (2006) argue that it is rare to see pure ischaemic changes without neuropathic changes and identify two common foot types in people with diabetes:

1. The *neuropathic* foot, in which peripheral neuropathy predominates but the arterial supply to the foot is not affected. Typical clinical features are varying degrees of deficit to (a) touch, (b) vibration, (c) temperature and (d) pain sensation within the foot and lower limb.
2. The *neuroischaemic* foot, whereby peripheral neuropathy is coupled with a reduced arterial supply, often due to peripheral arterial disease. Typical clinical features are a cold foot on palpation which may be pale or cyanosed in colour and pulses may be weak or absent.

Identifying the underlying aetiology of diabetic foot ulceration is essential to inform management planning, as management of neuropathic ulceration will differ significantly to that of neuroischaemic ulceration. Furthermore, the prognosis for wound healing differs for neuropathic and neuroischaemic ulceration. Zimny *et al.* (2002) found that healing times in diabetic foot ulcers predominantly depended on the aetiological cause of the ulcer, with the shortest healing times for neuropathic ulcers compared to ischaemic or neuroischaemic groups.

Both the nonspecialist and expert practitioner in diabetes care need to be competent in identifying key clinical indictors which may explain diabetic foot ulcer genesis and impact on effective wound healing. The issue of clinical competency is an important factor in diabetic foot ulcer management, as early recognition and management of risk factors can reduce the deterioration of diabetic foot ulcers and development of further episodes of ulceration. In recognition of the need for meeting standards in diabetes care, the Diabetes Nursing Strategy Group (2005) has devised a competency framework for diabetes nursing. This framework will assist nurses in developing knowledge and skills to support excellence in care for patients with diabetes.

(b) Assessment of general medical history (management of glycaemic levels)

Reporting of glucose levels from patient to practitioner is significant in wound assessment and wound management as the effect of uncontrolled hyperglycaemia (raised glucose levels) in the short term increases the risk of infection. Self-monitoring of blood glucose levels is advocated for people living with diabetes with a level of 7 mmol/L being an optimum figure (NICE, 2002).

Type 1 diabetes affects approximately 15 % of all people living with diabetes in England, primarily affecting the younger population (<30 years of age) (DH, 2001). For these patients insulin therapy is mandatory in an attempt to achieve as near normal glucose levels as possible.

Type 2 diabetes affects approximately 85 % of all people living with diabetes in England (DH, 2001). For these patients a number of strategies may be employed to normalize glucose levels: diet alone or a combination of diet and oral hypoglycaemic/s and sometimes insulin therapy. The UK Prospective Diabetes Study (UKPDS) (1998) found that three years after diagnosis 50 % of failing diet controlled patients required more than one glucose-lowering drug. Hence, use of combination therapy (treatment with more than one type of oral hypoglycaemic drug) for management of type 2 diabetes can optimize glycaemic control further by increasing sites of action of drug therapy, leading to reduced episodes of hyperglycaemia (NICE, 2002).

Relatively small elevations in blood glucose levels can detrimentally affect the normal functioning of a patient's white blood cell activity; hence normal immune response to bacterial invasion is impaired. Patients with prolonged uncontrolled hyperglycaemia can develop chronic damage to the vascular and neurological systems, further complicating wound management. These patients may require the input of a number of health care professionals to facilitate positive clinical outcomes in diabetic foot ulcer management. Health care professionals are recommended to measure the percentage concentration of glucose in red blood cells using a test called HbA1C; a level of 6.5–7.5 % is the recommended target (NICE, 2002).

In addition to managing glycaemic control, risk factors for arterial disease must also be controlled. The *National Service Framework for Diabetes* (DH, 2001) suggests that as many as 70 % of adults with type 2 diabetes have hypertension (high blood pressure) and more than 70 % have dyslipidaemia (raised level of lipids in the blood).

(c) Assessment of medication

It is not unusual for patients with diabetes to be prescribed a number of pharmacological agents, which may be for:

1. Pre-existing medical conditions that may be unrelated to diabetes
2. Identifiable complications associated with diabetes, commonly hypertension and dyslipidaemia (see below)
3. Reducing the risk of developing associated complications of diabetes, commonly peripheral arterial disease and neuropathy

Hypertension. UKPDS (1998) and NICE (2002) advocate tight control of blood pressure in diabetic patients, i.e. a target blood pressure of <140/<80 mmHg to reduce the risk of microvascular (small vessel) and macrovascular (large vessel) disease, which can lead to peripheral vascular disease, coronary heart disease, stroke and diabetes-related deaths. Provision of pharmacological agents, such as ACE inhibitors or beta blockers, have been found to reduce the risk of a number of vascular complications in diabetic patients when prescribed for blood pressure management. Provision of such medication may have a positive clinical benefit in preventing or treating nonresponsive diabetic foot ulcers, with arterial disease as the prime aetiological factor.

Dyslipidaemia in people with diabetes can increase the risk of macrovascular complications and hence some patients may be prescribed statin therapy to manage their lipid levels. PRODIGY knowledge (DH, 2006) guidance offers comprehensive practical suggestions on the management of lipids in people with type 2 diabetes, as outlined in the national guidelines (NICE, 2002). Hence stabilization of lipids may be a significant factor in diabetic foot ulcer management.

Additionally, a number of pharmacological agents can significantly increase the risk of ulceration and in established diabetic foot ulcers may interfere with the mechanisms of normal wound healing. Hence a thorough collection of current and past medication is vital for inclusion within a good assessment model. Significant medications to note, due to their impact on wound healing, are: steroid therapy, anticoagulant therapy, nonsteroidal anti-inflammatory drugs (NSAIDs) and immunosuppressant drugs.

> **?** Walter has a history of heart disease and hypertension. How can members of the multiprofessional team work together to control such risk factors for delayed wound healing and further episodes of diabetic foot ulceration?

(d) Assessment of nutritional factors

Good nutrition is an essential component for effective wound healing (Russell, 2001). However, this aspect of wound management is often overlooked.

Malnutrition and weight loss are prevalent among hospitalized and long-term care patients, particularly the elderly. Himes (1999) points to a correlation between nutritional status, body weight and the rate of wound healing, concluding that a greater understanding of the role of nutrition and weight gain in wound healing can result in more effective patient care.

It is crucial that the individual's nutritional status is properly assessed prior to advocating any special dietary intakes or reductions in food groups. In general the healthy diet for people with diabetes is low in fat, sugar and salt, high in fruit and vegetables and moderate in bread, potatoes, cereals, pasta and rice, which is also a good basis for effective wound healing. Everyone with diabetes should receive dietary information and support. A registered dietician can provide specific dietary advice (Diabetes UK, 2006).

(e) Assessment of social factors

Recognition and appropriate support mechanisms regarding socioeconomic status is important in diabetic foot ulcer management as low social status may result in poor access to health care and education (International Working Group on the Diabetic Foot, 1999). Consequently, in relation to wound care any delay in accessing health care may delay delivery of essential treatment, resulting in poor clinical outcomes for diabetic foot ulcer management.

Paile-Hyvarinen *et al.* (2003) report that depression is prevalent in people with diabetes. It is reported to be as high as 15 %, which is associated with a higher medical symptom burden, poor self-care and a higher number of micro- and macrovascular complications (Katon *et al.*, 2006). Lidfelt *et al.* (2005) highlighted negative health effects from living alone; this was explained by lifestyle conditions such as smoking, dietary habits and alcohol but was also due to social and mental conditions, e.g. low paid work and low occupational status. Agardh *et al.* (2004) found that established risk factors, such as obesity smoking and physical inactivity, were implicated in the development of type 2 diabetes; in men these factors are also associated with low socioeconomic position.

For this reason, in wound care management a number of scales may be used, e.g. the MOS 36-item Short-Form Health Survey (SF-36), to assess quality of life and depression, to determine whether this will impact on the physiological and metabolic management of the disease process and subsequently wound management (Walters *et al.*, 1999).

8.4.2 | "Hands On" Stage

(a) Skin assessment

A number of methods are recommended in the literature to allow the practitioner to make a simple assessment of the diabetic foot. Edmonds and Foster (1999) advocate the simple staging system, which covers the entire spectrum of diabetic foot disease:

Stage 1: normal foot
Stage 2: high-risk foot

Stage 3: ulcerated foot
Stage 4: infected foot
Stage 5: necrotic foot
Stage 6: unsalvageable foot

Changes to the skin can give an indication of the patient's vascular status, neurological status, and ulceration risk and will allow early identification of the presence of bacterial and fungal skin infection. The skin on both legs and feet should be assessed as subtle differences in colour and temperature may become apparent.

Dermatological problems are common in people with diabetes; approximately 30% of diabetic patients will experience skin problems during the course of their disease (Ahmed and Goldstein, 2006). Chapter 3 explores skin changes secondary to diabetes mellitus in greater depth, but it is pertinent within this chapter briefly to discuss the increased risk of infection in diabetic patients.

Skin infections are commonly observed in the foot in individuals with diabetes (Lipsky and Berendt, 2000). Edmonds (2005) suggests that infection alone is rarely a sole factor, but a factor that can complicate diabetic foot ulcers leading to considerable tissue necrosis in the neuropathic and neuroischaemic foot.

Falanga (2005a) suggests a number of reasons why individuals with diabetes mellitus are more prone to infection:

1. Hyperglycaemia has a detrimental effect on the immune system.
2. Tissue hypoxia due to underlying vascular disease.
3. Compressive forces from daily activities such as walking can affect the function of white blood cells involved in the normal immune response.

Infection of diabetic foot ulcers is primarily caused by bacteria, but the effect of fungal infection on diabetic foot ulceration is also recognized as a risk factor for delayed healing in diabetic foot ulcers by Missoni *et al.* (2006). They recommend that routine bacteriological tests should be supplemented with targeted mycologic tests to test for the presence of fungal species in diabetic foot ulcers. Figure 8.2 shows an interdigital ulcer with evidence of bacterial and fungal infection (note the skin condition).

Cutting *et al.* (2005) were involved in identifying criteria for infection in different wound types. Using a Delphi approach, whereby consensus opinion was sought from a multiprofessional team of wound care experts, criteria for identifying infection in the diabetic foot were produced (Table 8.2).

Identification of infection in wounds can be challenging, particularly so in diabetic foot ulcers. Chapter 4 provides a comprehensive guide to the assessment and management of infected wounds.

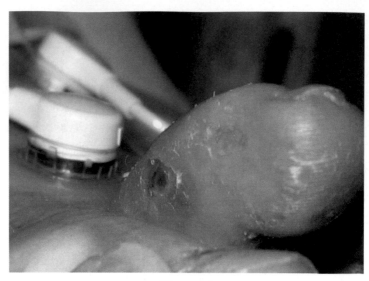

Figure 8.2
Diabetic foot ulcer affected by bacterial and fungal infection

- Cellulitis

- Lymphangitis

- Phlegmon

- Purulent exudate

- Pus/abscess

- Crepitus in the joint

- Erythema

- Increase in exudate volume

- Localized pain in a normally insensate (neuropathic) foot

- Malodour

- Probe to bone

Table 8.2
Criteria for identifying infection in diabetic foot ulcers (Cutting *et al.*, 2005)

? **Consider Walter's ulcers (Figure 8.1) in respect of the criteria suggested by Cutting *et al.* (2005) in Table 8.2. Does the clinical appearance and description indicate the presence of infection?**
Examination of the soiled dressing can also offer clues as to the presence of infection. Walter's dressing was soiled with a blue/green exudate (Figure 8.3). What type of infection does this suggest?

Edmonds (2005) suggests that the classic signs of infection may not always be present in diabetic patients. Only half of infection episodes show signs of infection (Edmonds and Foster, 2006). In the presence of neuropathy and ischaemia signs of infection can be diminished as the normal inflammatory response is impaired. Always remain extra vigilant when assessing the diabetic foot for signs of infection. If the wound is critically colonized or infection is present, refer the patient to the diabetic foot care team who will initiate antimicrobial therapy and/or systemic antibiotics.

(b) Foot deformity

The manifestation of peripheral neuropathy in the diabetic foot is complex. Loss of sensation is a major contributory factor for diabetic foot ulceration. However, Zimny *et al.* (2004) suggest that there is often a complex interplay between multiple factors:

- Limited joint mobility
- Glycosylation of collagen

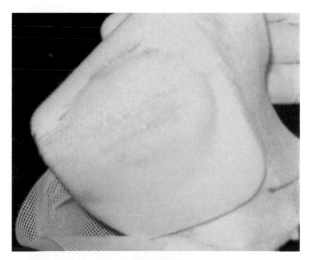

Figure 8.3
Soiled dressing

- Altered foot pressures
- Ethnic background
- Autonomic neuropathy
- Motor neuropathy

Limited joint mobility in the foot is well documented within published literature (Zimny *et al.*, 2004; Ledoux *et al.*, 2005). This is mainly associated with glycosylation of collagen that results in thickening of the skin and periarticular structures: tendons, ligaments and joint capsules (Dinh and Veves, 2005). In the foot limited joint mobility can give rise to elevated plantar pressures, mainly in the forefoot, a prime site for neuropathic ulceration.

There appears to be some ethnic variation in terms of limited joint mobility with patients of Caucasian background having significantly less joint mobility than patients of Afro-Caribbean background (Dinh and Veves, 2005).

Autonomic neuropathy is a common problem in patients with a long duration of diabetes, which can result in loss of vasomotor control to the bones in the feet. If the blood supply to bones is altered this can result in demineralization of bone. This pathological process can cause Charcot's osteopathy, a disease process where the bones in the foot become weak and prone to spontaneous fracture which can give rise to severe deformity. Bony changes are most common at the midfoot (tarsal–metatarsal region of the foot) (Figure 8.4) but can also occur at the ankle (Watkins, 2003).

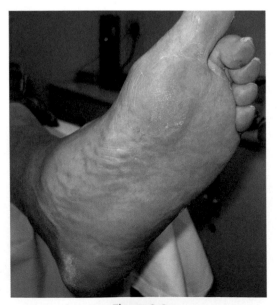

Figure 8.4
Charcot's osteopathy

Motor neuropathy in the diabetic foot can cause muscle weakness and wasting of intrinsic muscles which typically results in clawing of the digits and plantar flexion of the metatarsal heads. These structural changes cause bony prominences which become prime sites of pressure during gait, particularly when coupled with sensory loss (Dinh and Veves, 2005).

(c) Wound characteristics

Accurate assessment of foot ulcers is essential to monitor outcomes and establish treatment effectiveness. Successful management of diabetic foot ulceration relies on effective communication between all members of the multiprofessional team, yet despite the need for practitioners frequently to liaise with one another there are currently no agreed standardized systems for describing diabetic foot ulcers. Macfarlane and Jeffcoate (1998) suggest that the following factors should be considered and documented within patient records to ensure that an accurate account of healing is recorded and legal implications of accurate record keeping are addressed:

- Wound location
- Wound dimensions (height, width, surface area, depth)
- Nature of the wound bed (necrotic/sloughy/granulating/epithelializing)
- Volume of wound exudate (low/moderate/high)
- Consistency of wound exudate (serous/purulent)
- Wound margins (hyperkeratotic/rolled edges/undermined)
- Pain
- Presence of bony sequestrium or foreign bodies
- Presence of infection
- Condition of the peri-wound skin (e.g. macerated/dermatitis)
- State of surrounding skin (e.g. erythema, inflammation)

Wound measurement is an important component of wound assessment that allows baseline measurements to be recorded for future comparison and allows healing times to be monitored and outcomes to be predicted. Accurate assessment of wound dimensions can be challenging in clinical practice; there are many methods that can be employed to measure a wound, ranging from simple techniques, such as linear measurement, through to highly sophisticated computerized systems, which may not be readily available in everyday clinical practice (McIntosh, 2006).

There are a number of wound classification systems in existence, e.g. the Wagner Scale (Boulton *et al.*, 2004), which assesses ulcer depth and the presence of osteomyelitis and gangrene. However, there is no one system that has been accepted universally. Some classification systems are specific to the diabetic foot. Perhaps the most widely recognized classification system employed to classify diabetic foot ulcers is the Texas Classification System (Armstrong *et al.*, 1998), illustrated in Figure 8.5.

STAGE	GRADE			
	0	**1**	**2**	**3**
A	Pre- or post-lesion – intact	Superficial wound	Penetrating to tendon or capsule	Penetrating to bone or joint
B	+ Infection	+ Infection	+ Infection	+ Infection
C	+ Ischaemia	+ Ischaemia	+ Ischaemia	+ Ischaemia
D	+ Infection and ischaemia	+ Infection and ischaemia	+ Infection and ischaemia	+ Infection and ischaemia

Figure 8.5
The University of Texas Classification System (Armstrong *et al.*, 1998)

?   **Considering Walter's ulcers (Figure 8.1), classify the ulcers using the University of Texas Classification System as detailed above.**

(d) Vascular assessment

All individuals with diabetes should receive annual assessment by trained personnel as part of ongoing care (NICE, 2004). This should identify any risk factors and complications, such as neuropathy or vascular disease, that may significantly increase the potential for generation of diabetic foot ulcers (Scottish Intercollegiate Guidelines Network (SIGN), 2001).

An accurate prognosis for healing can be determined by a comprehensive vascular assessment. Hence the staged elements of vascular assessment are:

1. Clinical observation for signs of arterial insufficiency
2. Palpation of foot pulses
3. Doppler assessment
4. Ankle brachial pressure index

1. Clinical observation. The neuroischaemic foot is usually cold to touch and pale or cyanosed. Edmonds and Foster (1999) suggest that as many as 50% of people with diabetes attending a diabetic foot clinic will have neuroischaemic feet. The combination of peripheral vascular disease coupled with neuropathy can prove to be limb threatening for individuals with diabetes (McIntosh and Newton, 2005). It is imperative that practitioners are able to promptly identify

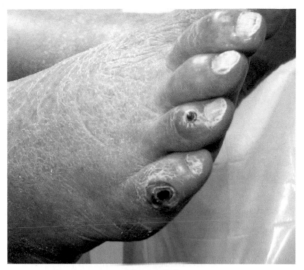

Figure 8.6
The neuroischaemic foot

the neuroischaemic foot and implement management strategies rapidly to prevent adverse outcomes. Neuroischaemic foot ulcers frequently occur on the margins of the foot, on the toes, as in Figure 8.6, and under thickened toenails (subungual ulceration) (Edmonds and Foster, 2006).

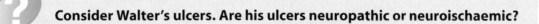

Consider Walter's ulcers. Are his ulcers neuropathic or neuroischaemic?

2. Palpation. Palpation of foot pulses (dorsalis pedis and posterior tibial) is an important aspect of vascular assessment, but the presence or absence of foot pulses should not be used alone as an indicator of the presence or absence of arterial disease (Vowden and Vowden, 2002). Palpation of foot pulses will not provide sufficient information to allow the clinician to make an informed judgement of the patient's vascular status and further tests are often required (Baker *et al.*, 2005a).

3. Doppler assessment. Doppler ultrasound is commonly used in practice to identify the presence or absence of arterial disease in the diabetic foot and is particularly useful for finding nonpalpable foot pulses. Auditory evaluation of Doppler sounds can provide the skilled practitioner with a great deal of information regarding the strength, rhythm and phasicity of the pulse and the extent of arterial disease. However, accurate interpretation of sounds requires a considerable amount of practitioner skill. Vowden and Vowden (2002) further discuss interpretation of Doppler sounds.

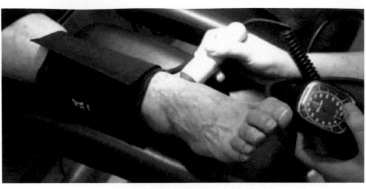

Figure 8.7
Measuring ankle systolic pressure using Doppler ultrasound

4. The ankle brachial pressure index (ABPI). The ankle brachial pressure index is a further clinical adjunct that allows quantification of the vascular status of the diabetic foot. This involves measuring systolic pressures in the upper and lower limbs (Figure 8.7) and calculating a ratio. The ankle brachial pressure index provides an objective measure of severity of vascular disease in the lower limb and can be used to inform wound management decisions, i.e. whether the wound has adequate perfusion for wound healing or whether referral or revascularization is indicated (Marshall, 2004).

A limitation of the ankle brachial pressure index in the prediction of wound healing in diabetic patients is the increased incidence of calcification of lower limb arteries. This can result in falsely high values and more reliable methods are suggested to be toe brachial pressure readings (Vowden and Vowden, 2002; Marshall, 2004) and measurement of transcutaneous oxygen (Kalani *et al.*, 1999; Baker *et al.*, 2005a).

Toe brachial pressure index (TBPI) measurement is similar to the ankle brachial pressure index measurement but involves measuring systolic pressure at the toe where the incidence of calcification is rare.

Measurement of transcutaneous oxygen tension (tcPO2), as seen in Figure 8.8, is a noninvasive, simple method of measuring cutaneous hypoxia, where electrochemical transducers are attached to the skin, allowing segmental readings to be taken from the lower limb and foot, hence identifying the level of arterial disease impacting on wound healing.

Kalani *et al.* (1999) investigated the predictive value of transcutaneous oxygen tension and toe brachial pressure index results for the healing of chronic diabetic foot ulcers. Findings indicate that transcutaneous oxygen tension is a better predictor for ulcer healing than the toe brachial pressure index in diabetic patients with chronic foot ulcers and that the probability of ulcer healing is low when transcutaneous oxygen tension is <25 mmHg, a figure corroborated by Frykberg *et al.* (2006). However, transcutaneous oxygen tension measurements may be falsely low in the presence

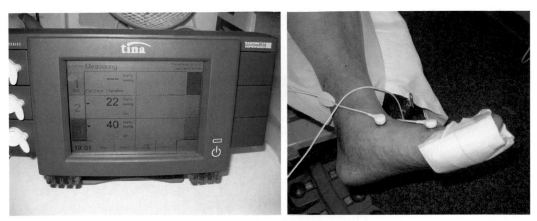

Figure 8.8
Measuring transcutaneous oxygen tension

of infection, as this impairs oxygen diffusion in the neuroischaemic foot. After the infection has been resolved, values may rise even without vascular intervention (Edmonds, 2005).

When vascular assessment indicates ischaemia a rapid referral should be made to the vascular team as revascularization will be required for wound healing.

(e) Neurological assessment

Reports indicate that approximately 50 % of people who present at diabetic foot clinics have peripheral neuropathy (Edmonds and Foster, 1999). When assessing the neurological status in individuals with diabetes clinical observation is essential. Classic visual changes may be observed in the lower limbs and feet which are typical of sensory, autonomic and/or motor neuropathy.

The clinical presentation of sensory neuropathy is complex. The patient may present with complete sensory loss or they may experience neuropathic pain. Neuropathic pain typically presents as a burning pain in the foot or leg, frequently at night. This should not be confused with nocturnal ischaemic pain, which is relieved by movement; painful neuropathy is not relieved by rest. Hence, neuropathic pain can be debilitating for the individual and pharmacological intervention may often be required to obtain relief. Referral should be made to the diabetologist for further assessment as good glycaemic control may also help reduce symptoms.

Autonomic neuropathy can cause decreased activity of sweat glands in the feet, visibly distended veins and dry skin (anhydrosis), which increases the risk of skin fissures (Dinh and Veves, 2005). The foot tends to be warm, pink in colour, as seen in Figure 8.9, with palpable foot pulses.

Motor neuropathy in the foot can cause wasting of small intrinsic muscles. This leads to characteristic structural changes in the diabetic foot: clawing of toes and prominent metatarsal heads (Figure 8.9). When this is coupled with sensory loss these areas become prime sites of tissue damage.

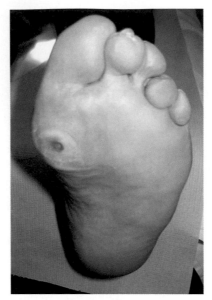

Figure 8.9
Digital deformity and prominence of the first metatarsal with resultant ulceration

Neuropathic foot ulcers primarily occur on the plantar aspect of the foot (sole of the foot) under the metatarsal heads, as in Figure 8.9, or on the toes, and are associated with repetitive mechanical forces. Skin lesions, such as a callus or corns, can also cause high plantar pressures. Edmonds and Foster (2006) describe a callus as a pre-ulcerative lesion that must be managed appropriately by a podiatrist. If calluses are neglected haematomas can form underneath the hardened skin which can lead to tissue necrosis and ulceration.

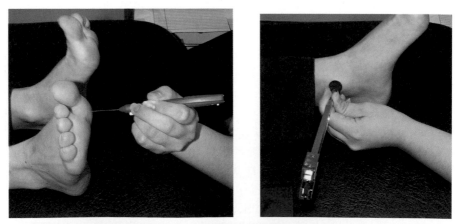

Figure 8.10
Testing neurological status with (a) a 10 g monofilament and (b) a 128 Hz tuning fork

Quantifying the neurological status of individuals presenting with diabetic foot ulceration allows accurate diagnosis of the wound aetiology. A number of methods are recommended in practice to test for sensory loss. The use of 10 gram monofilaments (Figure 8.10(a)) to detect light touch (NICE, 2004) and 128 Hz tuning forks (Figure 8.10(b)) or a neurosthesiometer to assess vibration perception are said to be the most reliable methods in practice (Baker *et al.*, 2005b).

> **Consider the information provided in Walter's case study. What findings might be expected from neurological assessment?**

8.5 | Wound Management Model for Diabetic Foot Ulcers

This model has two recommended stages which should be sequenced as follows:

1. The *"hands off"* stage involves verbal *information giving* consisting of:

   (a) Patient-centred approach
   (b) Education/prevention
   (c) Multiprofessional team
   (d) Nutritional factors
   (e) Social factors

2. The *"hands on"* stage involves *physical intervention* for:

   (a) Wound bed preparation
   (b) Management of infection
   (c) Antimicrobials
   (d) Offloading diabetic foot ulcers
   (e) Charcot's osteopathy
   (f) Future wound healing

8.5.1 | *"Hands Off"* Stage

(a) Patient-centred approach

The patient must remain central to any wound care plan if positive outcomes are to be achieved. Diabetes care providers should ensure that they manage the patient holistically, taking into account the patient's feelings associated with living with a chronic disease and foot ulceration. Previous studies have investigated diabetic patients' perceptions of the care they receive (Callaghan and Williams, 1994; Ribu and Wahl, 2004). Findings suggest that patients prefer a patient-centred approach from carers who are highly knowledgeable and skilled and show an interest in them and value them as an individual.

(b) Management of education/prevention of wounds

The *National Service Framework for Diabetes* recommends structured education to improve patients' knowledge and understanding of their condition, enabling them to undertake more effective self-care (DH, 2001). In terms of foot health this would focus on the patient and practitioner partnership in attempting to reduce the factors that may contribute to the generation and chronicity of diabetic foot ulcers.

A number of programmes have been introduced to educate and encourage those living with diabetes to manage their own diabetes (including foot care) independently:

* The expert patient programme
* DAFNE (dose adjustment for normal eating) programme for type 1 diabetes (DAFNE Study Group, 2002)
* DESMOND (diabetes education and self-management for ongoing and newly diagnosed) programme for type 2 diabetes (DESMOND collaborative, 2002)

For health care professionals, supporting good self-care is an essential element of diabetes care and as part of a wound care package can facilitate successful clinical outcomes in diabetic foot ulcer management.

Care planning with patients who have diabetic foot ulcers should be an inclusive process. The process of agreeing a wound care plan enables a patient to be actively involved in deciding how their wound will be managed.

> **Consider Walter's case. How can members of the multiprofessional team work together to identify risk factors for delayed wound healing and target educational strategies to improve the outcome in this case?**

(c) Multiprofessional team in wound care

Individuals living with diabetes will require the support of numerous health care professionals at differing stages of the condition: e.g. at the first diagnosis there is an immediate need to obtain good metabolic control (7 mmol/L). For medium- and long-term diabetes management, maintaining good metabolic control can help reduce or eliminate the risk of complications, which are often aetiological factors in the genesis of diabetic foot ulcers.

The need for a multiprofessional team approach in diabetes care is clearly outlined within section 12 of the *National Service Framework for Diabetes* (DH, 2001) and within the NICE (2004) and SIGN (2001) guidelines. A report by the DH (2005), *Improving Diabetes Services – The NSF Two Years On,* reiterates the principles of the NSF as (a) patient-centred care, (b) working together and (c) support for service delivery. These principles should ensure that people with diabetes receive integrated health care with effective communication between health care providers in order to achieve optimal individualized care.

Multiprofessional involvement is essential in diabetic foot ulcer management as it enables:

- Mechanical control of foot function and offloading of pressure with provision of specialist footwear and insoles. Podiatrists and orthotists will play a crucial role in the implementation of offloading strategies
- Wound control, with the use of managed wound dressing products appropriate to the stage of the wound. Nurses and podiatrists must liaise regarding dressing choice and frequency of dressing change.
- Microbiological control, with the use of wound dressing products, superficial and deep wound swabbing and the provision of antibiotic therapy. All members of the multiprofessional team must liaise with the diabetologist.
- Vascular control, staged via provision of pharamacological agents, lifestyle changes such as smoking cessation, increased activity, revascularization and surgery.
- Metabolic control: self-monitoring and maintenance of glucose levels within narrow parameters of good control.
- Educational control using a patient-centred approach and considering social factors, diet and behaviour (Edmonds *et al.*, 2004a). All members of the multiprofessional team will be involved in the delivery of patient education.

(d) Management of nutritional factors in wound care
A number of programmes have been reported that focus on management of glycaemic levels in order to reduce the onset and effects of long-term complications that may adversely affect wound healing.

With regards to wound healing Russell (2001) identifies key nutritional elements:

1. Glucose for generating deposition of new tissue
2. Fatty acids for generation of new cell structure
3. Protein for collagen formation
4. Vitamin C for development of healthy granulation tissue

Krook *et al.* (2003) implemented a lifestyle modification programme in order to assess the benefits on glycaemic control for 304 patients with type 2 diabetes. Exercise training, nutrition and stress management were offered and the conclusions were a significant reduction in glycaemic and blood pressure levels. High glucose levels and uncontrolled hypertension may significantly delay healing; hence this is clinically valuable in wound care management.

Dhindsa *et al.* (2003) implemented a very low calorie diet on cardiovascular and metabolic variables in a group of obese type 2 diabetic patients. A lack of control group limits the conclusions, but some positive indicators were achieved in terms of reducing the cardiovascular and metabolic variables by reducing the body mass index. Reducing the body mass index can have positive effects on reducing overall lipid levels, which may impact positively on halting the progression of peripheral vascular disease and therefore improve wound healing times in diabetic foot ulcer management.

A dietician can provide specific dietary advice for individuals with diabetic foot ulcers that will take into account individual lifestyle and cultural preferences (Diabetes UK, 2006).

(e) Management of social factors in wound care

Diabetes is a psychologically and behaviourally demanding disease (Delamater *et al.*, 2001) and may therefore impact on the management of diabetic foot ulcers.

Research suggests that gender may play a part in these social factors. Lidfeldt *et al.* (2005) found that women with existing IFG (impaired fasting glucose) living alone had a 2.6-fold increased chance of developing type 2 diabetes. In addition, psychosocial factors such as low decision latitude at work and low sense of coherence was associated with type 2 diabetes in women. Depression is more common in patients with chronic diseases such as diabetes and this is associated with worse glycaemic control and health complications and decreased quality of life. Explanations from the literature identify a number of socially related risk factors such as smoking, lifestyle, dietary factors and alcohol intake between the genders, which should be considered for successful management of diabetic foot ulcers.

Delamater *et al.* (2001) suggest that methods of effective intervention should be established to improve psychosocial therapies, i.e. encouraging self-management skills and patient empowerment. Patients should be instructed on how to undertake their own foot care safely and manage their own diabetes, where possible. In Walter's case his wife is eager to assist Walter. Advice can therefore be targeted at both Walter and his wife.

8.5.2 | "Hands On" Stage

This section will explore the use of clinical guidelines and the best available evidence to generate a thorough systematic protocol-based approach. The use of a protocol-based approach to the management of diabetic foot ulcersis is not a new concept; in fact Brem *et al.* (2004) suggested the following protocol for patients with diabetic foot ulcers:

1. Measurement of the wound by planimetry
2. Optimal glucose control
3. Surgical debridement of all hyperkeratotic, infected and nonviable tissue
4. Systemic antibiotics for deep infection, drainage and cellulitis

5. Offloading
6. Moist wound environment
7. Treatment with growth factors and/or cellular therapy if the wound is not healing after 2 weeks with this protocol

However, point 7, treatment with growth factors, has significant cost implications and may not be readily accessible in everyday practice.

For health care professionals development of protocols should outline a realistic clinical pathway for diabetic foot ulcer management considering locality and resources covering initial diagnosis, identification of clinical action points, key advice, multiprofessional consultation and evaluation, and referral mechanisms. These measures should ensure clear and auditable standards of care are offered when managing diabetes-related foot ulceration.

A suggested systematic protocol-based approach to the management of diabetic foot ulcers has been identified in Figure 8.11.

The "Hands on" stage involves the following:

(a) Wound bed preparation

The wound bed preparation model has been suggested as a tool to assist the healing of chronic wounds, including diabetic foot ulcers. This model has the suggested acronym "TIME" to heal.

Falanga (2004) suggests that the TIME framework aims to optimize the local wound environment for healing by addressing four key areas:

Tissue management. Assess the amount of viable and nonviable tissue. Necrotic tissue and slough can delay wound healing so wound debridement should be undertaken to facilitate healing (Watret, 2005).

Inflammation and infection control. Diabetic foot ulcers are prone to bacterial and fungal infection. Steps should be taken to minimize infection risk.

Moisture balance. Exudate assessment is an important aspect of wound assessment to ensure that the moisture balance is achieved.

Epithelial (edge) advancement to achieve closure of diabetic foot ulcers can be delayed due to the presence of callus. Frequent debridement by a skilled practitioner is essential to promote healing (Watret, 2005).

Wound debridement is an essential aspect of diabetic foot ulcer management that facilitates wound healing (Edmonds *et al.*, 2004b). Sharp debridement, by a skilled practitioner as seen in Figure 8.12, serves many functions:

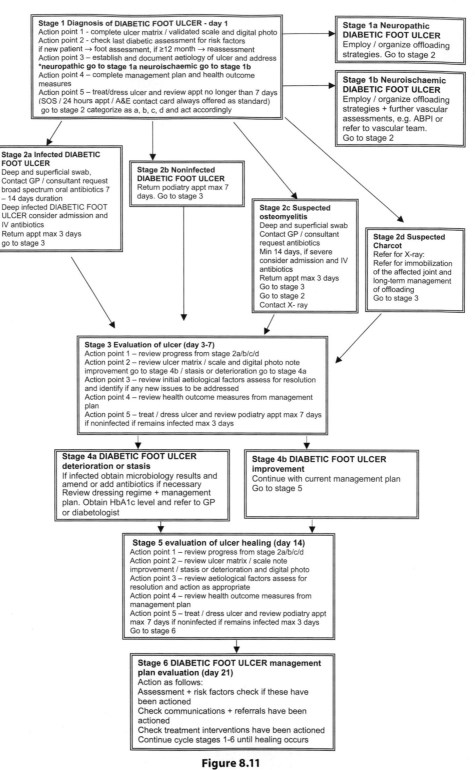

Figure 8.11
Suggested protocol for diabetic foot ulcer management

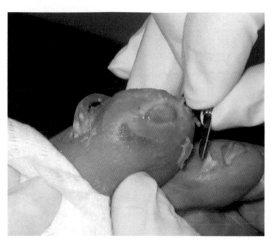

Figure 8.12
Sharp debridement of a diabetic foot ulcer

- Removes callus from the wound periphery to reveal the true extent of the wound margins
- Removes dead or devitalized tissue from the wound bed
- Reduces pressure on the wound bed
- Facilitates drainage
- Stimulates healing

There are a number of factors that should be considered prior to undertaking sharp debridement on the diabetic foot. It is imperative that sharp debridement is only undertaken by practitioners who have received specific training in the technique. It is also essential to distinguish correctly between the neuropathic foot and the neuroischaemic foot. In the presence of a good blood supply neuropathic ulcers can undergo aggressive debridement to healthy, bleeding tissue. However, while it is recognized that neuroischaemic ulcers benefit from the removal of nonviable tissue, extreme caution must be exercised during sharp debridement to avoid trauma to viable tissue (Edmonds *et al.*, 2004b).

Although sharp debridement is generally considered to be the gold standard treatment for diabetic foot ulcers (Leaper, 2002; Edmonds *et al.*, 2004b) there may be occasions when it is not appropriate. If the foot is painful, particularly when wounds are primarily due to ischaemia, the patient may not tolerate sharp debridement and alternative methods should be considered.

Larvae therapy is one such alternative that has been suggested by Edmonds *et al.* (2004b). Although there is limited evidence from large prospective clinical trials to establish the effectiveness of larvae therapy for diabetic foot ulcers, Sherman (2003) undertook a small study (*n*=18) on nonhealing diabetic foot ulcers compared to conventional treatment (described only as surgical or nonsurgical intervention). Findings suggest wounds treated with larvae were better debrided, showed hastened growth of granulation tissue and had greater healing times, but in the absence of a standardized control group the reliability of these findings is questionable. In a climate of evidence-based practice further quality randomized controlled studies are warranted to ascertain the clinical effectiveness of larvae therapy for diabetic foot ulcer management.

Moisture balance is essential to promote healing and protect the peri-wound tissues from maceration. The concept of moist wound healing has long been established (Winter, 1962), but despite a plethora of modern moist dressings there is currently no evidence to suggest that any one dressing is superior for diabetic foot ulcers. Dressing selection will depend on a number of factors:

- Volume of wound exudate and the ability of the dressing to absorb fluid
- Condition of the surrounding skin
- Nonadherent properties of the dressing
- Patient-related factors such as mobility levels, footwear and desire to bathe should be considered
- Bacterial burden
- Local wound care formularies

(b) Management of infection in the diabetic foot

Infection in the diabetic foot can spread rapidly, resulting in devastating consequences. Infection is implicated as a causative factor for major amputation (Edmonds, 2005). The diabetic patient presenting with a foot infection must be assessed promptly and managed aggressively. Cavanagh *et al.* (2005) suggest that the initial treatment should include wound cleansing, debridement of nonviable tissue and probing, with a blunt sterile instrument, to ascertain depth and identify foreign bodies or exposed bone. If a sterile probe inserted into the wound reaches bone, osteomyelitis (bone infection) is indicated. Figure 8.13 shows a diabetic foot ulcer on the medial aspect of the first metatarsophalangeal joint. On probing this wound exposed bone was felt. If osteomyelitis is suspected, plain X-rays can assist diagnosis, but initially reports may prove normal and evidence of

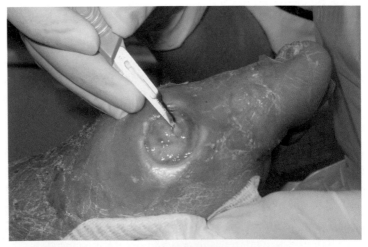

Figure 8.13
Diabetic foot ulcer with osteomyelitis

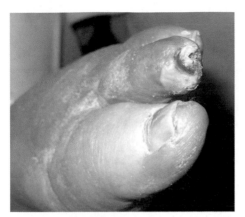

Figure 8.14
Osteomyelitis of the digit

osteomyelitis may not be apparent for 14 days (Edmonds *et al.*, 2004b). Figure 8.14 illustrates osteomyelitis in a digit characterized by a classic sausage toe appearance.

(c) Use of antimicrobials for diabetic foot ulcers

With the emergence of antibiotic resistant strains of bacteria a variety of modern wound dressings
have been developed that claim to restore the bacterial burden of the wound to acceptable levels
while promoting wound healing. Silver, iodine and honey impregnated dressings are commercially
available antimicrobial dressings.

Silver has been shown to be an effective antimicrobial, due to its ability to bind to bacterial DNA,
reducing their ability to replicate (Cooper, 2004). Silver impregnated dressings are widely used
in clinical practice to manage diabetic foot ulcers. However, a Cochrane review on the use of
silver dressings for treating diabetic foot ulcers revealed that there are currently no randomized
or controlled trials that evaluate their clinical effectiveness (Bergin and Wraight, 2006). A systematic review of the evidence for antimicrobial interventions for diabetic foot ulcers generally
concluded that the current evidence base is too weak to recommend any particular antimicrobial
agent (Nelson *et al.*, 2006).

Edmonds *et al.*, (2004a) stress that systemic antibiotic therapy is always indicated if the patient
shows signs of cellulitis, lymphangitis and osteomyelitis. Topical antimicrobial therapy alone will
not suffice in the management of cellulitis, lymphangitis and osteomyelitis; however, they may be
used in conjunction with systemic therapy. Lipsky and Berendt (2000) suggest that antibiotics are
usually selected empirically initially and then modified depending on results of culture and sensitivity tests. Therefore, if infection is suspected swabs should be taken to identify the infecting
organism, as suggested in Figure 8.11, stage 2a, of the suggested protocol for diabetic foot ulcer
management. In the case of severe infection the patient will require urgent hospital admission
for intravenous (IV) antibiotics. On admission the foot should be urgently assessed to ascertain
whether surgical drainage and debridement is required (Edmonds, 2005).

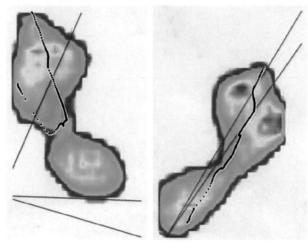

Figure 8.15
Elevated foot pressures

It is imperative that all members of the diabetes foot care team work collaboratively when managing an infected diabetic foot ulcer in order to promote a positive clinical outcome.

(d) Offloading strategies for diabetic foot ulcers

Due to the effects of sensory, motor and autonomic neuropathy, the diabetic foot is often subject to elevated plantar pressures. This can be a contributory factor to the development of diabetic foot ulceration and can delay wound healing if left unaddressed. Figure 8.15 illustrates elevated plantar pressures over the forefoot of a diabetic patient (the red areas illustrate areas of high plantar pressure).

Standard wound management models for diabetic foot ulcer management therefore include aggressive pressure offloading strategies (Marston, 2004), as highlighted in Figure 8.11, stages 1a and 1b, of the suggested protocol for diabetic foot ulcer management.

Armstrong *et al.* (2005) undertook a randomized controlled trial investigating the effectiveness of different offloading strategies for diabetic foot ulcers. The total contact cast healed a higher proportion of diabetic foot ulcers in a shorter time than removable cast walkers and half-shoes. Findings suggest that total contact casts reduce pressure at the site of ulceration by 84–92% and therefore the total contact cast has been suggested as the gold standard in pressure reduction.

However, this form of offloading may not be appropriate for all patients with foot ulceration. In the presence of ischaemia and/or infection the total contact cast may be contraindicated and an alternative strategy that allows regular assessment of the wound should be considered (McIntosh, 2006). Several removable devices are available: removable walkers (Figure 8.16), half shoes, simple insoles, total contact insoles, temporary footwear with forefoot or rearfoot adaptations (such as Darco Heelwedge shoes (Figure 8.17)), felt padding (Figure 8.18) and the use of crutches or wheelchairs.

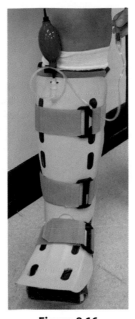

Figure 8.16
Removable walker

? Offloading foot ulcers are often challenging and options must be explored with the patient. Walter felt he could not manage with a removable device and due to the presence of infection the total contact cast was not appropriate in this instance. Following discussion with Walter and his wife, felt padding was applied to his foot (Figure 8.18) and a temporary Darco boot was provided to redistribute pressure from the ulcers.

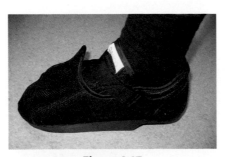

Figure 8.17
Darco Heelwedge shoe

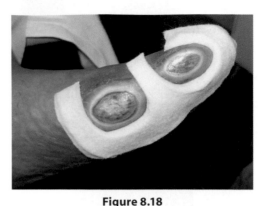

Figure 8.18
Felt padding was applied to Walter's foot to redistribute pressure from the two areas of ulceration

Zimny *et al.* (2003) evaluated the effects of felted foam on wound healing in neuropathic diabetic foot ulcers compared to standard offloading (half-shoe). Findings suggest that felted foam is at least as effective as half-shoes and therefore is a useful alternative, especially when other offloading devices are not deemed suitable, as in Walter's case.

As Walter's wounds showed signs of infection, broad-spectrum antibiotics were initiated and a topical silver impregnated hydrofiber® dressing was applied (Figure 8.19).

Unfortunately, a major disadvantage of removable devices is reliance on patient compliance. Armstrong *et al.* (2003) explored activity patterns of patients with diabetic foot ulceration. Findings suggest that patients issued with removable pressure-relieving modalities only use these devices for a minority of steps taken each day. One factor practitioners should consider is the fact that neuropathic patients cannot feel pain and are therefore often reluctant to curtail their activities and so do not comply with pressure-relieving devices (McIntosh, 2006).

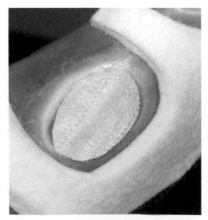

Figure 8.19
Application of a silver-impregnated dressing on Walter's ulcer

Therapeutic footwear can also act as a useful adjunct for healing diabetic foot ulceration. Maciejewski *et al.* (2004) reviewed current evidence for the effectiveness of therapeutic shoes in preventing diabetic foot ulcers and found that several studies reported statistically significant protective benefits from therapeutic footwear. However, therapeutic footwear used alone will not provide sufficient pressure relief and they should therefore be used in conjunction with pressure-relieving insoles for the management of foot ulceration.

All patients presenting with diabetic foot ulcers should be assessed by a member of the diabetes foot care team for provision of a pressure-relieving modality tailored to meet the needs of the individual.

(e) Management of the Charcot foot

The Charcot joint is often reported as a gradual and destructive manifestation of neurosensory damage in the patient with diabetes (Shapiro *et al.*, 1998). The development of the Charcot changes in the diabetic foot can increase the likelihood of developing deformity, increased risk of skin breakdown and lower limb amputation (Sinacore, 1998). Consequently, it is common for practitioners to have to manage a diabetic foot ulcer (Figure 8.20), or pre-ulcerative changes (Figure 8.21) and Charcot foot in combination.

Therefore, management of the Charcot foot and its associated complications, such as diabetic foot ulceration, is either directed at partial weight-bearing strategies, offloading high-pressure areas or employment of complete immobilization techniques, as highlighted in Figure 8.11, stage 2d, of the suggested protocol for diabetic foot ulcer management.

Exact intervention is often influenced by:

1. Stage of development of Charcot
2. Complications such as the presence of ulceration
3. In the absence of a foot ulcer instigation of offloading measures to prevent their occurrence

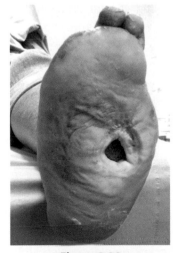

Figure 8.20
Charcot foot with plantar ulceration

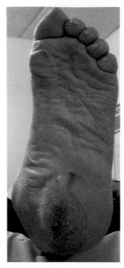

Figure 8.21
Charcot foot with pre-ulcerative lesion on the heel secondary to pressure

(f) The future of diabetic foot ulcer management

As the science of wound healing and the identification of the critical components of the healing process are further understood, advanced therapeutic products are constantly evolving (Falanga, 2005b).

Negative pressure wound therapy has emerged as a treatment for complex wounds. It is thought that negative pressure promotes healing by accelerating wound debridement, removing excess fluid that can inhibit wound healing, decreasing localized oedema and increasing blood flow (Thomas, 2001).

Evidence from randomized controlled clinical trials supports the use of negative pressure wound therapy for diabetic foot ulcers (McCallon *et al.*, 2000; Armstrong and Lavery, 2005). Armstrong and Lavery (2005) undertook a large multicentre study to investigate whether negative pressure wound therapy (VAC) improves the proportion and rate of wound healing after partial diabetic foot amputation. Control patients received standard moist wound care according to consensus guidelines. Findings demonstrate that more patients healed in the negative pressure wound therapy group (56%) than in the control group (39%), with the rate of wound healing faster in the negative pressure wound therapy group. Although research is ongoing it has been suggested that negative pressure has a significant role to play in wound care (Banwell and Teot, 2003).

Other newer initiatives for managing diabetic foot ulcers include active treatment modalities such as topical application of growth factors and living human skin equivalent (Marston, 2004). A large multicentre study evaluated the effect of platelet-derived growth factors (PDGF) on the healing of neuropathic diabetic foot ulcers. Results suggest that daily application of PDGF increased healing rates when compared to placebo (Steed, 2006). Currently these treatments are costly and further research is needed to develop a rational strategy for the effective use of such products before they can be introduced into standard practice (Falanga, 2005b).

8.6 | Case Scenario Revisited

Consider the initial questions posed:

1. **How was this ulcer caused?**

   The cause of this ulcer was multifactorial; the underlying aetiology of the wound was a combination of sensory neuropathy and ischaemia. The cause of the ulcer was identified as mechanical forces during ambulation. The patient had recently purchased new foot-wear. Pressure and friction from new shoes during his daily activities had caused a blister which rapidly ulcerated.

2. **What assessments should be undertaken before implementing a management plan?**

   Using the suggested assessment model for diabetic foot ulcers, the assessment process was split into two sections: the "hands off" and "hands on" stages.

   Medical history, medication, social factors and nutritional factors were considered to assist in identifying wound aetiology. The patient was unable to feel pain, indicative of sensory neuropathy. He has a history of ischaemic heart disease suggestive of the possibility of peripheral arterial disease. His diabetes control is currently unstable, increasing ulcer risk and delayed healing.

   The "hands on" stage involved assessing the condition of the skin, the presence of deformity, wound characteristics and vascular and neurological assessments. Assessment findings confirmed sensory deficit and a reduced arterial supply to the feet and lower limbs.

3. **Which management strategies are the most appropriate for this case?**

   The suggested protocol for diabetic foot ulcer management was used to ensure a systematic approach to wound assessment. At the initial consultation sharp debridement of dead and devitalized tissue was undertaken by a podiatrist. Due to the presence of purulent exudate, green/blue exudate on the soiled dressing (Figure 8.3) and localized erythema around the wound margins infection (Figure 8.1). *Pseudomonas* infection was suspected. Swabs were taken to identify the infecting organisms and broad-spectrum antibiotics were initiated. To control moisture balance and prevent maceration of the surrounding tissues and offer an antimicrobial role, a silver-impregnated Hydrofiber dressing was applied. Due to the presence of infection and ischaemia the total contact cast was contraindicated. Felt padding was applied (Figure 8.16) and a Darco shoe was issued. Foot health education was provided and a review appointment was made for two days later.

4. **Who should be involved in this patient's care?**

   Management of diabetic foot ulcers requires a team approach. Central to the team is the patient, Walter. The diabetologist will assume overall care for Walter, addressing glycaemic control and microbiological control to manage infection. The diabetes specialist nurse will assist in the management of glycaemic control and nutritional status as well as working collaboratively with specialist podiatrists to provide optimum wound care. Podiatrists and orthotists will be involved to assess the mechanics of the foot and implement offloading strategies and footwear advice. Community nurses and podiatrists will be involved to provide regular wound dressings. Walter and his wife are pivotal to successful treatment and care must be tailored to meet their needs. Walter's wife was initially concerned regarding Walter's lack of care. This largely stemmed from the fact that Walter's glycaemic control was poor and she was frustrated with his new treatment regime. Once this had been discussed and she had a better understanding her initial concerns were reduced.

? Reflection

Take time to reflect upon your learning from this chapter. Ask yourself:

1. **What knowledge did I possess prior to reading this chapter?**

2. **How has my knowledge developed?**

3. **How will I implement this into my future practice?**

References

Agardh, E.E., Ahlbom, A. and Andersson, T. (2004) Explanations of socioeconomic differences in excess risk of type 2 diabetes in Swedish men and women. *Diabetes Care*, **27**(3), 716–21.

Ahmed, I. and Goldstein, B. (2006) Diabetes mellitus. *Clinics in Dermatology*, **24**(4), 237–46.

Armstrong, D.G. and Lavery, L.A. (2005) Negative pressure wound therapy after partial diabetic foot amputation: a multicentre, randomised controlled trial. *The Lancet*, **366**, 1704–10.

Armstrong, D.G., Lavery, L.A. and Harkless, L.B. (1998) Validation of a diabetic wound classification system. *Diabetes Care*, **21**(5), 855–59.

Armstrong, D.G., Lavery, L.A. and Kimbriel, H.R. (2003) Activity patterns of patients with diabetic foot ulceration. *Diabetes Care*, **9**, 2595–7.

Armstrong, D.G., Lavery, L.A., Wu, S. *et al*. (2005) Evaluation of removable and irremovable cast walkers in the healing of diabetic foot wounds. *Diabetes Care*, **28**(3), 551–4.

Baker, N., Murali-Krishnan, S. and Fowler, D. (2005a) A user's guide to foot screening. Part 2: peripheral arterial disease. *The Diabetic Foot*, **8**(2), 58–70.

Baker, N., Murali-Krishnan, S. and Rayman, G. (2005b) A user's guide to foot screening. Part 1: peripheral neuropathy. *The Diabetic Foot*, **8**(1), 28–37.

Banwell, P. and Teot, L. (2003) Topical negative pressure (TNP): the evolution of a novel wound therapy. *Journal of Wound Care*, **12**(1), 22–8.

Bergin, S.M. and Wraight, P. (2006) Silver based wound dressings and topical agents for treating diabetic foot ulcers. *The Cochrane Database of Systematic Reviews*, Issue 1, Article No. CD005082. pub2. DOI: 1002/14651858 CD005082.pub2.

Boulton, A.J.M., Connor, H. and Cavanagh, P.R. (2004) *The Foot in Diabetes*, 3rd edn, John Wiley and Sons, Ltd, Chichester, pp. 66.

Brem, H., Sheenan, M. and Boulton, A. (2004) Protocol for treatment of diabetic foot ulcers. *American Journal of Surgery*, **187**(5), Suppl. 1, 1–10.

Callaghan, D. and Williams, A. (1994) Living with diabetes: issues for nursing practice. *Journal of Advanced Nursing*, **20**(1), 132–9.

Cavanagh, P.R., Lipsky, B.A., Bradbury, A.W. *et al*. (2005) Treatment for diabetic foot ulcers. *The Lancet*, **366**, 1725–35.

Cooper, R. (2004) A review of the evidence for the use of topical anti-microbial agents in wound care, in *World Wide Wounds* (online), Available at: http://www.worldwidewounds.com/2004/february/cooper/Topical-Antimicrobial-Agents.html, Accessed 20 October 2006.

Cutting, K.F., White, R.J., Mahoney, P. *et al*. (2005) Understanding wound infection, in *Identifying Criteria for Wound Infection*, European Wound Management Association (EWMA) Position Document, MEP Ltd, London, pp. 2–5.

DAFNE Study Group (2002) Training in flexible, intensive insulin management to enable dietary freedom in people with type 1 diabetes: dose adjustment for normal eating (DAFNE) randomised controlled trial. *British Medical Journal*, 2002, **325**, 746.

Delamater, A.M., Jacobson, A.M., Anderson, B. *et al*. (2001) Psychosocial therapies in diabetes. *Diabetes Care*, **24**, 1286–92.

Department of Health (2001) *National Service Framework for Diabetes: Standards*, Department of Health (online), Available at: `http://www.dh.gov.uk/PublicationsAndStatistics/Publications/PublicationsPolicyAndGuidance/PublicationsPolicyAndGuidanceArticle/fs/en?CONTENT_ID=4002951andchk=09Kkz1`, Last accessed 09 September 2006.

Department of Health (2005) *Improving diabetes Services – The NSF two years on* (online), Available at: `http://www.dh.gov.uk/prod_consum_dh/groups/dh_digitalassets/wdh/wen/documents/digetalasset/dh_4`, Last accessed 27 June 2007.

Department of Health (2006) Diabetes type 2 lipid management, in *Prodigy Knowledge* (online), Available at: `http://www.prodigy.nhs.uk/diabetes_type_2_lipid_management`, Last accessed 29 September 2006.

DESMOND Collaborative (2002) Desmondweb (online), Available at: `http://www.desmond-project.org.uk/`, Last accessed 22 October 2006.

Dhindsa, P., Scott, A.R. and Donnelly, R. (2003) Metabolic and cardiovascular effects of very low calorie diet therapy in obese patients with type 2 diabetes in secondary failure; outcomes after 1 year. *Diabetic Medicine*, **20**, 319–24.

Diabetes Nursing Strategy Group (2005) *An Integrated Career and Competency Framework for Diabetes Nursing* (online), Available at: `http://www.diabetesnurse.org.uk/Downloads/Competency-Framework.pdf`, Last accessed 27 September 2006.

Diabetes UK (2006) *Eating Well* (online), Available at: `http://www.diabetes.org.uk/Guidediabetes/Treatment__your_health/Eating_Well/`, Last accessed 20 October 2006.

Dinh, T.L. and Veves, A. (2005) A review of the mechanisms implicated in the pathogenesis of the diabetic foot. *Lower Extremity Wounds*, **4**(3), 154–9.

Edmonds, M. (2005) Infection in the neuroischaemic foot. *Lower Extremity Wounds*, **4**(3), 145–53.

Edmonds, M. and Foster, A. (1999) *Managing the Diabetic Foot* (ed. M. Edmonds), Blackwell Science, Oxford.

Edmonds, M. and Foster, A.V.M. (2006) ABC of wound healing diabetic foot ulcers. *British Medical Journal*, **332**, 407–10.

Edmonds, M., Foster, A. and Sanders, L. (2004a) *A Practical Manual of Diabetic Foot Care*, Blackwell Publishing, London.

Edmonds, M., Foster, A.V.M. and Vowden, P. (2004b) Wound bed preparation for diabetic foot ulcers, in *Wound Bed Preparation in Practice*, European Wound Management Association (EWMA) Position Document, MEP Ltd, London.

Falanga, V. (2004) Wound bed preparation: science applied to practice, in *Wound Bed Preparation*, European Wound Management Association (EWMA) Position Document, MEP Ltd, London, pp. 2–5.

Falanga, V. (2005a) Wound healing and its impairment in the diabetic foot. *The Lancet*, **366**, 1736–43.

Falanga, V. (2005b) Advanced treatments for non-healing chronic wounds, in *World Wide Wounds* (online), Available at: http://www.worldwidewounds.com/2005/april/Falanga/Advanced-Treatments-Chronic-Wounds.html, Accessed 20 October 2006.

Frykberg, R.G., Zgonis, T., Armstrong, D.G. *et al.* (2006) Diabetic foot disorders: a clinical practice guideline. *The Journal of Foot and Ankle Surgery*, **45**(5), Suppl., 1–65.

Himes, D. (1999) Protein-calorie malnutrition and involuntary weight loss: the role of aggressive nutritional intervention in wound healing. *Osteomyelitis and Wound Management*, **45**(3), 46–51, 54–5.

International Working Group on the Diabetic Foot (1999) International Consensus on the Diabetic Foot, International Working Group on the Diabetic Foot, Amsterdam, The Netherlands.

Kalani, M., Brismar, K., Fagrell, B. *et al.* (1999) Transcutaneous oxygen tension and toe blood pressure as predictors for outcome of diabetic foot ulcers. *Diabetes Care*, **22**(1), 147–51.

Katon, W., Unutzer, J., Fan, M.Y. *et al.* (2006) Cost effectiveness and net benefit of enhanced treatment of depression for older adults with diabetes and depression. *Diabetes Care*, **29**(2), 265–70.

Krook, A., Holm, I., Pettersson, S. *et al.* (2003) Reduction of risk factors following lifestyle modification programme in subjects with type 2 (non-insulin dependent) diabetes mellitus. *Clinical Physiology and Functional Imaging*, **23**(1), 21–30.

Leaper, D. (2002) Sharp technique for wound debridement in *World Wide Wounds* (online), Available at: http://www.worldwidewounds.com/2002/december/Leaper/Sharp-Debridement.html, Last accessed 22 October 2006.

Ledoux, W.R., Shofer, J.B., Smith, D.G., *et al.* (2005) Relationship between foot type, foot deformity, and ulcer occurrence in the high-risk diabetic foot. *Journal of Rehabilitation Research and Development*, **42**(5), 665–72.

Lidfeldt, J., Nerbrand, C., Samsioe, G. *et al.* (2005) Women living alone have an increased risk to develop diabetes, which is explained mainly by lifestyle factors. *Diabetes Care*, **28**, 2531–6.

Lipsky, B.A. and Berendt, A.R. (2000) Principles and practice of antibiotic therapy of diabetic foot infections. *Diabetes Metabolism Research Review*, **16**, Suppl. 1, S42–S46.

McCallon, S.K., Knight, C.A., Valiulus, J.P. *et al.* (2000) Vacuum-assisted closure versus saline-moistened gauze in healing of postoperative diabetic foot wounds. *Ostomy Wound Management*, **46**(8), 28–32.

Macfarlane, R. and Jeffcoate, W. (1998) How to describe a foot lesion with clarity and precision. *The Diabetic Foot*, **1**(4), 135–44.

Maciejewski, M.L., Reiber, G.E., Smith, D.G. *et al.* (2004) Effectiveness of diabetic therapeutic footwear in preventing reulceration. *Diabetes Care*, **27**(7), 1774–82.

McIntosh, C. (2006) *Diabetic Foot Ulcers: An Educational Booklet* (sponsored by Smith and Nephew), Wounds UK Publishing, Aberdeen.

McIntosh, C. and Newton, V. (2005) Superficial diabetic foot ulcers, in *Skin Care in Wound Management: Assessment, Prevention and Treatment* (ed. R. White), Wounds UK Publishing, Aberdeen, pp. 47–73.

Marshall, C. (2004) The ankle: brachial pressure index. A critical appraisal. *British Journal of Podiatry*, **7**(4), 93–5.

Marston, W.A. (2004) Dermagraft®, a bioengineered human dermal equivalent for the treatment of chronic nonhealing diabetic foot ulcer. *Expert Review of Medical Devices*, **1**(1), 21–31.

Missoni, E.M., Kalenić, S., Vukelić, M. *et al.* (2006) Role of yeasts in diabetic foot infection. *Acta Medica Croatia*, **60**(1), 43–50.

National Institute for Clinical Excellence (2002) *Clinical Guidelines for Type 2 Diabetes Management of Blood Glucose.*

National Institute for Clinical Excellence (2004) *Clinical Guidelines for Type 2 Diabetes: Prevention and Management of Foot Problems, Clinical Guideline 10.*

Nelson, E.A., O'Meara, S., Golder, S. *et al.* (2006) Systematic review of antimicrobial treatments for diabetic foot ulcers. *Diabetes Medicine*, **23**(4), 348–59.

Paile-Hyvarinen, M., Wahlbeck, K. and Eriksson, J.G. (2003) Quality of life and metabolic status in mildly depressed women with type 2 diabetes treated with paroxetine: a single blind randomised placebo controlled trial. *BMC Family Practise*, **4**(7), available at: `http://www.pulmedcentral.nih.gov/articlerender.fcgi?tool=pulmed&pubmedid=12747810`, Accessed 2 July 2007.

Ribu, L. and Wahl, A. (2004) How patients with diabetes who have foot and leg ulcers perceive the nursing care they receive. *Journal of Wound Care*, **13**(2), 65–8.

Russell, L. (2001) The importance of patients' nutritional status in wound healing. *British Journal of Nursing*, **10**(6), Suppl., S42, S44–S49.

Scottish Intercollegiate Guidelines Network (SIGN) (2001) Management of diabetic foot disease, in *Management of Diabetes: A National Clinical Guide* (online), Available at: `http://www.sign.ac.uk/guidelines/fulltext/55/index.html`, Last accessed 12 June 2006.

Shapiro, S.A., Stansberry, K.B., Hill, M.A. *et al.* (1998) Normal blood flow response and vasomotion in the diabetic Charcot foot. *Journal of Diabetes and Its Complications*, **12**, 147–53.

Shearer, A., Scuffham, P., Gordois, A. *et al.* (2003) Predicted costs and outcomes of reduced vibration detection in the UK. *The Diabetic Foot*, **6**(1), 30–7.

Sherman, R.A. (2003) Maggot therapy for treating diabetic foot ulcers unresponsive to conventional therapy. *Diabetes Care*, **26**, 446–51.

Sinacore, D.R. (1998) Acute Charcot arthropathy in patients with diabetes mellitus: healing times by foot location. *Journal of Diabetes and Its Complications*, **12**, 287–93.

Singh, N., Armstrong, D.G. and Lipsky, B.A. (2005) Preventing foot ulcers in patients with diabetes, *Journal of the American Medical Association*, **293**, 217–28.

Steed, D. (2006) Clinical evaluation of recombinant human platelet-derived growth factor for the treatment of lower extremity ulcers. *Plastic Reconstruction Surgery*, **117**(7), Suppl., 143s–149s.

Thomas, S. (2001) An introduction to the use of vacuum assisted closure, in *World Wide Wounds* (online), Available at: http://www.worldwidewounds.com/2001/may/Thomas/Vacuum-Assisted-Closure.html, Last accessed 20 October 2006.

UK Prospective Diabetes Study (UKPDS) (1998) Intensive blood-glucose control with sulphonylureas or insulin compared with conventional treatment and risk of complications in patients with type 2 diabetes (UKPDS 33). *The Lancet*, **352**(9131), 837–53.

Valk, G.D., Kriegsman, D.M.W. and Assendelft, W.J.J. (2006) Patient education for preventing diabetic foot ulceration (review), in *The Cochrane Collaboration*, John Wiley and Sons, Ltd, Chichester.

Vowden, K. and Vowden, P. (2002) Hand-held Doppler ultrasound: the assessment of lower limb arterial and venous disease (Suppl.), Huntleigh Healthcare Ltd.

Walters, S.J., Morrell, C.J. and Dixon, S. (1999) Measuring health-related quality of life in patients with venous leg ulcers. *Quality of Life Research*, **8**(4), 327–36.

Watkins, P.J. (2003) ABC of diabetes: the diabetic foot, *British Medical Journal*, **326**, 977–9.

Watret, L. (2005) Wound bed preparation and the diabetic foot. *The Diabetic Foot*, **8**(1), 18–26.

Wild, S., Roglic, G., Green, A. *et al.* (2004) Global prevalence of diabetes. *Diabetes Care*, **27**, 1047–53.

Winter, G. (1962) Formulation of the scab and the rate of epithelialisation in the skin of the domestic pig. *Nature*, **193**, 293–4.

Zimny, S., Schaltz, H. and Pfohl, M. (2002) Determinants and estimation of healing times in diabetic foot ulcers. *Journal of Diabetes and Its Complications*, **16**, 327–32.

Zimny, S., Schatz, H. and Pfohl, U. (2003) The effects of applied felted foam on wound healing and healing times in the therapy of neuropathic diabetic foot ulcers. *Diabetic Medicine*, **20**, 622–5.

Zimny, S., Schatz, H. and Pfohl, M. (2004) The role of limited joint mobility in diabetic foot patients with an at-risk foot. *Diabetes Care*, **27**(4), 942–6.

Deborah Turner, Jill Firth and Heidi Davys

Chapter 9

Foot Ulceration in Rheumatoid Arthritis

9.1 | Introduction

Rheumatoid arthritis (RA) is the most common inflammatory arthritis, affecting more than 350 000 people in the UK (Symmons, 2002). RA is primarily a disease that is associated with the inflammation and destruction of synovial joints, but has additional extra-articular features that vary from one individual to another. Features that may affect tissue viability include anaemia, nodules, cutaneous vasculitis and peripheral neuropathy. More recently it has also been demonstrated that RA is associated with an increased prevalence of peripheral vascular disease. Wound healing in these patients is often severely impaired and immunosuppressant medication required to control the disease process predisposes patients to infection. The foot remains a neglected area in rheumatology and as a consequence the pathogenesis of foot ulceration in patients with RA is poorly researched and the risk factors for ulceration are unclear.

It should be recognized that the morbidity associated with foot ulceration in RA is less than that for diabetes and rarely leads to amputation. However, foot ulceration is not a trivial clinical problem in RA; it is often a chronic, recurrent and painful complication of the disease and its importance may be underestimated. Estimating the prevalence of foot ulceration in RA and identifying factors that are both predictive and prognostic are currently under investigation by this team and many others. The intention of this chapter is to use current research where available, and in those instances where evidence is lacking the authors will write from their extensive clinical practice and experience. Effective management of the painful chronic ulcers often seen with RA will require knowledge of the general principles of wound care, along with a good understanding of the disease process of rheumatoid arthritis and its extra-articular features and a basic understanding of lower limb mechanics.

9.2 | Prevalence of Foot Ulceration in RA

In recent research 10–13 % of patients with RA were found to have a history of foot ulceration and 4–5 % reported open ulceration at the time of investigation (Firth *et al.*, 2006; Matricali *et al.*, 2006). Foot ulceration was found to be associated with long-standing disease duration, greater use of specialist footwear and a higher prevalence of previous foot surgery. In this study, 52 % of patients reported multiple episodes of ulceration, with the most common sites being the dorsal aspect of hammer toes, the metatarsal heads and hallux valgus (Firth *et al.*, 2006).

An audit of patient records in the Rheumatology Foot Clinic at Leeds General Infirmary, UK, found 80 new cases of foot ulceration per year, representing 10 % of the podiatry workload. In a three year audit period of the same clinic, a total of 149 patients attended for wound care. Of these patients 73 % had RA and cases of ulceration were predominantly found in female RA patients (79 % female) with long-standing disease (Davys *et al.*, 2006). In keeping with the findings of others, 64 % of patients experienced more than one episode of ulceration in the three year period and recurrent episodes did not always occur at the same foot site. Ulceration was found most frequently on pressure-vulnerable bony sites located on the plantar forefoot in the region of the metatarsal heads and the dorsal toes at the interphalangeal joints.

Diabetes-related foot ulceration has been shown to have a major negative effect on the quality of life of both patients and their families (Carrington *et al.*, 1996). RA, like diabetes, is a chronic disease and even early/mild foot involvement in rheumatic diseases has been shown to impact negatively on health-related quality of life (Wickman *et al.*, 2004). Foot ulceration associated with RA is usually long-standing and painful, limits choices in footwear and affects social participation; therefore it is likely to impact negatively on the quality of life and psychological well-being. The recurrent nature of this problem and its associated comorbidity warrants further investigation to establish risk factors for ulceration in order to be able to develop strategies for prevention and to improve the level of care for patients who develop ulcers.

9.3 | Case Scenario

Case Scenario 9

Steve, a 48-year-old male patient with a 12-year history of RA was referred to the rheumatology foot ulcer clinic by the rheumatology specialist registrar. He was attending the RA therapy resistant clinic (as his RA had failed to respond to many disease-modifying antirheumatic drug (DMARD) therapies) and his current medication included Prednisolone (corticosteroid), Methotrexate (a DMARD) and Etanercept injections (anti-TNFα biologic therapy). He presented with ulceration over the second metatarsal head on both feet. Steve had severe foot deformity including pesplanovalgus deformity, hallux valgus, lesser toe retraction and subluxation at the metatarsolphalangeal (MTP) joint, most notably over both second MTP joints. He reported that the wound had been present for approximately three months. The ulcers were undermined; the right had a granular base and the left was probing down to the bone (Figure 9.1).

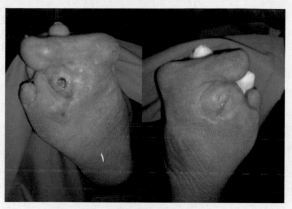

Figure 9.1
Bilateral plantar ulceration

The ulcers were painful on weight bearing and during debridement of the surrounding callus. He reported that the pain associated with the ulcers was severely limiting the types of daily activities he could undertake; therefore he spent longer periods of rest, which he thought exacerbated stiffness and discomfort in other joints (knee and hips).

As you read on, consider the following questions. This chapter will enable you to assess and treat this patient's chronic painful ulceration appropriately.

1. **What other information would you need to gather about Steve's medical history?**

2. **Which assessments should be undertaken in order to obtain a full understanding of the nature of the wound?**

3. **What is the effect of Etanercept on both the wound and healing?**

4. **What assessments and referrals to members of the multiprofessional team are required to ensure that Steve's foot is accommodated adequately in footwear and high-pressure areas offloaded effectively?**

5. **Consider strategies for managing Steve's pain.**

The information provided within the following sections should enable you to answer the five questions posed above. The answers to these will be considered towards the end of the chapter.

9.4 | Causation

The causation of lower limb ulceration in patients with RA (like other disease states) has been found to be multifactorial. Studies of ulceration in RA have focused on leg ulcers, but some researchers include the foot as a site although it is poorly defined. Several aetiological factors have been identified in the literature and include venous and arterial insufficiency, trauma and pressure (Thurtle and Cawley, 1983; McRorie et al., 1998; Pun *et al.*, 1990). The salient risk factors for foot ulceration in diabetes (peripheral neuropathy, peripheral vascular disease, foot deformity, raised plantar pressures and trauma from footwear; for further details refer to Chapter 8) also have the potential to affect RA patients (Kumar *et al.*, 1994; Macfarlane and Jeffcoate, 1997; Abbott *et al.*, 2002). It must be recognized that ulceration associated with RA in the foot is more likely to be caused by increased tissue stress at sites of deformity, but this factor should not be considered in isolation. Observations in clinical practice suggest that all of the above factors often play a significant role in the development of foot ulcers. In addition, patients with RA have reduced self-care capacity and often have impaired nutritional status and complex immunosuppressant treatment regimens, all of which contribute to delayed wound healing. Therefore, as the possible causes are examined it is important to remember that comprehensive assessment is essential as more than one factor may need to be addressed to promote wound healing and prevent recurrence.

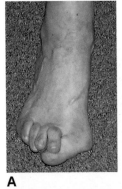

A

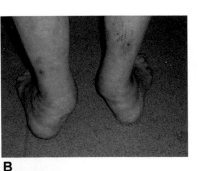

B

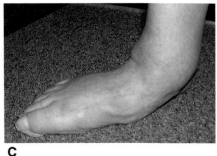

C

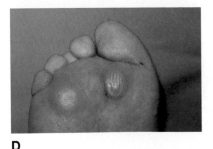

D

Figure 9.2
Typical foot deformities associated with RA: A, hallux valgus (bunion), note that the second toe is overriding and the lesser toes are retracted; B, severe valgus heel deformity; C, pes plano valgus foot deformity; D, prominent metatarsal heads with overlying callus

9.4.1 | Foot Structure and Function

Foot involvement in RA is very common, affecting 16% at diagnosis and 90–100% in patients with long-standing disease (Jacobs, 1984; Geppert *et al.*, 1992; Michelson *et al.*, 1994). In a study of 200 patients with RA, 86% had radiological changes in the feet. The metatarsophalangeal (MTP) joints were found to be the most frequently involved joints in the feet, affecting 77% of patients (Vidigal *et al.*, 1975). In RA the damage caused to the joint by inflammation (synovitis) can result in erosions of the cartilage and bone in the joint. Erosive changes commonly occur at the MTP joints and can occur very early in the disease process.

Deformities of the foot occur frequently in patients with RA and typically include hallux valgus (bunions), valgus heel deformity, pes plano valgus (flat arch and valgus heel), lesser toe deformities and prominent metatarsal heads (Figure 9.2).

Foot deformities, bony prominences and eroded MTP joints tend to focus stress on to a smaller area of distribution, thereby increasing the pressure. Callus forms in areas of high mechanical stress, initially as a protective response but ultimately it may further increase the pressure and concentrate the stress to underlying soft compliant tissue (Thompson, 1988). The plantar metatarsal heads and dorsal aspects of the lesser toes are common sites for pressure-induced lesions such as callosities and adventitious bursae formation, and are subsequent risk sites for ulceration (Vidigal *et al.*, 1975). Figure 9.3 shows the typical foot deformities that occur in long-standing RA and the areas at risk of ulceration.

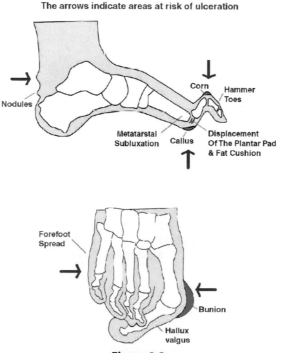

Figure 9.3
Areas at risk of developing ulceration in patients with RA (produced by J.Firth and B.Holliday, reprinted by kind permission of the Tissue Viability Society)

The skin and soft tissue serve as a mechanical protective medium, shielding the body from external stresses (Thompson, 1988). Soft tissue failure (ulceration) occurs as a result of an abnormal interaction between an environmental stress and soft tissues over a given period of time. Under normal circumstances, the soft tissue under the foot is very strong and extremely resilient to failure under stress. In RA, the amount of soft tissue between the skin and the bones may be decreased in many areas of the foot, thus increasing the risk of ulceration. It has been shown that peak pressures under the metatarsal heads in patients with RA are between two to three times greater than that of normal subjects (Minns and Craxford, 1984). Figure 9.4 shows typical peak pressure profiles in RA patients.

Higher peak pressures have been identified at MTP joints that have an overlying callus compared to those without a callus (Woodburn and Helliwell, 1996). Davys et al. (2005) revealed that MTP joints with an overlying callus were more eroded than those without a callus, suggesting that a relationship may exist between local stresses, joint damage and callus formation. This finding is further supported by the work of Tuna et al. (2005) who reported an association between joint erosions and plantar pressure distribution. In this study patients with high joint erosion scores had higher static forefoot peak pressures. It is important therefore when assessing patients with RA to establish how active the disease is at the present time and also how the disease has progressed

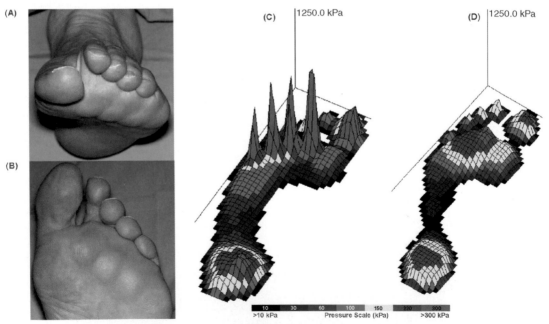

Figure 9.4

Typical peak pressure profiles seen in patients with RA with age-matched control: A and B, forefoot clinical features showing lesser toe deformities, prominent metatarsal heads, with overlying callus formation; C, peak pressure profile for corresponding pictures (A and B); note the high focal pressures over the lesser MTP joints; D, peak pressure profile for an age- and gender-matched healthy person (reprinted by kind permission of Churchill Livingstone, Edinburgh, Helliwell, P., Woodburn, J., Redmond, A., Turner, D. and Davys, H. (2006). *The Foot and Ankle in Rheumatoid Arthritis: A Comprehensive Guide*)

over time. Those patients with more aggressive disease are those who are likely to have more joint erosions, foot deformity and are at a greater risk of developing ulceration.

RA has also been shown to alter foot function during walking. Limited joint movement at the ankle, subtalar and MTP joints, and muscle weakness can result in changes to the normal loading transfer in the foot. It has been shown that patients with RA will typically have a delayed heel lift and loss of propulsion in the forefoot, which is likely to be a compensation strategy to avoid loading painful MTP joints in the forefoot (Turner *et al.*, 2005, 2006; Semple *et al.*, 2007). Those patients with a valgus heel deformity have been shown to exhibit a shift in peak pressures from the central to the medial metatarsal heads and these changes in loading are associated with an increased prevalence of callosities, which are potential risk sites for ulceration (Woodburn and Helliwell, 1996).

9.4.2 | Vascular Disease

Peripheral vascular disease (PVD) affects tissue viability by reducing the amount of oxygen reaching the tissues and impairing the removal of carbon dioxide and waste products. Evidence is now emerging that peripheral arterial disease is common in patients with RA (Alkaabi *et al.*, 2003; del Rincón *et al.*, 2005). It has been suggested that RA is associated with premature and accelerated atherosclerosis without the presence of traditional risk factors for atherosclerosis, although these may coexist (Van Doornum *et al.*, 2002). The same inflammatory process that drives RA is thought to drive the development of atheroma. In relation to the lower limb patients with RA have been found to have a higher prevalence of peripheral arterial obstructive disease as measured by the ankle brachial pressure index (Alkaabi *et al.*, 2003). Figure 9.5 shows a patient with RA with coexistent PVD and a long previous history of smoking, resulting in painful ischaemic necrotic digits.

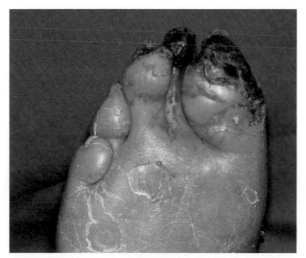

Figure 9.5

Clinical picture of PVD in a patient with long-standing RA and a history of smoking. Note the dusky red appearance of the limb associated with critical ischaemia and the dry necrosis on apical digits

RA is known to be the third most common underlying disease in patients affected by lower limb ulceration (Callam *et al.*, 1985, 1987). It is estimated that 9% of rheumatology outpatients have a leg ulcer at any one time (McRorie *et al.*, 1994). Leg ulceration in RA is likely to be multifactorial; vasculitis, arterial disease, venous insufficiency, peripheral oedema and infection have all been cited as possible causes. RA patients may be at an increased risk of venous disease through immobility, muscle atrophy and restricted ankle mobility (McRorie *et al.*, 1998). Arthritis affecting the ankle joint causes loss of movement, which impairs the venous muscle pump, increasing venous pressure and the possibility of damage to the veins. In addition, one to two thirds of RA patients are also affected by an anaemia that is associated with chronic disease (Wilson *et al.*, 2004). This further depletes the quality of the blood supply to the peripheral tissues and, unlike iron-deficiency anaemia, cannot be corrected.

Vasculitis, or inflammation of the blood vessels, is often suspected in this client group, particularly in ulcers of sudden, unexplained onset. Vasculitis is an uncommon of feature of RA; the clinical prevalence has been reported to be about 1–5% of patients with RA (Luqmani *et al.*, 1994). Blood vessels of all sizes can be affected, but usually involvement of the small arteries is a characteristic feature of rheumatoid vasculitis. The outcome of the inflammation depends on the size and location of the vessels involved. The most common clinical manifestation is small infarcts along the nail bed (Figure 9.6).

Cutaneous vasculitis involving the skin only affects around 3.6% of RA patients (Cimino and O'Malley, 1999; Turreson *et al.*, 2003) and it is difficult to ascertain the proportion of these cases that proceed to ulceration. Less frequently, involvement of the small or medium sized arteries can lead to peripheral neuropathy or more severe organ failure (Breedveld, 1997). Characteristically, vasculitic ulcers are often multiple, extremely painful, they are sharply demarcated with punched-out edges, are slow to heal and can deteriorate very quickly (Figure 9.7).

Common sites are the lower leg and the dorsum of the foot, although skin lesions can appear on areas of local pressure and previously traumatized skin (Cawley, 1987; Mat *et al.*, 1997). If vasculitis is suspected a rheumatology opinion should be sought and a biopsy is sometimes necessary.

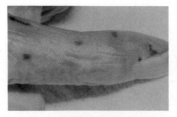

Figure 9.6
Clinical picture showing the most common clinical manifestation of cutaneous vasculitis (small infarcts along the nail bed) (reprinted by kind permission of Churchill Livingstone, Edinburgh, Helliwell, P., Woodburn, J., Redmond A., Turner, D. and Davys, H. (2006). *The Foot and Ankle in Rheumatoid Arthritis: A Comprehensive Guide*)

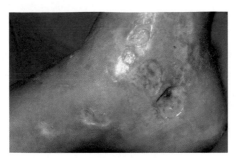

Figure 9.7
Vasculitic ulcers around the ankle, with scar tissue from a previous episode of vasculitis.
Note the sharply demarcated, punched-out edges, a characteristic feature of this type of
ulcer, and the surrounding erythema associated with the underlying inflammation

A vasculitic ulcer, although less common, requires a different approach to the management of the patient's overall disease state and will not heal with wound care alone. Systemic treatments are usually needed to control the inflammatory process and a major part of the treatment is focused on pain management. High doses of oral steroids are generally given and may be accompanied with intravenous cyclophosphamide. Due to the immunosuppressive nature of these drugs patients need to be monitored carefully for signs of infection (which may be masked).

9.4.3 | Neurological Impairments

In RA, severe symptomatic loss of sensation is less common than in diabetes. However, it is vital that this is not overlooked as neuropathy is an established complication of RA. Peripheral neuropathy is said to be a frequent complication associated with RA, but its clinical relevance remains poorly defined. The most common disorders are mononeuritis, sensorimotor neuropathy and entrapment neuropathy. RA patients may have electrophysiological findings of peripheral neuropathy, even in the absence of clinical evidence (Lanzillo *et al.*, 1998; Sankini *et al.*, 2005).

Several papers have identified an association between medication used to treat RA and the development of neuropathy, most notably leflunomide and infliximab (Bharadwaj and Haroon, 2004; Jarand *et al.*, 2006). A significantly higher incidence of peripheral neuropathy has been reported in patients with RA treated with leflunomide. The typical onset occurred about three months after the leflunomide was initiated and all patients who were found to have neuropathy by nerve conduction studies had reported symptoms of paraesthesia (Bharadwaj and Hardoon, 2004). Therefore, clinicians should be aware of the possibility of peripheral neuropathy in patients treated with leflunomide, especially when other risk factors (diabetes, pernicious anaemia) are present (Martin *et al.*, 2005).

Although it has been shown that patients with RA may have electrophysiological evidence of neuropathy, only a small proportion of patients will develop a loss of protective sensation which would mean that they were unable to detect injury. Plantar sensitivity (determined using Semmes–Weinstein monofilaments) has been shown to be significantly reduced in patients with RA compared to age- and gender-matched controls (Rosenbaum *et al.*, 2006). In this study, which had a small sample size ($n = 25$), seven patients with RA were reported to have loss of protective sensation defined as the inability to detect the 10 g monofilament.

It has been noted that patients with RA can be slow to report sensory impairment (Good, *et al.*, 1965; Lanzillo *et al.*, 1998) and as a result it is important that loss of sensation is not ignored as a possible contributory factor to ulceration and delayed healing. An additional consideration is the fact that as these patients are used to pain they tend to have high pain thresholds, so although the protective sensation may be intact foot pain is commonplace and only a marked change in the level or nature of pain may alert an individual to the possibility of tissue damage.

9.4.4 | Ability to Self-Care

A lack of self-care of the feet by patients with RA can have severe implications. Self-examination of the feet may be compromised by upper or lower limb joint pain, stiffness or deformity, and impaired manual dexterity of the hands may limit the ability of patients to perform their own basic foot care. Patients with RA frequently experience difficulty using nail clippers to cut their toenails because of hand deformity and limited grip strength (Figure 9.8).

Complex foot deformities which may be fixed may make it impossible for patients to examine regions of the foot that are at risk of developing an ulcer, e.g. in between the toes. It is also worth considering that this client group tend to have a high pain threshold because they have to adapt to

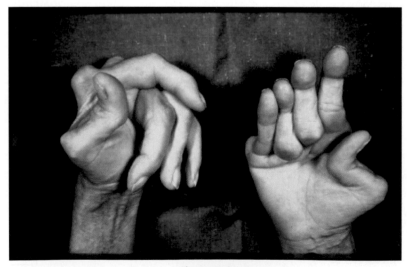

Figure 9.8
Clinical picture of the typical types of hand deformities seen in patients with RA

living with a painful, chronic disease. Foot pain is commonplace and only a marked change in the level or nature of pain may alert an individual to the possibility of tissue damage.

9.4.5 | Nutrition

A reduced self-care capacity is a factor that also affects nutrition in this client group in terms of the ability to shop, prepare and consume food. Assessment by an occupational therapist is often valuable as the provision of adapted cutlery and modification of the kitchen environment can go a long way to addressing these problems. The problem can be exacerbated by pain and restricted jaw opening as a result of arthritis affecting the temporomandibular joint, which makes eating painful. Some patients with RA are also affected by secondary Sjogren's syndrome, which impairs saliva production, reduces lubrication of food and may require the provision of artificial saliva or additional medication. Poor appetite may result from pain, inactivity, fatigue, depression or the side effects of medication. If this is the case, referral to a dietician to assess nutritional intake and address deficits is vital to prevent malnutrition and will help promote tissue viability.

It should be noted that while a marked weight loss is often a notable feature of RA it does not necessarily reflect malnutrition. Researchers have found impaired nutritional status and reduced body mass index without differences in dietary intake (Helliwell *et al.*, 1984; Gomez-Vacuero *et al.*, 2001). While good, well-balanced dietary intake may not correct weight loss in RA, wound healing places added demands upon resources that should be taken into account in the assessment process.

9.4.6 | Previous History of Ulceration

Many patients with RA have recurrent episodes of ulceration, and for this reason a previous history of ulceration must be considered as a leading risk factor for future ulceration. It has been suggested that altered mechanics of the scar tissue may increase the risk for ulceration. Scar tissue is not as strong as normal tissue and is thought to be more vulnerable to the shearing forces during walking and is more likely to break down (Levin, 1995). It has been suggested that the scar tissue is less able to dissipate mechanical stress and transmits large concentrated loads to the underlying softer tissue (Cavanagh *et al.*, 2001). Recurrent ulceration is a particular concern in those patients vulnerable to acute infection, including those patients receiving therapies such as biologics (which are discussed in more detail below).

9.5 | Drugs Used in the Treatment of RA. What Are the Possible Effects on Healing and Infection Rates?

The benefits of early aggressive treatment of RA are now well documented, so that now instead of the traditional progressive approach to treatment (where treatment is "stepped up" according to

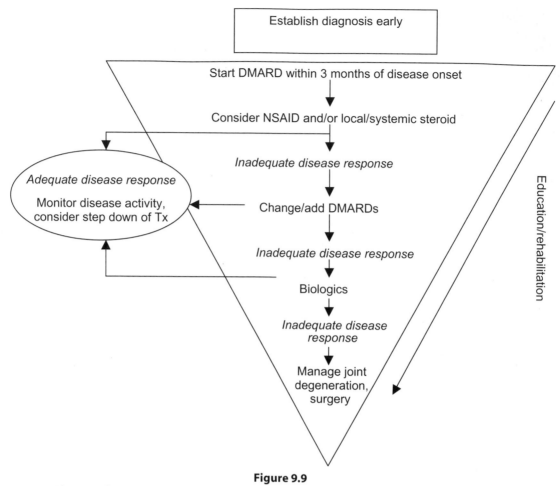

Figure 9.9
The step-down approach to the medical management of RA (reprinted by kind permission
of Churchill Livingstone, Edinburgh, Helliwell, P., Woodburn, J., Redmond, A., Turner, D. and
Davys, H. (2006). *The Foot and Ankle in Rheumatoid Arthritis: A Comprehensive Guide*)

the patient's response), treatment is often given with multiple disease-modifying antirheumatic
drugs (DMARDs) initially and then "stepped down" as the patient responds (Figure 9.9).

Disease-modifying drugs, such as sulphasalazine and methotrexate, are used not only to simply
relieve symptoms but also to delay progression of the disease. A full discussion of the medical
management of RA is beyond the scope of this chapter, and can be found elsewhere (Helliwell
et al., 2006). The groups of drugs commonly used and their impacts on tissue viability can be found
in Table 9.1.

Some patients who have failed to respond to conventional DMARD therapy may be treated with
the newly developed drugs, which have been designed to block specific components of the
inflammatory process in RA (the biologics). The most common drugs are the agents active against
tumour necrosis factor α (TNF α), marketed as Infliximab, Etanercept and Adalimumab, and those

Medication	Impact on tissue viability
Nonsteroidal anti-inflammatory drugs, e.g. diclofenac, naproxen	Inhibit platelet aggregation and proper coagulation. The risks of bruising, bleeding and haematoma formation (an excellent medium for micro-organism growth) may be increased
Cytotoxic drugs, e.g. methotrexate, azathioprine	May impair wound healing and increase the risk of infection
Steroids, e.g. prednisolone	Result in a thinned abnormal dermis and epidermis; interfere with both the inflammatory and proliferative stages of tissue repair and inhibit wound contracture
Anti-TNF drugs, e.g. Infliximab, Etanercept	Little is known about the effect on tissue viability and wound healing; increase the risks of infection

Table 9.1
The impact of medication on tissue viability in RA

that block the action of a protein called interleukin-1 (IL-1), which is marketed as Anakinra. These agents have been in widespread use for the treatment of RA for several years. Rituximab (CD20+ B-cell antibody) and abatacept (the CD4 cell co-stimulation) are newer biologic therapies and have only recently had approval for treatment of RA (Winthrop, 2006).

Drugs can either assist or inhibit the wound healing process. Most knowledge regarding the impact of these drugs on tissue viability in RA is gleaned from studies of surgical wounds. The implications for health professionals caring for a foot ulcer are less clear-cut.

The antiplatelet effects of nonsteroidal anti-inflammatory drugs (NSAIDs) commonly used for the treatment of RA can inhibit proper coagulation and platelet aggregation, which increases the risk of haematoma and seroma formation following trauma. This can provide an ideal environment for micro-organism growth and infection.

In the past concerns regarding the possible effect of methotrexate on wound healing have led to the common practice of discontinuation of the drug one week prior to elective surgery and the medication is restarted once sutures are out, providing that the wound is healing satisfactorily. Whether methotrexate should be continued or discontinued during the pre-operative period has been controversial. The actual evidence for the impact of methotrexate on wound healing is weak, with the larger studies showing no increase in early wound complications (Sany *et al.*, 1993; Escalante and Beardmore, 1995). Indeed, more recent reports show that it is unlikely that the continued use of low-dose methotrexate treatment increases the risk of post-operative complications in patients with RA and provides support in favour of not discontinuing methotrexate in the pre-operative period. In a study of RA patients undergoing reconstructive foot and ankle surgery, the use of methotrexate, glucocorticosteroids, NSAIDs, gold or hydroxychlorquine were not found to contribute to post-operative healing and infection complications (Bibbo *et al.*, 2003). In relation to the management of a chronic wound, the discontinuation of a cytotoxic drug for a longer period would have a significant impact on the patient's disease and may result in a disease flare, which would negate the possible benefits for wound healing.

The impact that corticosteroids have on tissue viability is well documented. Corticosteroids affect almost every stage of wound healing and their effects are most notable in the inflammatory phase (Karukonda *et al.*, 2000a). Vasoconstriction induced by corticosteroids results in localized hypoxia and reduced supply of nutrients, which impairs cell proliferation, collagen synthesis, suppression of wound contraction and reduced resistance to bacterial infection (Karukonda *et al.*, 2000b). It is not uncommon during a flare of the disease for a patient with RA to be given an intra-muscular or intra-articular injection of glucocorticosteroids as these are not associated with the same risks of continuous oral therapy when used intermittently.

Many of the DMARD therapies commonly used to treat RA have no significant defined inhibition on the wound healing process per se (Karukonda *et al.*, 2000b). However, they are associated with an increased susceptibility for infection which can be an important cause for delayed wound healing. Patients with an inflammatory arthritis are twice as likely than the general population to develop an infection and there is a further increase in infection risk in patients taking DMARDs (Edwards *et al.*, 2004; Olsen and Stein, 2004). Emerging data suggest that biological agents pose an increased risk to infection, particularly when used in combination with corticosteroids or methotrexate (Winthrop, 2006). The reported rates of infection are higher for those treated with the newer biologic therapies than those not treated with biologics (Neven *et al.*, 2005). However, there is also evidence that a higher risk for infections occurs with a higher disease activity in RA (Doran *et al.*, 2002) and the use of biological agents is often associated with RA severity, which makes it difficult to separate infection risk due to severity of disease activity or the biological agent (Winthrop, 2006).

Risk factors for developing an infection will be dependent on a number of factors including:

- Disease activity
- Medication and immunosuppression
- Presence of comorbidity (diabetes, PVD)
- Self-care ability and compliance

It is important that the practitioner managing foot wounds in patients with RA has a good knowledge of the drug therapies used to treat the underlying disease and their implications for wound healing. Extra vigilance is required when monitoring wounds for infection as frequently the classic clinical signs of infection may be masked by the therapeutic benefits of the drugs, but also the infection may be exacerbated when the patient's disease is in a state of active flare.

It is widely accepted that anti-tumour necrosis factor (anti-TNF) drugs should not be given in the pre-operative period, largely because these drugs are powerful immunosuppressant therapies associated with an increased risk of infection. Thus far, a single small study has failed to show any increase in post-operative infections and delayed healing rates (Bibbo and Goldberg, 2004), but as these drugs are relatively new these results may not be applicable to nonsurgical wounds and therefore, further work is needed in this area. Certainly, chronic leg ulceration is a contraindication to treatment with anti-TNF therapies because of the infection risks, and there has been a drive to ensure that any potential portal for infection is addressed promptly. The problem with nonsurgical wounds, however, is that it is difficult to predict healing time, and the suspension of immunosuppressant medication for upwards of a month would be expected to precipitate a flare of arthritis that in itself may delay healing. Hence, any decision to suspend cytotoxic or anti-TNF therapies should be made either according to local protocols or in consultation with a rheumatologist. The authors of this chapter have also experienced incidences where patients have been very reluctant to report the development of foot ulcers or even refused to stop taking their biologic therapy because of the dramatic improvement that this type of medication made to their quality of life when started. Clear concise explanations of the risks of severe rapidly progressing infections should be given to the patient to ensure that they do not continue with biologic therapy when advised to suspend it by the medical team. It is not common practice to suspend NSAIDs, which the majority of RA patients rely upon for the relief of pain and stiffness, and any interruption in steroid therapy is dangerous and may precipitate Addisonian crisis.

Iloprost is an example of a medication that can be used to facilitate the healing process and is usually administered via intravenous infusion. Iloprost infusions improve the vascular perfusion of the limb and, in selected cases, may be an important therapeutic tool for the care of ulcerative lesions (Mirenda et al., 2005). In patients with RA, Iloprost may be a particularly beneficial adjunct therapy to the normal immunosuppressant therapy used in the treatment of vasculitic ulcers (Veale et al., 1995).

9.6 | Patient Assessment

As previously described, RA is a multisystem disease and as such requires a comprehensive assessment of the vascular, neurological and musculoskeletal systems. It is important to also acknowledge patient perception and psychosocial issues when assessing an individual who has developed RA-related foot ulceration. This enables a holistic approach to wound management and allows care plans to be tailored to meet individual needs.

9.6.1 | Foot Assessment

When assessing the foot it is important to use a systematic approach and it is convenient to examine the foot in three regions: the rearfoot, midfoot and forefoot (including toes). Table 9.2 provides a suggested outline for assessment of the foot in patients with RA.

Foot component	
All areas	**Examine skin**
	Ulceration
	Necrosis
	Scarring (previous ulceration)
	Signs of arterial/venous insufficiency
	Nodules
	Corns/callus
	Haemorrhage into callus
	Blisters
	Skin infection (fungal/bacterial infections)
	Thinning of the skin/bruising (associated with long-term steroid use)
	Examine the nails
	Nail deformity (thickened nails)
	Fungal nail infections
	Splinter haemorrhages/nail fold infarcts
	Ingrowing toenails
	Evidence of poor self-care/neglect
Rearfoot	Valgus heel deformity
	Ankle swelling
Midfoot	Collapse of the arch (flat foot)
Forefoot	Hallux valgus
	Lesser toe deformity
	Interdigital ulceration/maceration/corns/fungal infection
	Prominent metatarsal heads
	Corns/callus

Table 9.2
Foot assessment outline

9.6.2 | Footwear Assessment

Examination of the footwear is an essential part of the patient assessment. It has been shown that a high proportion of patients wear ill-fitting footwear. Burns *et al.* (2002) found that a high proportion (72 %) of elderly patients on a general rehabilitation ward wore the wrong sized shoes. Patients with foot deformities like those seen in RA find it very difficult to buy footwear that can accommodate their deformities. Pressure from footwear can result in the development of ulceration, particularly on dorsal toe areas and over bunions. When assessing footwear it is important to examine overall fit and wear marks (a suggested footwear assessment checklist can be found in Table 9.3).

Footwear component	
Upper	Look for deformation of the upper around the toe and hallux valgus deformities Look at the shoe for medial bulging Feel inside the upper for abrasion of the lining
Outer sole	Look for excessive wear patterns
Insole	Look for areas of heavy wear and indentations as these will give an indication of high-pressure areas
Assess fit	Check the length and the width of the shoe

Table 9.3
Suggested footwear assessment

It is also important to ask patients about their usual footwear (the type they may wear on a regular basis). Some patients may come to clinic appointments in their "best" or smart shoes. Some patients may spend most of the day in slippers; therefore it is important that you assess them for fit and suitability.

9.6.3 | Vascular Assessment

The presence of vascular disease is evaluated by a combination of clinical signs and symptoms plus abnormal results from a noninvasive vascular test. Signs and symptoms of vascular disease are:

- Cold feet
- Blue toes
- Intermittent claudication
- Rest pain
- Night cramps
- Poor healing
- Sparse hair growth on the lower limb
- Skin atrophy
- Muscle wasting
- Thickened nails

When assessing patients with RA it is important to remember that muscle wasting may be present, but it is often related to disuse atrophy. Furthermore, the sedentary lifestyle as a consequence of joint pain and deformity may mean that exercise-induced ischaemic symptoms such as intermittent claudication may not be reported by patients.

An elaborate vascular examination is generally not required for routine screening (Cavanagh and Ulbrecht, 1991) and is somewhat dependent on the availability of vascular testing equipment in the outpatient setting. Initial screening based on palpation of pulses, appearance of limb and patient's symptoms should be undertaken in every patient, and if an abnormality in vascular status is suspected, further investigation is indicated. Cold extremities, absent pulses, pallor on elevation and rubor on dependency are all indicative of significant peripheral vascular disease (Levin, 2001). It must be noted that palpation of pulses is susceptible to variation between observers and the pulses may be difficult to palpate in the presence of swelling that may be related to a disease flare or ankle oedema. When assessing the temperature gradient in this patient group, it must also be noted that inflammation of joints and soft tissues may elevate the temperature in the lower limb.

Noninvasive measurement of blood pressure in peripheral arteries using Doppler ultrasound provides an objective measurement of vascular status. The most commonly used measurements are the ankle brachial pressure index (ABPI) and the toe pressure index. Caution should be exercised when applying the blood pressure cuff to a lower limb where oedema is present and the skin appears friable. It may be necessary to apply a protective layer of soft bandage to prevent trauma and bruising, especially if the patient is on steroid therapy. The presence of arterial stiffness has been found to be more prevalent in patients with RA than those without RA (Roman *et al.*, 2005). The relative incompressibility of the arteries associated with arterial stiffness will influence the blood pressure recorded and this should be taken into consideration when performing and interpreting an ABPI in this group of patients.

9.6.4 | Neurological Assessment

There is a general lack of published material on neurological assessment in patients with RA. Joint deformities and associated soft-tissue contractures can make assessment of reflexes difficult. In cases where patient history and brief examination suggests some neurological deficit, a detailed neurological assessment should be performed. In order to establish areas with loss of protective sensation and those areas at risk of developing ulceration, the use of the 10 g Semmes–Weinstein monofilament is recommended on any pressure-vulnerable site of the foot.

9.6.5 | Clinical Scenario

The left foot was failing to improve and discharge was exuding from the ulcer site, no other classic clinical signs of infection were noted. The ulcer was swabbed for culture and sensitivity and following a case conference with the rheumatology clinical nurse specialist and rheumatologist it was decided to commence a course of antibiotics and to suspend his Etanercept injections. Steve was commenced on 7 days of Flucloxicillin 500 mg QDS. As the ulcer was probing down to the bone with a potential risk for osteomyelitis an X-ray was arranged.

Questions

1. How would you monitor the subtle changes of such a small open ulcer?

2. Should the antibiotics be continued in this case when underlying bone is exposed?

3. In addition to antibiotics, what other drugs could be given to provide an optimum healing environment and encourage healing?

4. Should Steve restart his biologic therapy?

9.7 | Wound Assessment

Foot ulceration like that often seen in RA is a challenge to continuously monitor and evaluate because the process of healing/deterioration can often be quite subtle. Generic wound care monitoring systems and those developed for the diabetic foot may be employed but many ulcers associated with RA are small and can be superficial, so these instruments can lack the sensitivity to detect the subtle changes during the healing process.

Scaled photography is one of the best methods to document an ulcer and can allow analysis of the ulcer bed for slough, assess the state of surrounding tissue and permit the assessment of the effectiveness of debridement and measure the rate of healing (Vowden and Vowden, 2001). This method may not always be practical in community clinic settings and as a minimum the external dimensions of the ulcer should be recorded on each occasion to monitor the wound healing progress. In RA, foot ulcers are commonly undermined, which makes it difficult to assess the wound volume. Gentle probing may be necessary to assess the nature of structures involved (bone, joints, tendons), but is often too painful to undertake in patients with RA. There is a risk of osteomyelitis especially when the ulcer extends down to bone/joints. The presence/absence of osteomyelitis should be determined using radiographs or other imaging modalities. In cases where joint deformities and erosions are present it is often difficult to detect the subtle changes of osteomyelitis and serial radiographs may need to be undertaken.

The typical clinical signs of infection can be masked by the immunosuppressive medication used to treat RA, which can make it difficult to establish whether a wound has become infected. In addition, key clinical indicators for the presence of infection (pain and inflammation) are also present with synovitis, which can occur with a disease flare. Indicators that an ulcer has become infected include: an increase in pain at the site, increased erythema of the surrounding skin, a rapid increase in size or deterioration of the ulcer (this can also indicate the presence of vasculitis), purulence, heat and oedema surrounding the ulcer. If there is a clinical suspicion of an infection, the wound should be swabbed. All cutaneous wounds are contaminated with bacteria, but there needs to be in excess of 100 000 bacteria per gram of tissue for a clinical infection (Krizek and Robson, 1975). Contamination is the presence of nonreplicating bacteria within the wound and is a normal condition in chronic wounds. The fact that wounds are contaminated does not contribute to impairment in healing. Critical colonization is where there are no systemic signs of infection, but rather subtle local signs. In critical colonization the bacteria are competing with the host for oxygen and nutrients, contributing to delayed healing. In these instances antibiotic therapy may be warranted.

Blood can be useful in monitoring disease activity and help determine if an infection is present. An elevation in inflammatory markers without deterioration in the patient's arthritis disease activity may provide additional evidence of infection. When caring for patients on immunosuppressant therapies it is also important to monitor for systemic signs of infection, such as pyrexia and fever, as infection can progress rapidly and prompt intervention is required.

9.8 | Treatment Options

The principles and goals for treating ulceration are simple:

- Find the cause(s) of the ulcer where possible and treat accordingly.
- Identify factors affecting tissue viability.
- Heal the ulcer itself.
- Prevent infection in active ulcers.
- Manage the painful ulcer.
- Monitor progression and determine the outcome (healed (yes/no), time to heal in weeks, and so on).
- Prevent further episodes of ulceration at the same site when healed or at new sites.

9.9 | Management of Underlying Disease

The importance of a team approach to the effective management of patients with RA is well documented (Vliet Vlieland, 2004) and this is also the case when managing wounds in this client group. A clear understanding of RA, its manifestations, progression and treatment is essential, combined with a comprehensive knowledge of the elements of care, which their fellow professionals can contribute to the overall management package. Understanding and utilizing the skills of the team in a timely fashion can contribute significantly to helping patients reach an "optimum level of good health" and to heal wounds (Stamp, 1998).

The importance of the team approach in rheumatology has been described by Stamp (1998). Figure 1.3 in Chapter 1 highlights the major role each member of the team may play for management of those with foot wounds. Pain is often a predominate feature of the types of ulcers associated with RA; therefore pain reduction must be considered to be one of the major objectives of management.

Steve was reviewed a week later; the swab report revealed enteric skin flora only and the X-ray report was inconclusive for osteomyelitis. The surrounding callus was macerated and a high strike-through of exudate was noted on the dressing.

The patient was referred for an Aircast offloading boot but was unable to wear it. The boot was too heavy and aggravated his already swollen, tender knees. He was also not able to put it on by himself due to his existing hand deformity with additional synovitis, as his RA was flaring since his medication had been stopped and he lived on his own.

Questions

1. Which dressings would be the most appropriate for Steve to manage the wound himself at home?

2. Should debridement of the surrounding callus be carried out?

3. What other measures could be utilized to offload the forefoot area effectively?

9.10 | Local Wound Management

9.10.1 | Debridement

The rationale and therapeutic benefit of sharp scalpel debridement for the management of ulceration is well established in diabetes. In this patient group, callus has been identified as a positive predictor of subsequent ulceration and debridement of plantar callosities has been shown to reduce peak pressures, and facilitate wound healing (Young *et al.*, 1992; Murray *et al.*, 1996). In patients with RA, the effect of callus debridement surrounding or overlying ulceration has not been tested under controlled conditions. In RA, ulceration frequently occurs under heavy callus. Tissue damage may be hidden by callus formation and the well-trained eye may detect clues to an ulcer that is not necessarily obvious on initial examination, such as an area of haemorrhage under thick callus (Figure 9.10) or increased pain (Edmonds *et al.*, 1986; Cavanagh *et al.*, 2001).

This is an area where nursing and podiatry practice can be at odds, as a nurse may consider the skin to be intact or healed whereas a podiatrist is more likely to debride callus formation to reveal

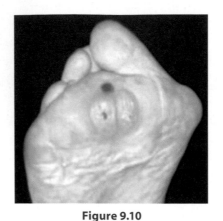

Figure 9.10
An area of haemorrhage under thick callus and evidence of wound exudate tracking distally from the site

an ulcer. Callus debridement is indicated where tissue damage is suspected and clinical experience suggests that debridement of forefoot plantar callosities significantly reduces pain and appears to facilitate healing of plantar ulceration. However, equally overzealous debridement of callus which leaves the remaining skin denuded and vulnerable to stress may result in tissue breakdown (Woodburn *et al.*, 2000).

As previously described, ulceration can occur under heavy callus and as such ulcers will often have callus formation around the edges. Tissue breakdown occurs underneath the callus and wound exudate from the site can track distally and often break through the skin (Figure 9.10). Clinical experience of the authors reveals that foot ulcers with large amounts of slough are not frequently seen in patients with RA. However, in cases where removal of slough is required sharp debridement is often too painful, and in those instances chemical debridement may be warranted. Hydrogels can be used to debride and to deslough a wound, rehydrating necrotic tissue, absorbing slough and wound exudates, and in nonresponding wounds larvae therapy (maggots) may be considered. A neuropathic rheumatoid foot is rarely seen, but ischaemia is an associated complication of RA, and therefore any form of debridement will be painful in the ischaemic foot and should be undertaken with extreme caution.

9.10.2 | Dressing Selection

When choosing a dressing for an ulcer on the foot of a patient with RA the authors recommend certain criteria should be reached. The dressing should be assessed for its ability to:

- Reduce pain and cushion prominent bony areas with high pressure without adding to pressure from the interface with footwear.

- Be removed without causing trauma to the wound and surrounding tissue, especially where tissue viability is reduced in patients on long-term steroid therapy.
- Be comfortable through wear time, e.g. bulky dressings should be avoided, especially for inter-digital areas, as they may serve to increase pressures further. Excessively bulky dressings further limit footwear choice and mean that patients may be less ambulant as a result.
- Absorb exudates so there is no strike-through during the wearing time or maceration to the surrounding tissue.

In clinical practice polyurethane foam dressings are a suitable choice as they meet the above criteria. These foam dressings have a soft silicone layer that does not stick to the wound surface or cause trauma to new tissue when removed. In addition, the dressings are slightly tacky, allowing patients to apply the dressings with ease, particularly when hand deformity is present. They have cushioning properties as well as the ability to absorb exudate, help in the mainte-nance of a moist healing environment while minimizing the risk of maceration. Thin variations of these dressings are also available which are particularly suitable for interdigital wounds where significant deformity is present. In addition, they can also be used as protection of compromised and/or fragile skin.

It is extremely important that dressings do not become too bulky and that the toes are not encircled with tape in order to attempt to hold dressings in place as this can limit the peripheral circulation further. Tubular gauze bandage can be used to secure toe dressings and can be applied easily with or without an applicator. Bulky dressings may also limit the room within footwear, causing discom-fort and making the patient less ambulant, and can cause additional pressures to prominent areas, which may result in further tissue breakdown.

In an attempt to minimize the risks of cross-infections it may be necessary to ask patients to avoid bathing and showers, thus keeping dressings dry and minimizing the need for frequent dressing changes, but the practical issues for patients must be considered. Patients with RA frequently report the therapeutic benefits of relaxing in a warm bath to ease their joints. Restricting bathing to keep a wound dry is not always necessary as dressings that temporarily seal an ulcer can be used. Unfortunately these are not always effective and therefore strategies such as waterproof protectors, frequently used for protecting plaster casts, can be used to keep the area dry and permit bathing.

9.10.3 | Offloading Strategies

In most cases of ulceration, high pressures over the site have been identified as a major contributory factor in pathogenesis of the ulcer. Therefore, reduction of pressure at the site must be seen as a prime objective in wound care management in order to facilitate wound healing. During the acute stages of a painful foot ulcer, particularly over the plantar MTP joints, traditional

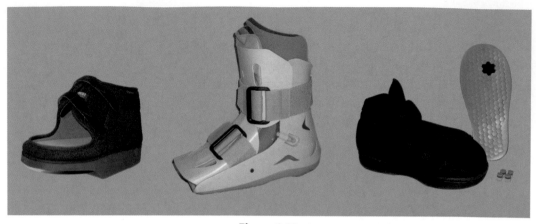

Figure 9.11
Offloading devices suitable for patients with RA. From left to right: lightweight forefoot "offloader" boot, Aircast short pneumatic walker and the DH walker shoe

methods of offloading high-pressure sites can be used and these include DH pressure relief walkers and the Aircast pneumatic walkers. These types of offloading strategies are effective in many instances, but they can present practical problems for patients with RA. Hand impairments (deformity and muscle weakness) can mean that patients struggle when they have to put these devices on and remove them. When muscle weakness is present in the lower limb, patients will often report that the devices feel heavy and cumbersome. Patients may also be experiencing a disease flare in response to suspension of medication and proximal joints (knees and hips) may be aggravated by the use of offloading devices. In these instances the devices, which are easier to use and made from light-weight materials, are useful. Devices that meet these criteria are the Aircast short pneumatic walker, lightweight forefoot "offloader" boots and DH walker shoes (Figure 9.11); the authors' clinical experience has shown that most patients with RA can successfully use these devices.

If an ulcerated site on the foot in patients with RA is successfully offloaded most will heal quickly. However, the major challenge is the prevention of future ulceration. A combination of appropriate footwear and foot orthoses are used to prevent ulcers reoccurring and fragile areas from breaking down. Additional depth and width footwear is available for patients to purchase, usually via mail order and internet resources; availability is still limited on the high street. RA patients with significant rearfoot or forefoot deformity will usually require specialist ready-made or bespoke footwear from the appliance/orthotics department to accommodate the deformity adequately, reduce pressure over the ulcerated area and allow healing to occur. The footwear pyramid (Figure 9.12) demonstrates how the need for footwear/specialist footwear alters with the extent of foot deformity.

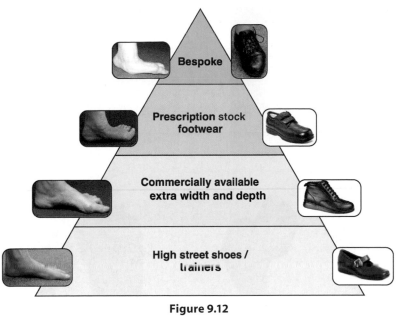

Figure 9.12
The footwear pyramid demonstrates how the need for specialist
footwear alters with the extent of foot deformity

The use of specialist footwear and orthoses have been shown to be effective at reducing levels of foot pain and high plantar pressures, which can lead to ulceration in patients with established forefoot disease (Fransen and Edmonds, 1997; Hodge *et al.*, 1999; Chalmers *et al.*, 2000). Despite the potential clear benefits of specialist footwear, low levels of patient satisfaction and poor compliance have been reported (Williams and Meacher, 2001). It has been shown that involvement of the patient in the decision-making process for footwear selection and providing adequate follow-up to monitor the effectiveness of footwear are key factors in ensuring higher levels of satisfaction, effective use of footwear and the optimum benefits of specialist footwear (Williams and Nester, 2006; Williams *et al.*, 2007). Orthotic devices are usually individually contoured to the patient's feet, to provide support in the arch, fully accommodate deformity and redistribute pressure away from prominent bony areas; they are commonly referred to as total contact inlays. A lightweight, supportive material with thermal properties is recommended for the shell, such as high-density plastazote, as this will successfully offload high pressures in the forefoot region into the arch. A cushioning covering is usually extended under the forefoot to reduce pressures further. Leather top covers are often utilized because they be easily cleaned, which is important for patients with active ulcers when there is the possibility of exudate leaking from the dressing (Figure 9.13 shows a typical total contact inlay and change in pressure with a total contact inlay).

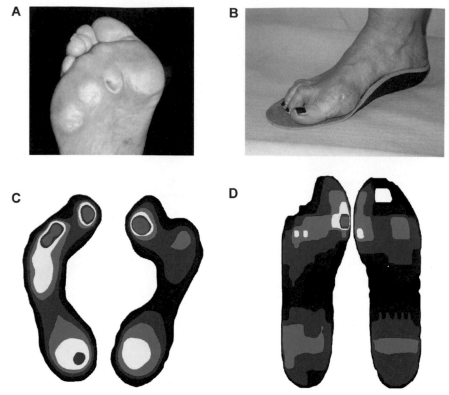

Figure 9.13
Example of using a total contact orthoses and specialist footwear to reduce pressure over an
area at risk of ulceration: A, callus with extravasation over the second plantar MTP joint; B, high-
density plastazote orthoses with a leather top cover; C, barefoot pressure profile (note the high
pressure over the second MTP joint and absence of toe loading); D, Inshoe pressure profile
with the orthoses (note the reduction in pressure and increased loading in the midfoot)

9.10.4 | Clinical Scenario

**Steve was admitted to the rheumatology ward on two occasions and
received a course of Iloprost infusions, which failed to improve the wound
states. With periods of rest from work and during hospital admissions the ulcers
improved, but when Steve recommenced normal activity further tissue breakdown was noted, even with appropriate offloading strategies in place. Surgical
intervention to the foot and ankle was discussed with the patient and other
members of the rheumatology team. The patient was keen to be considered
for foot surgery so he could get back to his normal level of activities. The rheumatologist was in agreement and a referral was sent to the specialist foot and
ankle surgeon.**

Question
Is surgical intervention warranted in managing Steve's foot health?

9.10.5 | Foot Surgery

Surgical intervention should be viewed as part of the total care package for management of RA patients with foot ulceration. In recent years there have been advances in orthopaedic techniques. Surgical intervention should be considered when pressure areas have developed, leading to intractable calluses or ulceration. In the forefoot, once the MTP joints have become subluxed, the surgical intervention is usually extensive and an excisional arthroplasty (the metatarsal heads are removed) (Figure 9.14) is usually undertaken (Harris and Carrington, 2006).

Criteria for surgical intervention in the foot in patients with RA have yet to be developed and the best way forward at the present time is to organize multiprofessional foot clinics so that conservative management can be optimized; if this fails, surgical options can be considered. Clinical experience shows that patients with ulcers that are failing to heal, those with recurrent episodes of ulceration (where medications to treat RA are regularly suspended) and those with intractable foot pain are ideal candidates for surgical intervention.

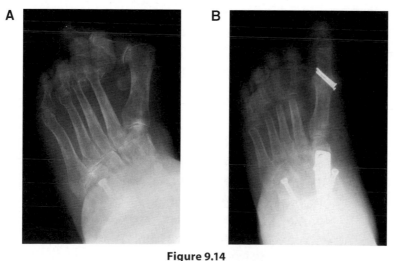

Figure 9.14
X-rays of excisional arthroplasty of subluxed MTP joints: A, subluxed MTP joints prior to surgical intervention; B, post-MTP joint excisional arthroplasty

9.11 | Case Scenario Revisited

1. **What other information would you need to gather about the patient's medical history?**

   RA is predominantly a disease that affects the musculoskeletal system (joints and soft tissues), but it is associated with many extra-articular features that can affect tissue viability. These include vascular disease (arterial and venous), neurological deficits, respiratory disease and reduced self-care capacity, and often patients with RA will have impaired nutritional status and complex immunosuppressant treatment regimens, all of which contribute to delayed wound healing. Steve had a 12-year history of RA and was attending the therapy-resistant clinic, which suggests that his RA has not responded well to medication and as such he is at a greater risk of developing vascular disease and the other extra-articular features. The effects of long-term treatment with steroids, thinning of the skin, easy bruising, muscle weakness and an increased risk of developing diabetes also need to be considered in this case.

2. **Which assessments should be undertaken in order to obtain a full understanding of the nature of the wound?**

   RA is a multisystem disease and as such requires a multisystem approach to assessment. An assessment of the vascular and neurological system should be undertaken. Foot ulcers commonly develop at sites of high pressure over foot deformities and therefore an assessment of foot structure, function and footwear is imperative to gain a full understanding of the nature of the wound. Those patients with more aggressive disease are those who are likely to have more joint erosions, foot deformity and are at a greater risk of developing ulceration. In this clinical case the ulcers were located over the second MTP joints (these were prominent and were likely to be eroded due to the aggressive nature of his long-standing RA).

3. **What is the effect of Etanercept on both the wound and healing?**

   Taking Etanercept, particularly in conjunction with methotrexate, increases the risk of developing infections that can delay wound healing. In cases where infection occurs, the normal clinical signs of infection can be masked. In the clinical case the patient's current medication (a steroid, methotrexate and biologic therapy) would place him at increased risk of developing a severe infection and as a consequence the Etanercept therapy was suspended.

4. **What assessments and referrals to members of the multiprofessional team are required to ensure that the patient's foot is accommodated adequately in footwear and high-pressure areas are offloaded effectively?**

   In this case an assessment to determine the magnitude and location of peak pressures under the foot would provide useful information to determine optimal strategy for offloading. Plantar pressure studies revealed high peak pressures over the sites of ulceration.

A referral was made to the orthotist for an offloading device and initially offloading was attempted using an Aircast boot. However, Steve was not able to wear it (he found the boot was too heavy and he had difficulty putting the boot on and removing it due to hand deformities), and so offloading was achieved with total contact orthoses and accommodative footwear.

5. **Consider strategies for managing the pain experienced by the patient.**

   In cases where drug management needs to be suspended (e.g. biologic therapy as in Steve's case), a flare in the disease may occur. It is essential to work with the rheumatology team for effective management of the RA and pain. Patients may be given stronger analgesics in these instances or it may be necessary for a referral to the pain management clinic. Dressings for foot ulcers should be carefully selected in order to minimize pain by cushioning prominent bony areas and be removed without causing pain/trauma during re-dressings. In the clinical case the foot ulcers were extremely painful, the patient was prescribed stronger analgesics and was advised to take some prior to coming into the clinic for re-dressing appointments.

6. **How would you monitor the subtle changes of such a small open ulcer?**

   Scaled photography is one of the best methods to monitor the subtle changes in wound status. When this is not possible objective measures of wound dimensions should be recorded. Foot ulcers are commonly undermined, which makes it difficult to assess the wound volume. Gentle probing may be necessary to assess the depth and whether the wound extends down to bone. In this case the ulcers were undermined, the extent to which the ulcer tracked under the skin's surface was determined by gentle probing and measurements were taken to monitor the wound. The level of wound exudate, the presence of slough and the quality of the surrounding tissues were also documented.

7. **Should the antibiotics be continued in this case when underlying bone is exposed?**

   Due to complex foot deformities that are often seen in patients with RA it can be quite common for even very superficial ulcers to extend down to bone, but it is not necessary for antibiotics to be used routinely in these cases. However, these patients have to be monitored very carefully for the presence of osteomyelitis. It is often hard to determine whether osteomyelitis is present from X-rays when deformities and erosions are present and in this clinical case the radiology report was inconclusive for the presence of osteomyelitis.

8. **Should the patient restart his biologic therapy?**

   Although Steve's RA has become very active biologic therapy should not be recommenced until the ulcer has healed, because the ulcer penetrated down to bone and there was an increased risk of developing a severe infection.

9. **Which dressings would be the most appropriate for this patient to manage the wound himself at home?**

   Steve has severe hand deformities and finds it difficult to put on fiddly dressings. Liaison with district nurses, the practice nurse and the occupational therapist can help to support patient re-dressings and bathing at home. Steve was unable to use scissors so he was supplied with a selection of pre-cut tape to secure his sterile dressing to his wound; the use of partially adhesive dressings can also be useful in these circumstances.

10. **Should debridement of the surrounding callus be carried out?**

    In this case Steve did not have any clinical evidence of vascular disease and the patient reported that when callus built up around the edges of the wound it became more painful. Although the process of callus debridement was painful, careful debridement was undertaken and it gave the patient some short-term pain relief.

11. **What other measures could be utilized to offload the forefoot area effectively?**

    There are many offloading devices available. Figure 9.11 shows some devices particularly suited for patients with RA as they are lightweight and use Velcro straps for securing, which are easier to use in the presence of hand deformity.

12. **Is surgical intervention warranted in managing the foot health of this patient?**

    In this case, despite offloading, the foot ulcers remained static. Steve was unable to recommence his biologic therapy and as a result his arthritis had started to flare. Urgent surgical intervention is warranted in this case.

9.12 | Summary

This chapter has highlighted the need for the foot health provider to have a good knowledge and understanding of the underlying disease process and its medical management, as well as being able to assess and treat foot ulcerations competently in patients with rheumatoid arthritis. The clinical scenario emphasizes the complex nature of ulceration and demonstrates the effectiveness of multidisciplinary working to provide appropriate and timely management of this patient. Multidisciplinary foot care is well established and of proven benefit in other disciplines such as diabetes (Edmonds *et al.*, 1986), but provision of multidisciplinary foot health services in rheumatology remains patchy and the benefits unclear. Effective multidisciplinary care can be provided by disciplines working independently, but relies on the knowledge and awareness of the key health professionals involved in the patient's care and good lines of communication between team members. This model of connected but not integrated care probably reflects the most common model for what might be broadly considered multidisciplinary foot health input into rheumatology. Steve's clinical case scenario illustrates the potential complexity and severity of managing foot ulceration in RA. Better integration of care for both the assessment and management of ulceration in this client group has the potential to improve outcomes and reduce the recurrence rate.

> ## ? Reflection
>
> **Take time to reflect upon your learning from this chapter. Ask yourself:**
>
> 1. **What knowledge did I possess prior to reading this chapter?**
> 2. **How has my knowledge developed?**
> 3. **How will I implement this into my future practice?**

References

Abbott, C.A., Carrington, A.L., *et al.* (2002) The North-West Diabetes Foot Care Study: incidence of, and risk factors for, new diabetic foot ulceration in a community-based patient cohort. *Diabetic Medicine*, **19**(5), 377–84.

Alkaabi, J.K., Ho, M., Levison, R., Pullar, T. and Belch, J.J.F. (2003) Rheumatoid arthritis and macrovascular disease. *Rheumatology*, **42**, 292–7.

Bharadwaj, A. and Haroon, N. (2004) Peripheral neuropathy in patients on leflunomide. *Rheumatology*, **43**, 934.

Bibbo, C. and Goldberg, J.W. (2004) Infectious and healing complications after elective orthopaedic foot and ankle surgery during tumor necrosis factor-alpha inhibition therapy. *Foot and Ankle International*, **25**(5), 331–5.

Bibbo, C., Anderson, R.B., Davis, W.H. and Norton, J. (2003) Complications in rheumatoid foot and ankle reconstructive surgery: analysis of 718 procedures in 103 patients. *Foot and Ankle International*, **24**, 40–4.

Breedveld, F.C. (1997) Vasculitis associated with connective tissue disease. Baillieres Clinical Rheumatology, **11**(2), 315–34.

Burns, S.L., Leese, G.P. and McMurdo, M.E. T. (2002) Older people and ill fitting shoes. *Postgraduate Medical Journal*, **78**, 344–6.

Callam, M.J., Ruckley, C.V., Harper, D.R. and Dale, J.J. (1985) Chronic ulceration of the leg: extent of the problem and provision of care. *British Medical Journal*, **290**, 1855–6.

Callam, M.J., Harper, D.R., Dale, J.J. and Ruckley, C.V. (1987) Chronic ulcer of the leg: clinical history. *British Medical Journal*, **294**, 1389–91.

Carrington, A.L., Mawddsley, S.K., Morley, M., Kincey, J. and Boulton, A.J. (1996) Psychological status of diabetic people with or without lower limb disability. *Diabetes Research and Clinical Practice*, **32**, 19–25.

Cavanagh, P.R. and Ulbrecht, J.S. (1991) Biomechanics of the diabetic foot: a quantitative approach to the assessment of neuropathy, deformity and plantar pressure, in *Disorders of the Foot and Ankle: Medical and Surgical Management*, 2nd edn (ed M.H. Jahss), W.B. Saunders & Company, Philadelphia, Pennsylvania, pp. 1864–907.

Cavanagh, P.R., Ulbrecht, J.S. and Caputo, G.M. (2001) The biomechanics of the foot in diabetes mellitus, in *Levin and O'Neals The Diabetic Foot*, 6th edn (eds J.H. Bowker and M.A. Pfeifer), Mosby, St Louis, Missouri, pp. 125–96.

Cawley, M.I.D. (1987) Vasculitis and ulceration in rheumatic diseases of the foot, in *The Foot in Arthritis* (ed. M.I.V.S. Jayson), Baillière Tindall, London, pp. 315–331.

Chalmers, A.C., Busby, C., Goyert, J., Porter, B. and Schulzer, M. (2000) Metatarsalgia and rheumatoid arthritis – a randomized, single blind, sequential trial comparing 2 types of foot orthoses and supportive shoes. *Journal of Rheumatology*, **27**(7), 1643–7.

Cimino, W.G. and O'Malley, M.J. (1999) Rheumatoid arthritis of the ankle and the hindfoot. *Clinics in Podiatric Medicine and Surgery*, **16**(2), 373–89.

Davys, H.J., Turner, D.E., Helliwell, P.S., Conaghan, P.G., Emery, P. and Woodburn, J. (2005) Debridement of plantar callosities in rheumatoid arthritis, a randomized controlled trial. *Rheumatology*, **44**, 207–10.

Davys, H.J., Turner, D.E., Helliwell, P.S. and Emery, P. (2006) Foot ulcerations in patients with rheumatic diseases. *Annals of the Rheumatic Diseases*, **65**, Suppl. II, 669.

del Rincón I., Freeman, G.L., Haas, R.W., O'Leary, D.H. and Escalante, A. (2005) Relative contribution of cardiovascular risk factors and rheumatoid arthritis clinical manifestations to atherosclerosis. *Arthritis and Rheumat*, **52**(11), 3413–23.

Doran, M.F., Crowson, C.S., Pond, G.R., O'Fallon, W.M. and Gabriel, S.E. (2002). Predictors of infection in rheumatoid arthritis. *Arthritis and Rheumatism*, **46**, 2294–300.

Edmonds, M.E., Blundell, M.P., Morris, M.E., Thomas, E.M. and Cotton, L.T. (1986) Improved survival of the diabetic foot: the role of a specialised foot clinic. *Quarterly Journal of Medicine*, **60**, 763–71.

Edwards, J., Szczepanski, L., Szechinski, J., *et al.* (2004) Efficacy of B-cell-targeted therapy with Rituximab in patients with rheumatoid arthritis. *New England Journal of Medicine*, **350**, 2572–81.

Escalante, A. and Beardmore, T.D. (1995). Risk factors for early wound complications after orthopedic surgery for rheumatoid arthritis. *The Journal of Rheumatology*, **22**(10), 1844–51.

Firth, J., Hale, C.A., Helliwell, P.S. and Hill, J. (2006) The prevalence of foot ulceration in rheumatoid arthritis. *Annals of the Rheumatic Diseases*, **65**, Suppl. II, 670.

Fransen, M. and Edmonds, J. (1997) Off-the-shelf orthopaedic footwear for people with rheumatoid arthritis. *Arthritis Care Research*, **10**, 250–6.

Geppert, M.J., Sobel, M. and Bohne, W.H. (1992) The rheumatoid foot: Part I. Forefoot. *Foot and Ankle*, **13**(9), 550–8.

Gomez-Vacuero, C., Nolla, J.M., Foter, J., *et al.* (2001) Nutritional status in patients with rheumatoid arthritis. *Joint Bone and Spine*, **68**, 403–9.

Good, A.E., Christopher, R.P., Koepke, G.H., Bender, L.F. and Tarter, M.E. (1965) Peripheral neuropathy associated with rheumatoid arthritis. *Annals of Internal Medicine*, **63**(1), 87–99.

Harris, N. and Carrington, N. (2006) The surgical management of the rheumatoid foot and ankle, in *The Foot and Ankle in Rheumatoid Arthritis: A Comprehensive Guide* (eds P. Helliwell, J. Woodburn, A. Redmond, D. Turner and H. Davys), Churchill Livingstone, Edinburgh, pp. 125–196.

Helliwell, M., Coombes, E.J., Moody, B.J., Batstone, G.F. and Robertson, J.C. (1984). Nutritional status in patients with rheumatoid arthritis. *Annals of the Rheumatic Diseases*, **43**, 386–90.

Helliwell, P., Woodburn, J., Redmond, A., Turner, D., Davys, H. (2006). *The Foot and Ankle in Rheumatoid Arthritis: A Comprehensive Guide*, Churchill Livingstone, Edinburgh.

Hodge, M.C., Bach, T.M. and Carter, G.M. (1999) Orthotic management of plantar pressure and pain in rheumatoid arthritis. *Clinical Biomechanics*, **14**, 567–75.

Jacobs, S.R. (1984) Rehabilitation of the person with arthritis of the ankle and foot. *Clinics in Podiatry*, **1**(2), 373–99.

Jarand, J., Zochodne, D.W., Martin, L.O. and Voll, C. (2006) Neurological complications of Infliximab. *The Journal of Rheumatology*, **33**, 1018–20.

Karukonda, A.R.K., Corcoran Flynn, T., Boh, E.E., McBurney, E.I., Russo, G.G. and Millikan, L.E. (2000a) The effects of drugs on wound healing: part I. *International Journal of Dermatology*, **39**, 250–7.

Karukonda, A.R.K., Corcoran Flynn, T., Boh, E.E., McBurney, E.I., Russo, G.G. and Millikan, L.E. (2000b). The effects of drugs on wound healing: part II. Specific classes of drugs and their effect on healing wounds. *International Journal of Dermatology*, **39**, 321–333.

Krizek, T.H. and Robson, M.C. (1975) Evolution of quantitative bacteriology in wound management. *American Journal of Surgery*, **130**, 579–84.

Kumar, S., Ashe, H.A., Parnell, L.N., Fernando, D.J.S., Tsigos, C., Young, R.J., Ward, J.D. and Boulton, A.J.M. (1994) The prevalence of foot ulceration and its correlates in type 2 diabetic patients: a population-based study. *Diabetic Medicine*, **11**, 480–4.

Lanzillo, B., Pappone, N., Crisci, C., di Girolamo, C., Massini, R. and Caruso, G. (1998) Subclinical peripheral nerve involvement in patients with rheumatoid arthritis. *Arthritis and Rheumatism*, **41**(7), 1196–202.

Levin, M.E. (1995) Preventing amputation in the patient with diabetes. *Diabetes Care*, **18**, 1383–94.

Levin, M.E. (2001) Pathogenesis and general management of foot lesions in the diabetic patient, in *Levin and O'Neals The Diabetic Foot*, 6th edn (eds J.H. Bowker and M.A. Pfeifer), Mosby, St Louis, Missouri, pp. 219–60.

Luqmani, R.A., Watts, R.A., Scott, D.G. and Bacon, P.A. (1994) Treatment of vasculitis in rheumatoid arthritis. *Annales de Medecine Interne*, **145**, 566–76.

Macfarlane, R.M. and Jeffcoate, W.J. (1997) Factors contributing to the presentation of diabetic foot ulcers. *Diabetic Medicine*, **14**, 867–70.

McRorie, E.R., Jobanputra, P., Ruckley, C.V. and Nuki, G. (1994) Leg ulceration in rheumatoid arthritis. *British Journal of Rheumatology*, **33**, 1078–84.

McRorie, E.R., Ruckley, C.V. and Nuki, G. (1998) The relevance of large vessel vascular disease and restricted ankle movement to the aetiology of leg ulceration in rheumatoid arthritis. *British Journal of Rheumatology*, **37**, 1295–8.

Martin, K., Bentaberry, F., Dumoulin, C., *et al.* (2005) Neuropathy associated with leflunomide: a case series. *Annals of the Rheumatic Diseases*, **64**, 649–50.

Mat, C., Yurdakul, S., Tuzuner, N. and Tuzun, Y. (1997) Small vessel vasculitis and vasculitis confined to the skin, in *Vasculitis* (eds H. Yazici and G. Husby), Bailliere Tindall, London, pp. 237–57.

Matricali, G.A., Boonen, A., Verduyckt, J., *et al.* (2006) The presence of forefoot problems and the role of surgery in patients with rheumatoid arthritis. *Annals of the Rheumatic Diseases*, **65**(9), 1254–5.

Michelson, J., Easley, M., Wigley, F.M. and Hellmann, D. (1994) Foot and ankle problems in rheumatoid arthritis. *Foot and Ankle International*, **15**(11), 608–13.

Minns, R.J. and Craxford, A.D. (1984) Pressure under the forefoot in rheumatoid arthritis, a comparison of static and dynamic methods of assessment. *Clinical Orthopaedics and Related Research*, **July/ August**, 235–42.

Mirenda, F., La Spada, M., Baccellieri, D., Stilo, F., Benedetto, F. and Spinelli, F. (2005) Iloprost infusion in diabetic patients with peripheral arterial occlusive disease and foot ulcers. *Chirurgia Italiana*, **57**, 31–5.

Murray, H., Young, M.J., Hollis, S. and Boulton, A.J. M. (1996) The association between callus formation, high pressures and neuropathy in diabetic foot ulceration. *Diabetic Medicine*, **13**, 979–82.

Neven, N., Vis, M., Voskuyl, A.E., *et al.* (2005) Adverse events in patients with rheumatoid arthritis treated with Infliximab in daily clinical practice. *Annals of the Rheumatic Diseases*, **64**, 645–6.

Olsen, N.J. and Stein, M. (2004), New drugs for rheumatoid arthritis. *New England Journal of Medicine*, **350**, 2567–79.

Pun, Y.L.W., Barraclough, D.R.E. and Muirden, K.D. (1990) Leg ulcers in rheumatoid arthritis. *Medical Journal of Australia*, **153**, 585–7.

Roman, M.J., Devereux, R.B., Schwartz, J.E., *et al.* (2005) Arterial stiffness in chronic inflammatory diseases. *Hypertension*, **46**, 194–9.

Rosenbaum, D., Schmiegel, A., Meermeier, M. and Gaubitz, M. (2006) Plantar sensitivity, foot loading and walking pain in rheumatoid arthritis. *Rheumatology*, **45**(2), 212–4.

Sankini, R.A., Abdul-Zehra, I.K. and Al-Nimer, M.S.M. (2005) Neuropathic manifestations in rheumatoid arthritis: a clinical and electrophysiological assessment in a small sample of Iraqi patients. *Annals of Saudi Medicine*, **25**, 247–9.

Sany, J., Anaya, J.M., Canovas, F., *et al.* (1993) Influence of methotrexate on the frequency of postoperative infectious complications in patients with rheumatoid arthritis. *Journal of Rheumatology*, **20**(7), 1129–32.

Semple, R., Turner, D.E., Helliwell, P.S. and Woodburn, J. (2007) Regionalised centre of pressure analysis in patients with rheumatoid arthritis. *Clinical Biomechanics*, **22**(1), 127–9.

Stamp, J. (1998) The team approach to mobility and self care, in *Rheumatology Nursing*, 1st edn (ed. J. Hill), Churchill Livingstone, Edinburgh, pp. 195–208.

Symmons, D.P.M. (2002) Epidemiology of rheumatoid arthritis: determinants of onset, persistence and outcome. *Best Practice and Research in Clinical Rheumatology*, **16**(5), 707–22.

Thompson, D.E. (1988) The effects of mechanical stress on soft tissue, in *The Diabetic Foot*, 4th edn (eds, M.E. Levine and L.W. O'Neal), Mosby, St Louis, Missouri, pp. 91–103.

Thurtle, O.A. and Cawley, M.I.D. (1983) The frequency of leg ulceration in rheumatoid arthritis. *The Journal of Rheumatology*, **10**(3), 507–9.

Tuna, H., Birtane, M., Tastekin, N. and Kokino, S. (2005) Pedobarography and its relation to radiologic erosion scores in rheumatoid arthritis. *Rheumatology International*, **26**(1), 42–7.

Turner, D.E., Davys, H.J. and Woodburn, J. (2005). Foot function following forefoot reconstruction in rheumatoid arthritis. *Australian Journal of Podiatric Medicine*, **39**, 83–9.

Turner, D.E., Helliwell, P.S., Emery, P. and Woodburn, J. (2006) The impact of rheumatoid arthritis on foot function in the early stages of disease: a clinical case series. *BMC Musculoskeletal Disorders*, **21**, 102.

Turreson, C., O'Fallon, W.M., Crawson, C.S., Gabriel, S.E. and Matteson, E.L. (2003) Extra-articular disease manifestations in rheumatoid arthritis: incidence trends and risk factors over 46 years. *Annals of Rheumatic Diseases*, **62**, 722–7.

Van Doornum, S., McColl, G. and Wicks, I.P. (2002) Accelerated atherosclerosis: an extraarticular feature of rheumatoid arthritis? *Arthritis and Rheumatism*, **46**(4), 862–73.

Veale, D.J., Muir, A.H., Morley, K.D. and Belch, J.J. (1995) Treatment of vasculitic leg ulcers in connective tissue disease with Iloprost. *Clinical Rheumatology*, **14**, 187–90.

Vidigal, E., Jacoby, R.K., Dixon, A.S., Ratliff, A.H. and Kirkup, J. (1975) The foot in chronic rheumatoid arthritis. *Annals of the Rheumatic Diseases*, **34**(4), 292–7.

Vliet Vlieland, T.P. (2004). Multidisciplinary team care and outcomes in rheumatoid arthritis. *Current Opinion in Rheumatology*, **16**, 153–6.

Vowden, P. and Vowden, K. (2001) Investigations in the management of lower limb ulceration. *British Journal of Community Nursing*, **6**, Profore Suppl., 4–11.

Wickman, A.M., Pinzur, M.S., Kadanoff, R. and Juknelis, D. (2004), Health-related quality of life for patients with rheumatoid arthritis foot involvement, *Foot and Ankle International*, **25**(1), 19–26.

Williams, A. and Meacher, K. (2001) Shoes in the cupboard: the fate of prescribed footwear. *Prosthetics and Orthotics International*, **25**(1), 53–9.

Willams, A.E. and Nester, C.J. (2006) Patient perceptions of stock footwear design features. *Prosthetics and Orthotics International*, **30**, 61–71.

Willams, A.E., Rome, K. and Nester, C.J. (2007) A clinical trial of specialist footwear for patients with rheumatoid arthritis. *Rheumatology*, February, **46**(2), 302–7.

Wilson, A., Yu, H., Goodnough, L.T. and Nissenon, A.R. (2004) Prevalence and outcomes of anemia in rheumatoid arthritis: a systematic review of the literature. *The American Journal of Medicine*, **116**, 50s–57s.

Winthrop, K.L. (2006) Serious infections with anti-rheumatic therapy: are biologics worse? *Annals of the Rheumatic Diseases*, **65**, Suppl. III, 55–7.

Woodburn, J. and Helliwell, P.S. (1996) The relationship between valgus heel deformity and the distribution of forefoot plantar pressures and callosities in rheumatoid arthritis. *Annals of the Rheumatic Diseases*, **55**, 806–10.

Woodburn, J., Stableford, Z. and Helliwell, P.S. (2000) Preliminary investigation of debridement of plantar callosities in rheumatoid arthritis. *Rheumatology*, **39**, 652–4.

Young, M.J., Cavanagh, P.R., Thomas, G., Johnson, M.M., Murray, H.J. and Boulton, A.J.M. (1992) The effect of callus removal on dynamic plantar foot pressures in diabetic patients. *Diabetic Medicine*, **9**, 55–7.

Caroline McIntosh and Steve Hancox

Chapter 10

Nail Surgery Wounds

10.1 | Introduction

Ingrowing toenails (onychocryptosis) requiring surgical intervention are a common, debilitating problem observed in clinical practice. It has been estimated that 0.02% of the population in the UK will develop onychocryptosis requiring treatment each year (Cumming et al., 2005). Onychocryptosis is often encountered in young people, with a male predominance of 3:1 (Sugden et al., 2001), but while it is recognized that the incidence of onychocryptosis reduces with increasing age females experience onychocryptosis twice as often as males in individuals over the age of 60 (Weaver et al., 2004). The most common site for onychocryptosis is the great toe (hallux); lesser digits can also be affected but it is less commonly observed in the second to fourth digits (DeLauro, 1995). Typically the patient will present with acute pain and swelling around the nail, as observed in Figure 10.1. The condition can cause a number of problems for individuals affected: patients may develop infection, be unable to participate in sporting activities and experience difficulties in wearing footwear, which can impact on daily living and, in some cases, occupational activities.

Often surgical intervention is required to resolve onychocryptosis and facilitate wound healing. There are numerous surgical techniques, invasive and noninvasive, that can be performed to resolve the problem. The aim of this chapter is to consider chemical cautery resolution of onychocryptosis or other toenail pathologies requiring surgery, and the management of these wounds.

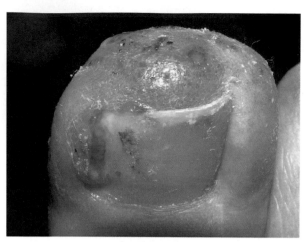

Figure 10.1
Pre-surgical wound

10.2 | Case Scenario

Consider the image and information provided for Case Scenario 10. All information provided is based on a case seen in a podiatry clinic.

Case Scenario 10

Paul is a 16-year-old man who underwent a partial nail avulsion with matrix phenolization of his right hallux (Figure 10.2). He initially presented to the podiatry clinic with onychocryptosis. Paul's mother had previously attempted to remove the corner of the nail without success and Paul had then received regular conservative treatment, basic nail care and footwear advice,

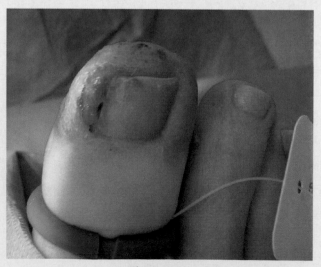

Figure 10.2
Post-surgical wound following removal of the nail and chemical cautery

from a private podiatrist. However, the problem was recurrent, affecting his ability to participate in sport. Paul is a keen rugby player and wanted to get back to playing sport. Following assessment and discussion with the patient a referral for surgery was made to remove the medial aspect of the nail plate (partial nail avulsion). The patient declared no major medical history and was able to follow instructions for post-surgical self-management of his wounds.

? Consider the following questions:

1. **How long would you expect this wound to take to heal?**

2. **What dressings should be used on a moist chemical burn wound of this type?**

3. **How often should the dressings be changed?**

4. **Describe the stages of healing that such a wound would have to take in order to heal fully.**

The information provided within the following sections should enable you to answer the questions posed above. The questions will be considered towards the end of the chapter.

10.3 | Anatomy and Physiology of the Nail

In order to gain an appreciation of nail surgery wounds it is pertinent to review the normal anatomy and physiology of the nail plate. The nail plate extends over the distal aspect of the digit, as observed in Figure 10.3.

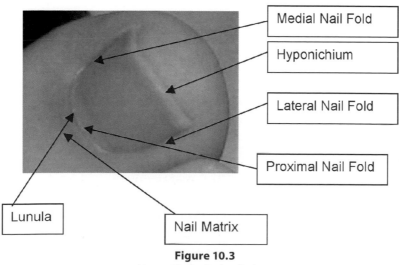

Figure 10.3
Nonpathological nail plate

The nail emerges from the proximal nail fold and is bordered on either side by the medial and lateral nail folds, and distally by the hyponichium (the section of the nail unit where the skin and nail meet). Nail is produced primarily by the nail matrix, which lies beneath the proximal nail fold. The distal matrix forms the inferior part of the nail plate and the proximal matrix forms the superficial layers of the nail plate. When the matrix extends distal to the proximal nail fold it appears as a white half-moon, the lunula. The nail bed appears as a pink area beneath the nail plate (Fleckman and Allan, 2001). Any damage to the matrix has the potential to permanently damage the nail (Rich, 2001) and hence regular repetitive trauma or an acute trauma can cause irreversible damage to the structure of the nail.

10.4 | Causation

The cause of ingrowing toenails is often multifactorial, including:

- Poor self-management can be a common contributing factor and is often related to improper nail cutting, especially cutting deep into the nail fold or leaving rough corners or pieces of nail within the nail fold (Weaver *et al.*, 2004).
- Nail shape and structure can increase the risk of onychocryptosis. Individuals with a curved nail plate and those with thin, soft nail plates that can easily split are predisposed to onychocryptosis (Rounding and Bloomfield, 2003).
- Acute trauma can result in damage to the nail which can consequently cause onychocryptosis.
- Poorly fitting footwear.
- Tight hosiery.
- Certain medications can increase the risk of secondary onychocryptosis. Onychocryptosis has been reported in conjunction with protease inhibitors used in treating HIV infection, oral retinoid used to treat a variety of dermatologic conditions, cyclosporine an immunosuppressant and oral antifungal treatments for onychomycosis (fungal nail infection) (Connelly *et al.*, 1999; Weaver *et al.*, 2004).

10.5 | Pathology of Onychocryptosis

Essentially onychocryptosis is initiated by the nail plate irritating the adjacent soft tissue of the medial or lateral nail folds. Once inflammation begins the accompanied swelling tends to exacerbate the condition by pressing further on to the nail and a cycle ensues with further swelling causing even more soft tissue irritation. This can lead to a skin breach, exudate production, bleeding and possibly infection.

Weaver *et al.* (2004) suggest a staging system for onychocryptosis:

Stage 1: characterized by inflammation and redness. Pain may be experienced with direct pressure on the nail. At this stage the condition can spontaneously resolve or be resolved by appropriate nail care.

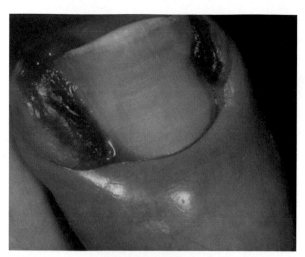

Figure 10.4
Infected onychocryptosis

Stage 2: characterized by inflammation and exudate production. Pain is usually experienced with slight pressure and during walking. Infection may be present at this stage and surgical intervention is often required.

Stage 3: characterized by granulation tissue formation. Granulation overhangs the edge of the nail plate and readily bleeds (Figure 10.1). Infection is common at this stage, as seen in Figure 10.4. Surgical intervention is required to cure the condition.

> **?** **How would you stage Paul's onychocryptosis? Also consider the lateral nail fold. Are there any signs of potential future problems?**

10.6 | Other Nail Pathologies Requiring Surgical Intervention

Onychocryptosis is one of the commonest toenail pathologies seen in clinical practice and remains a common reason for elective toenail surgery (Blake, 2005). However, other toenail pathologies may also require surgical intervention.

10.6.1 | Onychomycosis (Fungal Nail Infection)

This is a common condition affecting the nails, usually of adults, with a particular peak prevalence in the older population, as illustrated in Figure 10.5. Nearly 50% of all nail dystrophies are thought to be due to onychomycosis, with nearly 50% occurring in the toes (Bristow, 2004). Increasing age, family history and the presence of tinea pedis (athlete's foot) are associated with onychomycosis. Certain systemic diseases also increase the susceptibility of onychomycosis, namely diabetes, peripheral vascular

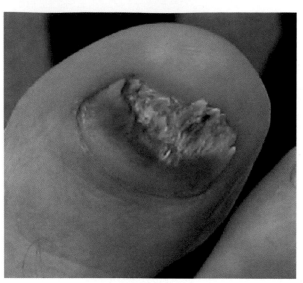

Figure 10.5
Onychomycosis of the nail

disease and immune disorders such as HIV and AIDS (Vender *et al.*, 2006). This is largely because affected individuals are immunocompromised and therefore at greater risk of opportunistic infection.

Onychomycosis can cause cosmetic distress to the individual affected with published reports, suggesting that onychomycosis can impact on the quality of life (Lateur, 2006). Treatment for onychomycosis includes topical and oral anti-fungal therapies with surgical avulsion sometimes considered as a last resort (Bristow, 2004).

10.6.2 | Onychauxis

Thickening or hypertrophy of the nail plate (onychauxis), as seen in Figure 10.6, may on occasion require surgical intervention. Changes are frequently observed in the first and fifth toenails as a

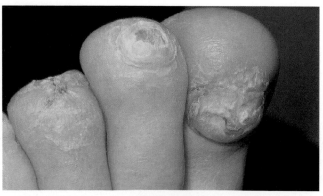

Figure 10.6
Onychauxis of the toenails

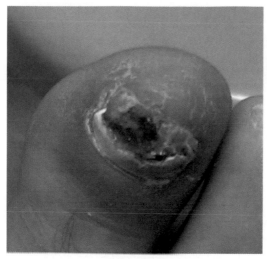

Figure 10.7
Subungual ulceration

result of damage from footwear over time or from an acute sudden trauma (de Berker *et al.*, 2002). Usually regular podiatric care, including nail cutting and drilling, can reduce nail thickness, maintain patient comfort and prevent further problems.

However, onychauxis can prove aesthetically concerning for individuals, particularly as secondary fungal infection can occur (de Berker *et al.*, 2002). Individuals may therefore opt for toenail avulsion to eradicate the problem. Onychauxis can, in certain cases, cause ulceration of the nail bed (subungual ulceration) due to increased pressure, particularly if tissue viability is compromised. Figure 10.7 shows an infected subungual ulceration under an onychauxic toenail in a patient with diabetes.

10.6.3 | Other Disorders

Nail disorders, including onychomycosis and onychauxis, are particularly common in the older population due to a number of factors, including impaired circulation, biomechanical changes and systemic disease (Singh *et al.*, 2005).

A less common presentation of nail thickening and deformity can be related to subungual exostosis, a benign bone tumour of the distal phalanx that occurs under the nail plate. Subungual exostosis most frequently occurs in the toes, with the hallux the most common site (Letts *et al.*, 1998), as illustrated in Figure 10.8. Lesions most often present in the second to third decade of life. Although rare in children, there are reports of exostoses occurring in children in the medical literature (Lokrec *et al.*, 2001). Surgical intervention is often required to treat the exostosis successfully.

10.7 | Surgical Procedure

Surgical procedures for nail pathologies, such as onychocryptosis, are routinely carried out under local anaesthetic by general practitioners, general surgeons, orthopaedic surgeons, podiatric

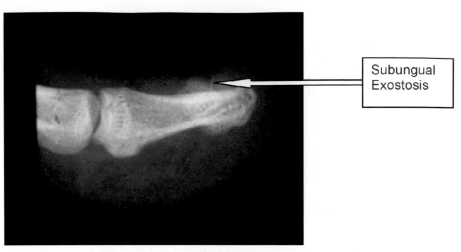

Subungual
Exostosis

Figure 10.8
Subungual exostosis visible on X-ray (reproduced with kind permission of Jim Pickard)

surgeons and podiatrists (Rounding and Bloomfield, 2003). There are a number of different surgical procedures used in practice, both noninvasive and invasive methods.

Chemical cautery, with phenol, is a frequently employed surgical method for the management of onychocryptosis (and other pathological nail conditions) that has been found to have the highest success rate (Rounding and Bloomfield, 2003; Aksakal *et al.*, 2004; Weaver *et al.*, 2004). This involves the removal of the entire nail plate (total nail avulsion), as seen in Figure 10.9, or a section of the nail plate with chemical cautery of the nail matrix using phenol, preventing future re-growth, as seen in Paul's case (Figure 10.2).

Podiatrists commonly use phenol for chemical ablation of the nail matrix (Rounding and Bloomfield, 2003). However, due to the potentially unpleasant nature of phenol (Health and Safety Executive, 2000), sodium hydroxide is gaining in popularity, particularly with emerging evidence supporting its use as a viable alternative to phenol (Cumming *et al.*, 2005). Other professionals, particularly orthopaedic surgeons and general surgeons, may opt for invasive methods, such as Zadik's procedure, whereby an incision is made at the base of the nail, the matrix is excised and then the skin is sutured and left to heal by primary intention.

10.7.1 | Chemical Cautery Surgery

In order to gain a greater appreciation of the healing process in chemical cautery wounds it is important to have an awareness of the surgical technique frequently employed. The procedure usually involves administering local anaesthetic into the base of the toe to achieve a digital block. Thus pre-surgical assessment must establish the patient's suitability for local anaesthesia as well as their potential for post-operative healing. The surgical procedure usually involves removal of

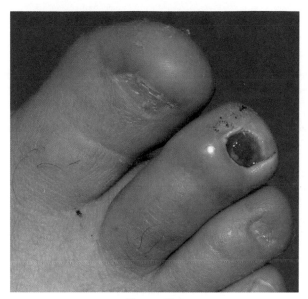

Figure 10.9
Total nail avulsion two days post-operative

the entire toenail (total nail avulsion) (Figure 10.9) or sections of nail from either side of the nail plate (partial nail removal) (Figure 10.2). While the toe is exanguinated with a tourniquet, as seen in Figure 10.2, a sterile pipette or sterile swab is used to introduce 80% phenol into the open wounds. Phenol is worked into each wound for a total of 3 minutes. This causes a chemical burn that destroys the nail matrix (nail-producing cells) and stops re-growth of the offending nail. Some practitioners use 80% sodium hydroxide for 20 seconds to achieve similar results. The use of cryotherapy such as liquid nitrogen is also documented as an effective management strategy (Blake, 2005).

> **?** **Prior to surgery it is important to assess Paul's suitability for local anaesthesia and his potential for post-operative healing. What assessment strategies should be undertaken in Paul's case?**

Unlike many other surgical wounds, which largely heal by primary intention, chemical cautery nail surgery wounds heal by secondary intention and although they are described as acute wounds they do not necessarily follow the orderly pattern of healing outlined in Chapter 2. Healing in these wounds is often prolonged due to the corrosive nature of phenol (Thomson *et al.*, 2002). Recent randomized controlled studies (Marshall *et al.*, 2005; McIntosh and Thomson, 2006) have investigated the time taken to heal following chemical ablation toenail surgery. Reports indicate that mean healing times varied; after total nail avulsion healing time ranged from 30 to 52 days and after partial avulsion surgery 18 to 31 days. Additionally, a randomized controlled trial examined the effectiveness of toenail surgery performed by podiatrists in the community and surgeons in the hospital setting (Thomson *et al.*, 2002). Findings suggest that podiatric surgery was more effective in all outcomes, with the exception of healing times, which were faster in the surgeons' group. This was attributed to the corrosive nature of the chemical, phenol, used by podiatrists versus the invasive technique requiring healing by primary intention in the surgeons' group.

As healing is often prolonged due to the corrosive nature of phenol used during surgery, it is imperative that a comprehensive, systematic patient assessment is undertaken prior to the surgical procedure. It is essential to identify potential contraindications for surgery, identify factors that impede tissue viability, increase infection risk and ultimately inform a prognosis for wound healing.

10.8 | Pre-surgical Assessment

Nail surgery is generally considered a minor surgical procedure. However, the risks of complications should not be underestimated. Prior to undertaking nail surgery it is important to ascertain the patient's suitability for the procedure. This would include general medical status and medication and assessment of vascular status of the lower limb and foot. Good tissue viability is crucial to secondary intention wound healing.

10.8.1 | Medical History

Systemic conditions should be explored prior to proceeding with toenail surgery. As discussed throughout the various chapters within this book, certain medical conditions can predispose to infection and contribute to chronicity of wounds, specifically diabetes mellitus, rheumatoid arthritis, peripheral vascular disease, lymphoedema, and immunosuppression. While none are absolute contraindications to surgery the potential for post-operative healing must be established.

For efficiency and completeness it is helpful to divide the medical history into further subsections: pharmacological history, vascular, neurological and dermatological.

1. | Medication
It is important to establish any medication, prescribed or otherwise, that the patient is taking, as certain medication can negatively impact on wound healing potential. These include:

- Corticosteroids, nonsteroidal anti-inflammatory drugs (NSAIDs) and disease-modifying antirheumatic drugs (DMARDs) are drugs that are known to suppress inflammation and increase the likelihood of infection (Cooper, 2005). Other drugs such as beta-blockers can also indirectly impact on wound healing by causing peripheral vasoconstriction (British National Formulary (BNF), 2007).

2. | Vascular history
Due to the corrosive nature of phenol and the resultant tissue damage caused by phenolization during nail surgery, normal wound healing physiology can be prolonged. It is therefore essential

that pre-surgical assessment establishes vascular perfusion to the foot as adequate because arterial perfusion is an essential prerequisite for healing. Poor vascular status caused by blood vessel disease such as atherosclerosis, arteriosclerosis or vasospasticity may be contraindications to toenail surgery.

A staged approach to vascular assessment should be adopted:

Stage 1. Observation of the lower limbs can offer a valuable insight into vascular status. Chapter 3 identifies clinical markers of arterial and venous disease that are easily identified on observation and can inform the practitioner on the state of the circulation.

Stage 2. Palpation of foot pulses, dorsalis pedis and posterior tibial pulses is a useful test to ascertain the presence and strength of blood perfusion in the foot. In Paul's case foot pulses were strong on palpation; therefore further investigation was unnecessary. However, if pulses are weak or absent on examination further tests are required.

Stage 3. Doppler ultrasound, as seen in Figure 10.10, is a commonly utilized tool to assess vascular status (Vowden and Vowden, 2002) and is used in the pre-surgical assessment of the nail surgery patient. Interpretation of Doppler sounds or Doppler waveforms are often necessary to make any conclusions as to the suitability of a patient for nail surgery.

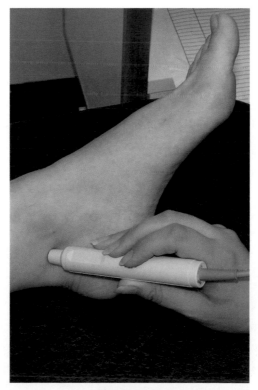

Figure 10.10
Doppler examination

Doppler devices inform the practitioner on the flow of blood in the arteries and give an indication of the patency of flow at the site of reference. This can be achieved by audible sounds or printable waveforms. Weak or irregular Doppler sounds require further investigation prior to ascertaining the patient's suitability for elective surgery.

Stage 4. The vascular status of any potential surgical candidate can be further investigated with Doppler ultrasound and ankle brachial pressure indices. This assessment helps to quantify lower limb perfusion by comparing systolic blood pressure in the arm with systolic pressure at the ankle to arrive at a ratio. An ankle brachial pressure index between 0.9 and 1.3 indicates viable tissues. Healing could be impaired in individuals with values lower than 0.9 or greater than 1.3, so the necessity of surgical intervention should be considered (Grasty, 1999).

Vascular disease is relatively common in certain populations, e.g. smokers, people with diabetes and the elderly. However, it should be noted that diabetes mellitus in itself is not a contraindication to podiatric nail surgery. It is important to make note of blood sugar control and in particular the HbA1c level indicator, which should ideally be below 6.5 mmol (International Diabetes Federation, 2005). In addition to the ankle brachial pressure index it is also advisable to perform a toe brachial pressure index as this is particularly useful if there is suspected small vessel disease (Marshall, 2004) (refer to Chapter 8 for further details).

3. | Neurological history

It is important to identify any deficits in sensation or muscle weakness which when coupled with vascular problems can reduce tissue viability and healing. In particular, diabetes can present with particular neurological deficits in the foot that may affect the vascular supply (refer to Chapter 8). Autonomic control of peripheral vessels may be affected, vessels can become calcified, affecting their elasticity, and atherosclerosis is more common. Small peripheral vessel disease specifically related to diabetes is well documented in the literature (Vowden and Vowden, 2002; Marshall, 2004).

4. | Dermatological

The condition of the skin is an important indicator of the healing capability of the underlying tissues, as discussed in Chapter 3. Skin quality should be assessed as atrophic and friable skin may be a contraindication to elective nail surgery and an indicator of underlying problems related to tissue viability in general. Consideration should be given to potential allergies to adhesives or tapes used to secure dressings in the post-operative period.

> **Following assessment, Paul did not have any significant medical history. What management strategies should now be implemented in Paul's case? What advice should be given to Paul in the post-operative period?**

10.9 | Post-operative Aftercare

Prior to the surgical procedure the patient should be made aware of healing times and potential for infection. Informed consent should be sought in line with local protocol.

Immediate post-operative care should include advice regarding appropriate footwear and general activity levels. Irritation from ill-fitting footwear and inappropriate activity levels will irritate a chemical cautery wound, delaying healing and causing local inflammation.

10.9.1 | Wound Dressing Regimens

Post-surgically the primary concern for the practitioner is to keep the surgical wound clean and free from infection. It is therefore important that practitioners involved in post-operative wound care adopt aseptic techniques to minimize infection risk at every redressing.

In published literature there is currently little in the way of well-designed controlled trials to investigate the most effective post-operative wound dressing regimen following toenail surgery. The choice of modern wound dressings is vast; the optimum dressing for this wound type is debatable. A study by Marshall *et al.* (2005) showed that dressing a nail surgery wound with a medicated honey dressing achieved a healing time similar to povidone iodine, although the subject numbers were small. Similarly, McIntosh and Thomson (2006) found there was no significant difference in healing times following surgery when comparing manuka honey and a paraffin tulle gras. Chemical cautery wounds tend to have moderate levels of exudate and a primary concern of the practitioner is to avoid adhesion of the dressing to the wound since this causes unnecessary pain for the patient and causes trauma to fragile granulation tissue during re-dressings. Furthermore, it is important to protect peri-wound skin from maceration. With this in mind it is recommended that nonadhesive, absorbent wound dressings are applied on a regular basis as determined by local policy. If critical colonization is suspected antimicrobials are recommended. If infection is suspected a swab should be taken to identify the infecting micro-organism and a referral should be made to a medical practitioner, or an advanced nurse or podiatrist with access to antibiotic therapy.

10.9.2 | Identifying Infection in the Post-surgical Wound

Chemical burns cause tissue damage that can lead to delayed healing and a delayed inflammatory response (Thomson *et al.*, 2002). This should be considered when assessing the wound following toenail surgery. It is possible that a delayed inflammatory response to the phenol or sodium hydroxide will occur, giving the false impression that an infection may be present. The misdiagnosis of post chemical cautery nail surgery infection is not surprising, especially for the inexperienced practitioner, although there are currently no epidemiological studies of the occurrence of infection misdiagnosis in this type of surgery.

In order to identify infection in chemical cautery wounds correctly it is important to monitor the wound for other signs of infection besides a localized inflammatory response. Cutting *et al.* (2005) undertook a Delphi study, whereby expert consensus was sought to identify clinical criteria for infection in various wound types. Acute wounds and partial thickness burns are categorized, but it could be argued that chemical cautery wounds might be classified as either. Identified signs of infection are subtly different for each wound type, further confusing the matter. It is the authors' opinion that the following criteria should be considered when assessing chemical cautery wounds for infection:

- Cellulitis
- Pus/abscess
- Malodour
- Increased exudate
- An increase in pain: nail surgery of this type is not particularly painful post-surgically and most patients report little or no discomfort (Marshall *et al.*, 2005; McIntosh and Thomson, 2006)
- Advancing inflammation and erythema moving away from the surgical site
- The wound stops healing or deteriorates
- Malodour: be conscious, however, that some chemical burn wounds can give a mild malodour in the absence of infection

Optimum local wound care, prevention of infection and pressure relief are all factors that should be addressed in the post-operative period to expedite wound healing. Pressure relief can be achieved with open footwear in the short term. Paul is keen to return to sport as soon as possible, but pressure relief and rest in the initial post-operative period was advised to promote rapid healing.

Figure 10.11 illustrates a healed wound following partial nail avulsion. It would be expected that Paul's wound, once healed, would have a similar appearance.

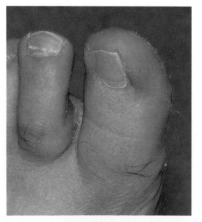

Figure 10.11
Healed wound following partial nail avulsion

10.10 | Case Scenario Revisited

Consider the initial questions posed:

1. **How long would you expect this wound to take to heal?**
   Limited evidence exists that provides a definitive time to healing for chemical cautery wounds. This largely depends on a number of variables, such as the presence of systemic disease, infection and extrinsic factors such as pressure from footwear. Evidence from two randomized controlled trials demonstrates that wound healing can take 18–31 days (approximately 2–5 weeks) following partial nail avulsion (Marshall *et al.*, 2005; McIntosh and Thomson, 2006). This should be brought to the attention of the patient prior to surgery.

2. **What dressings should be used on a moist chemical burn wound of this type?**
   Evidence demonstrates that a moist environment is required to facilitate healing of partial thickness wounds. However, there is little in the way of quality evidence to recommend the most effective wound dressing following toenail surgery. A nonadherent, absorbent dressing was applied to Paul's wound. This aims to minimize trauma to the nail bed on removal, preventing damage to fragile new granulation tissue and minimizing pain experienced by the patient. Dressing choice should also be dictated by exudate levels and any primary or secondary dressings selected should promote moisture balance.

3. **How often should the dressings be changed?**
   Frequency of required dressing change is largely determined by the level of wound exudate and the absorptive capacity of the dressings applied. Generally dressing change twice per week is sufficient for partial nail avulsion wounds. Paul is able to undertake his own re-dressings following advice.

4. **Describe the stages of healing that such a wound would have to take in order to heal fully.**
   As outlined in Chapter 2, there are four phases of wound healing. A nail avulsion wound will follow the normal pattern of healing; however, the inflammatory phase is often prolonged. This is thought to be due to the corrosive action of phenol used during the surgical procedure (Thomson *et al.*, 2002).

10.11 | Conclusion

This chapter has considered some of the commonest toenail pathologies that require surgical intervention and has briefly outlined the surgical procedure often employed by podiatrists. Pre-surgical assessment for chemical cautery toenail surgery has been considered and post-operative management explored. While podiatrists often undertake the surgical procedure, post-operative care is often multiprofessional. It is therefore important that all professionals involved in post-operative care of these wounds have an understanding of the healing process and treatment requirements of these unique wounds.

? Reflection

Take time to reflect upon your learning from this chapter. Ask yourself:

1. **What knowledge did I possess prior to reading this chapter?**

2. **How has my knowledge developed?**

3. **How will I implement this into my future practice?**

References

Aksakal, A.B., Oztas, P. and Atahan, C. (2004) Decompression for the management of onychocryptosis. *Journal of Dermatological Treatment*, **15**, 108–11.

Blake, A. (2005) A post-operative comparison of nail avulsion using phenol and cryotherapy. *British Journal of Podiatry*, **8**(4), 128–132.

Bristow, I. (2004) Onychomycosis: guide to management. *Podiatry Now*, **7**(10), Suppl., S1–S8.

British National Formulary (BNF) (2007) (online), Available at: http://www.bnf.org, Last accessed 29 January 2007.

Connelly, L.K., Dinehart, S.M. and McDonald, R. (1999) Onychocryptosis associated with the treatment of onychomycosis. *Journal of the American Podiatric Medical Association*, **89**(8), 424–6.

Cooper, R. (2005) Understanding wound infection, in *Identifying Criteria for Wound Infection*, European Wound Management Association (EWMA) Position Document, MEP Ltd, London.

Cumming, S., Stewart, S., Harborne, D. *et al.* (2005) A randomised controlled trial of phenol and sodium hydroxide in nail surgery. *British Journal of Podiatry*, **8**(4), 123–7.

Cutting, K.F., White, R.J., Mahoney, P. *et al.* (2005) Understanding wound infection, in *Identifying Criteria for Wound Infection*, European Wound Management Association (EWMA) Position Document, MEP Ltd, London, pp. 2–5.

de Berker, D., Bristoe, I., Baran, R. *et al.* (2002) *Nails Appearance and Therapy*, 2nd edn, Martin Dunitz, London, pp. 16–7.

DeLauro, T. (1995) Onychocryptosis. *Clinics in Podiatric Medicine and Surgery*, **12**(2), 201–13.

Fleckman, P. and Allan, C. (2001) Surgical anatomy of the nail unit. *Dermatology Surgery*, **27**, 257–60.

Grasty, M.S. (1999) Use of the hand-held Doppler to detect peripheral vascular disease. *The Diabetic Foot*, **2**(1), 18–21.

Health and Safety Executive (2000) *Chemical Hazard Alert – Phenol*. http://www.hse.gov.uk/ria/chemical/phenol.htm (12 September 2007).

International Diabetes Federation (2005) *Time to Act: Diabetes and Foot Care*, International Diabetes Federation, Brussels.

Lateur, N. (2006) Onychomycosis: beyond cosmetic distress. *Journal of Cosmetic Dermatology*, **5**(2), 171–7.

Letts, M., Davidson, D. and Nizalk, E. (1998) Subungual exostosis: diagnosis and treatment in children. *Journal of Trauma*, **44**(2), 346–9.

Lokrec, F., Ezra, E., Krasin, E. *et al.* (2001) A simple and efficient surgical technique for subungual exostosis. *Journal Pediatric Orthopaedics*, **21**(1), 76–9.

McIntosh, C. and Thomson, C.E. (2006) Honey dressing versus paraffin tulle gras following toenail surgery. *Journal of Wound Care*, **15**(3), 133–7.

Marshall, C. (2004) The ankle: brachial pressure index. A critical appraisal. *British Journal of Podiatry*, **7**(4), 93–5.

Marshall, C., Queen, J. and Manjooran, J. (2005) Honey vs. povidone iodine following toenail surgery. *Wounds UK*, **1**(1), 10–28.

Rich, P. (2001) Nail biopsy: indications and methods. *Dermatology Surgery*, **27**, 229–34.

Rounding, C. and Bloomfield, S. (2003) Surgical treatments for ingrowing toenails. *The Cochrane Database of Systematic Reviews*, Issue 1, Article NoCD001541.pub2. DOI:10.1002/14651858.CD001541.pub2.

Singh, G., Haneef, N.S. and Uday, A. (2005) Nail changes and disorders among the elderly. *Indian Journal of Dermatology Venereology and Leprology*, **71**(6), 386–92.

Sugden, P., Levy, M. and Rao, G.S. (2001) Onychocryptosis-phenol burn fiasco. *Burns*, **27**, 289–92.

Thomson, C.E., Paterson-Brown, S., Russell, I.T. and Russell, D.A. (2002) A clinical and economic evaluation of toenail surgery performed by podiatrists in the community and surgeons in the hospital setting: a randomised controlled trial, in Conference Proceedings of the 1st International Allied Health Professions on *Impacting on World Health*, Edinburgh.

Vender, R.B., Lynde, C.W. and Poulin, Y. (2006) Prevalence and epidemiology of onychomycosis. *Journal of Cutaneous Medical Surgery*, **10**, Suppl. 2, S28–S33.

Vowden, K. and Vowden, P. (2002) *Hand Held Doppler Ultrasound: The Assessment of Lower Limb Arterial and Venous Disease*, Huntleigh Healthcare Limited, Cardiff.

Weaver, T.D., Vy Ton, M. and Pham, T.V. (2004) Ingrowing toenails: management practices and research outcomes. *Lower Extremity Wounds*, **3**(1), 22–34.

About the Editors

Karen Ousey PhD MA BA DPPN PGDE RGN ONC
Principal Lecturer
University of Huddersfield, UK

Karen Ousey is a principal lecturer at the University of Huddersfield. Prior to this Karen lectured at the University of Salford. Her clinical background is within the speciality of orthopaedics and tissue viability. Karen has worked in numerous NHS trusts in the North West of England and in London. She has developed an interest in tissue viability issues throughout her nursing career and teaches the subject to both pre- and post-registration practitioners. Karen has edited the text *Pressure Area Care* (2005) published by Blackwell and has published various articles on issues relevant to tissue viability. Karen also has an interest in problem-based learning as a teaching and learning strategy and has published in this area.

Caroline McIntosh MSc BSc (Hons) Podiatry
Senior Lecturer
University of Huddersfield, UK

Caroline McIntosh is a senior lecturer in podiatry with a specialist interest in tissue viability. Prior to this Caroline worked as a senior podiatrist for a Trust in North Yorkshire. Caroline maintains a clinical role in an honorary capacity as a Specialist Podiatrist, working in diabetic foot ulcer clinics at Scarborough General Hospital. During her NHS employment Caroline established and acted as the lead podiatrist in a consultant-led vascular foot clinic. Caroline has published a number of papers in the field of tissue viability, particularly on the diabetic foot, and has presented at national and international conference. Caroline is also a member of the editorial advisory board for Wounds UK journal.

About the Authors

Kimberley Martin MSc BSc (Hons) Podiatry
Podiatry Team Leader
Gloucestershire PCT, UK

Kimberley Martin qualified as a registered general nurse in the early 1990s and worked in geriatrics in a range of primary and secondary care settings. She chose to pursue a career in podiatry and qualified from Wessex School of Podiatry, Southampton in 1998. She has worked as a senior podiatrist in Hull and more recently as a Podiatry Team Leader for Gloucestershire PCT. Kim completed her MSc in Podiatry in 2003 and has a specialist interest in the high-risk foot, specifically in relation to HIV and AIDS, and completed her thesis on the attitudes and knowledge of podiatrists on HIV and AIDS.

Nicoletta Frescos MPH B.Appl.Sci (Podiatry)
Clinical Education Coordinator/Lecturer
Department of Podiatry
La Trobe University
Victoria, Australia

Nicoletta Frescos is a clinical education coordinator and lecturer in the Department of Podiatry, La Trobe University, Australia and educator in the Masters and Postgraduate certificate course in Wound Care for Monash University. She is a podiatry consultant in the Wound Foundation Australia clinic at the Austin Hospital, where she also teaches medical, nursing, pharmacy and podiatry students on diabetic foot wound management.

She is currently a board member of the Podiatrist Registration Board Victoria, and a podiatry adviser for the Department of Veterans' Affairs.

Nicoletta has a keen interest in public health and health policy. She has been an active member of the Australian Podiatry Association, and in the past has held the position of President to the Victoria branch, and was executive member on the National board. Her research interests include the high-risk foot, wound management, chronic wound pain and interdisciplinary approach to wound care.

Tabatha Rando RN, Grad Dip CHN, Grad Cert STN, Cert Wound Mgt, Dip FLM, Cert IV WAT
Clinical Nurse Consultant – Wound Management
Royal Melbourne Hospital
Melbourne,
Victoria, Australia

Tabatha is a registered nurse who has worked as a Clinical Nurse Consultant in Wound Management and Tissue Viability since 1995 in community nursing and in the acute, subacute and aged healthcare sectors in Melbourne, Australia. She has a focus on improving standards of holistic, patient-focused, evidence-based care and is currently completing her Masters thesis.

Tabatha is committed to the provision of evidence-based wound management education, which is evident in her role as a lecturer in the education of the multidisciplinary team members at undergraduate and postgraduate levels. She is a course assessor for the Monash University Post Graduate Courses in Wound Management. She also works in two of the major chronic wound clinics in Melbourne. Tabatha has presented at various state, national and international wound management conferences, and is an invited international speaker in the Pacific region.

Her involvement in research to date has focused on hypergranulation, the use of advanced therapies in chronic wounds, pressure ulcer point prevalence and skin tear management. She has received various scholarships including an international travel fellowship to review wound management practices in the UK. She is an active member of the Australian Wound Management Association and a past president of the Wound Management Association of Victoria. Her major focus is upon wound prevention, management and improving practice.

Adrienne Taylor RGN RM DN DipHe MSc
Lead Nurse Tissue Viability
Salford Royal Hospitals NHS Trusts, UK

Adrienne's interest in leg ulcers developed when she questioned her own practice as a district nurse regarding leg ulcer management. This subsequently led to a small-scale research study and eventually a study at Masters level. Adrienne was involved in establishing a leg ulcer service in 1991 and has been involved in many studies. Her work undertaken for award of Master of Science was published in the Royal Society of Medicine Phlebology journal and has been included in the HTA health economics database. Her work was also instrumental in supporting the introduction of the four-layer bandage on FP10. During the last three years Adrienne has been involved in setting up a tissue viability service within a university teaching hospital.

Jacqui Fletcher RGN MSc Wound Healing and Tissue Repair BSc (Hons)
Healthcare Studies (Nursing), PG Cert (Education), ILT
University of Hertfordshire, UK

Jacqui Fletcher is currently the Programme Tutor for the BSc (Hons) Tissue Viability at the University of Hertfordshire and has an honorary contract as a Tissue Viability Nurse with East & North

Hertfordshire Acute Trust. Prior to this she worked as a Clinical Nurse Specialist in Tissue Viability in an integrated Trust in West Yorkshire from 1992–1996 and as Professional Development Leader from 1996–1997 at Salford Royal Hospitals NHS Trust.

She was the Chairperson of the Wound Care Society for four years and is an executive committee member for the European Pressure Ulcer Advisory Panel. Jacqui is also a member of the editorial advisory board for Wounds UK journal.

Veronica Newton MSc BSc (Hons) MChS
University of Huddersfield, UK

Veronica is senior Lecturer at the University of Huddersfield, Division of Podiatry where her academic responsibilities include teaching clinical management in diabetes care to podiatry and nursing students at undergraduate and postgraduate level. Veronica also holds a clinical specialist role undertaking a weekly session with the diabetes team at Calderdale and Huddersfield NHS trust treating a wide range of diabetic foot complications.

Deborah Turner PhD BSc (Hons) Podiatry

Debbie Turner qualified as a podiatrist in 1996 from the University of Huddersfield and worked as a community-based podiatrist in a local NHS trust. She studied for a PhD on a part-time basis while working as a podiatrist specialising in rheumatology and as a research assistant at the Academic Unit of Musculoskeletal Diseases at the University of Leeds. She is co-author on a book entitled *The Foot and Ankle in Rheumatoid Arthritis: A Comprehensive Guide.* This book focuses on management of common foot problems associated with rheumatoid arthritis.

Jill Firth RGN BSc (Hons)

Jill Firth qualified as a Registered General Nurse in 1989 and began work as Rheumatology Nurse Specialist for Bradford Teaching Hospitals NHS Trust in 1997. In 2004 Jill was awarded the Smith and Nephew Foundation Doctoral Nursing Studentship to undertake a study of the prevalence and possible predictors of foot ulceration in rheumatoid arthritis. She is studying for a full-time PhD at the University of Leeds.

Heidi Davys MSc BSc (Hons) Podiatry

Heidi graduated as a podiatrist from the University of Salford in 1998 and completed her Masters degree at the University of Huddersfield in 2004. She has been the lead rheumatology podiatrist in Leeds, West Yorkshire, for the last seven years and her role has included the implementation of a weekly foot ulcer clinic specifically for patients with rheumatic diseases. Heidi is also a research podiatrist in the Foot and Ankle Studies in Rheumatology (FASTER) programme at the University of Leeds and is a co-author of the book *The foot and Ankle in Rheumatoid Arthritis.*

Steve Hancox BSc (Hons) Podiatry
University of Huddersfield, UK

Steve graduated as a podiatrist from the University of Huddersfield in 1996. On qualification Steve worked as a podiatrist within the NHS prior to commencing his current post of senior lecturer in podiatry at the University of Huddersfield. In conjunction with his lecturing post Steve has managed a successful private practice for the last five years. Steve has specialist interests in pathomechanics, musculosketal podiatry and toenail surgery.

Index